THE ESOPHAGUS

Reflux and Primary Motor Disorders

(Formerly *Motor Disorders of the Esophagus*)

Dr. Frederick Gordon Kergin

Professor and Chairman, Department of Surgery.
University of Toronto 1957–66.

*This book is offered as a tribute to the late Frederick G. Kergin—
a dedicated teacher and a skilled thoracic surgeon.*

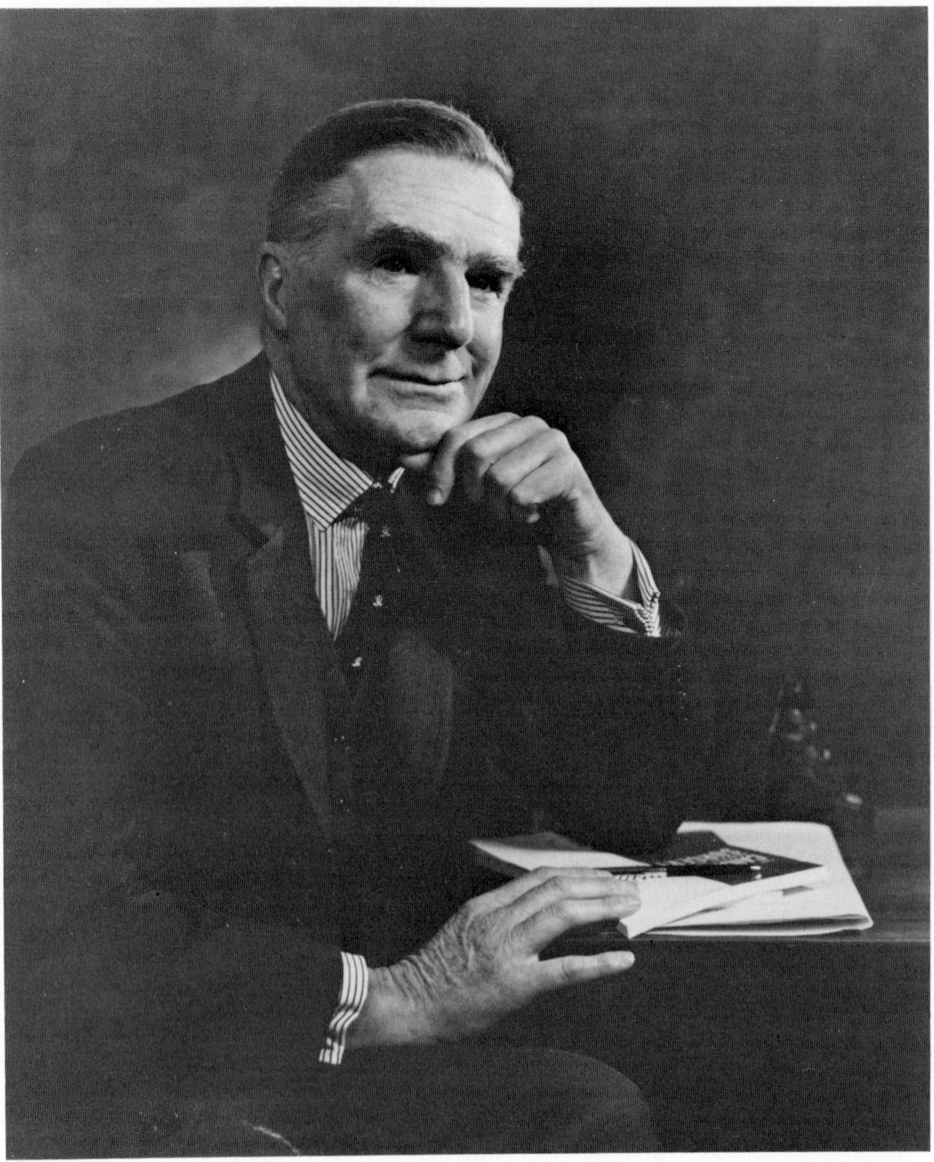

Photo by Karsh

THE ESOPHAGUS

Reflux and Primary Motor Disorders

(Formerly *Motor Disorders of the Esophagus*)

ROBERT D. HENDERSON,

M.B., F.R.C.S.(C)
Associate Professor of Surgery, University of Toronto;
Chief of Surgery, Women's College Hospital;
Consultant Surgeon, Toronto General Hospital
Toronto, Ontario, Canada

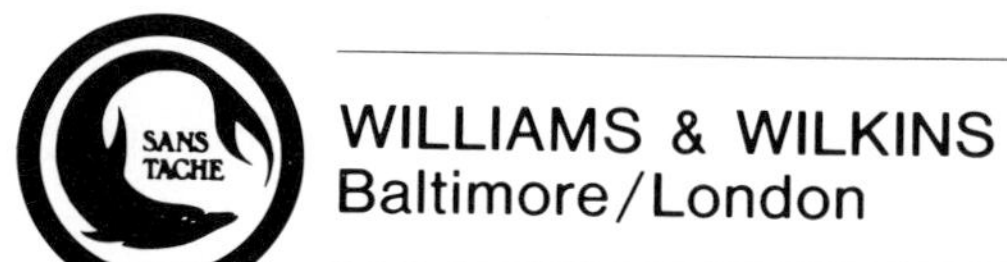

WILLIAMS & WILKINS
Baltimore/London

Made in the United States of America

Library of Congress Cataloging in Publication Data

Formerly *Motor Disorders of the Esophagus*

Henderson, Robert D
  The esophagus.

    Edition for 1976 published under title: Motor disorders of the esophagus.
    Includes index.
    1. Esophageal reflux. 2. Esophageal motility. 3. Hiatal hernia—Surgery. I. Title.
[DNLM: 1. Esophageal diseases—Physiopathology. 2. Esophagus—Physiopathology. 3. Esophageal reflux. 4. Gastrointestinal motility. WI250 H497m]
RC815.7.H46   1980   616.3′2   80-13210
ISBN 0-683-03948-2

Composed and printed at the
Waverly Press, Inc.
Mt. Royal and Guilford Aves.
Baltimore, Md. 21202, U.S.A.

Foreword

The indications for a revision of a textbook are in the main (a) that the first edition fulfilled a definite need and was therefore well received, (b) omissions and weaknesses became apparent that needed revision, (c) new information became available that needed presentation, and (d) further investigation and follow-up added support to the originally presented concepts.

It is apparent from reviewing the revision of *Motor Disorders of the Esophagus*, now retitled *The Esophagus: Reflux and Primary Motor Disorders*, that Doctor Robert D. Henderson has fulfilled all these criteria so that this edition adds to the armamentarium of us all—those who are interested in understanding the role of the esophagus in everyday teaching and practice and those who have a particular interest in the esophagus as their area of expertise.

Dr. Henderson is to be complimentd in pursuing his expertise and interest in this field and making his thoughts, backed up by well-defined studies and long-term follow-up, available to all.

Donald R. Wilson, M.D.
Professor and Chairman
Department of Surgery
University of Toronto

Preface

Interest in the esophagus has intensified over the past 20 years and we are now seeing a rapid improvement in our understanding of esophageal function in health and disease. Advances have taken place in the past four years making a revision of *Motor Disorders of the Esophagus* overdue.

The title of the book has been altered to *The Esophagus: Reflux and Primary Motor Disorders.* This title clarifies its content and recognizes the emphasis placed on reflux as an important etiologic factory in secondary motor spasm.

The text emphasizes the role of investigative procedures. In the author's opinion a careful history is the single most important study as in over 90 per cent of patients it will localize the disease to the esophagus. Other investigations are then used to differentiate between the various disorders and add precision to the diagnosis. Documentation of history, laboratory investigation, and response to treatment is based on 10 years of continuous analysis of new patients and long-term follow-up of those surgically treated.

Where possible the author's patient analysis is compared with the literature. The results of surgery are compared with those reported by other investigators and points of controversy are highlighted. While the present surgical approaches are regarded as optimal, undoubtedly further advances will be made and hopefully by slow evolution the most appropriate surgical approach will be selected.

Only by careful analysis of our clinical work can we hope to improve the quality of life of our patients.

Robert D. Henderson, M.B., F.R.C.S.(C), F.A.C.S.
Toronto, Ontario

Preface to *Motor Disorders of the Esophagus*

The steady expansion in knowledge, particularly during the past 20 years, has given the student of the esophagus a better understanding of its physiology and pathophysiology. However, this knowledge has not been made available to the general physician in convenient form, partly because it is scattered widely in the literature and also because a grasp of it requires some familiarity with basic investigative techniques. In this book Dr. Robert Henderson provides a practical summary of modern knowledge of esophageal dysfunction and disease and describes an approach to diagnosis and management based on his experience as a clinical investigator, a teacher, and a practicing surgeon. His evaluation of the esophageal literature is tempered by his broad experience, but in some instances his views of motor disorders are original.

The reader will recognize that the recommendations made in this book are the author's, but they are backed up by careful examination of and long familiarity with current methods of treatment. His recommendations are further supported by original basic and clinical research, and by extensive experience and careful follow-up. Where Dr. Henderson disagrees with current methods, he gives his reasons for preferring his own approach.

In the past decade, interest in esophageal disorders has begun to cross traditional specialist boundaries. For example, the cardiologist now recognizes that the esophagus is important in the differential diagnosis of "angina-like" and other cardiac pain. Respiratory physicians are now acutely aware that aspiration secondary to esophageal dysfunction is a major source of lung infection and may aggravate asthma. Similarly, otolaryngologists now recognize that they must learn more about disorders of the pharyngoesophageal junction, most of which are associated with a motor abnormality that, when recognized, can be treated.

The strong cross-specialty interest that has developed in esophageal disease has sparked a dramatic increase in investigative and therapeutic activity. For example, when Dr. Henderson started manometric studies at Toronto General Hospital seven years ago, few units existed in Canada. The manometry unit was opened to carry out investigations in the newly created division of general thoracic surgery, and in this undertaking the division's director, Dr. F. G. Pearson, provided much help and moral support. In the intervening years the demand for esophageal investigations has increased greatly. Patients are now referred by a wide variety of practitioners.

This book, *Motor Disorders of the Esophagus*, covers 90 per cent of all esophageal disease and is founded on a large and intensive experience. Presentations of the individual clinical entities are illustrated by characteristic case histories, and the symptoms, natural history, or results of therapy are usually grounded in a thorough personal review of large numbers of patients. The book presents original research into the pathogenesis of primary disordered motor activity (PDMA), organ replacement by bowel and stomach loops, scleroderma, the management of peptic strictures, and the application of gastroplasty to the complications of gastroesophageal reflux. Also the book supplies new data on the pharyngoesophageal junction and demonstrates the application of this knowledge to the management of dysphagia.

Motor Disorders will serve the reader best if he keeps in mind certain of Dr. Henderson's objectives. The general physician or surgeon will have a clearer view of motor disorders of the esophagus if:

- he adopts this book's practical classification of these disorders.
- he uses its precise terminology which clearly describes specific structures, phenomena, or concepts, and thus dispels the confusion and explodes some of the myths that still linger about esophageal function and disease. (The power of an inappropriate label to confuse can hardly be overestimated; e.g., *hiatal hernia* describes an anatomical defect but the symptoms associated with the defect, if any, are due to *gastroesophageal reflux*. Thus whenever he speaks about pathogenesis, the physician must name the cause: the *reflux*, not the *hernia*.)
- he accords to patient interview its pre-eminent place in the diagnosis of esophageal disease and recognizes the necessity of accurate diagnosis before any consideration is given to treatment.

Dr. Henderson and I first collaborated during the decade 1962–1972 when I was editor of the *Canadian Journal of Surgery* and when the late Frederick G. Kergin, one of the founders of the specialty of thoracic surgery in Canada, was chairman of the editorial board. Many of his concepts were new to the general surgeon and many, like those in his early papers on the high pressure zone (HPZ), required careful and exact exposition. Thus when he came in the fall of 1974 to discuss a review of motor disorders, in which he could share his experience with his residents, his students, and the many physicians who referred their "esophageal problems" to him, we set to work on a solid basis of respect for each other's talents, experience, and skills. The result of this collaboration is in this book.

As the acknowledgments bear witness, many people assisted Dr. Henderson, but, as will be clear to all who know him, *Motor Disorders* is his book. He offers it for the edification of every physician who wants a better understanding of that solid, hardworking and efficient organ, the esophagus. Through these physicians he seeks a better level of care for the many people who suffer from esophageal dysfunction.

John O. Godden, M.D. C.M., F.R.C.P. (C)
Commerce Court Medical Centre, Toronto

Acknowledgments

The author would like to thank the following people for their help in compiling the manuscript: Dr. J. Godden's editorial assistance in the preparation of the first edition was invaluable. Mrs. Joy Duran has supplied secretarial services. Mr. Gary Marryatt has assisted in compiling clerical research data necessary for the publication of the text. Artwork was again prepared by Mrs. Rasa Skudra of the Department of Art as Applied to Medicine and photography was by the Department of Photography, University of Toronto.

Financial support was obtained from the Women's College Hospital Research Fund.

Contents

SECTION III

ACHALASIA AND PRIMARY DISORDERED MOTOR ACTIVITY

SECTION IV

SCLERODERMA

SECTION V

THE PHARYNGOESOPHAGEAL JUNCTION

SECTION VI

ESOPHAGEAL DIVERTICULA AND MIXED MOTOR DISORDERS

SECTION I

Structure and Function

CHAPTER 1

Functional Anatomy of the Esophagus

For continued survival, growth and reproduction the human requires a constant supply of calories, which he obtains by eating a wide variety of animal and vegetable matter. The conversion of food to calories begins in the mouth, where the food is broken down to small particles, lubricated with saliva and propelled through the pharynx and esophagus into the stomach. Esophageal function plays no part in the digestive process but is limited to the transport of food from the mouth to the stomach. Transport is materially assisted by coordinated motor activity in the pharynx, cricopharynx and esophagus. This book concerns motor activity and the alterations produced in it by disorders of function and injury.

Anatomy and Embryology

It is assumed that the reader has some understanding of basic anatomy and embryology, and hence these subjects will be reviewed only briefly to point out the application of specific facts to the appraisal of normal function and disease.

Familiarity with the anatomy of the esophagus is essential to any clear understanding of its function in the normal subject and in the presence of disease. The composition and disposition of the muscles in this organ illustrate the relationship of structure to function; for example, its upper one-third is subject to disorders which do not affect the lower (smooth muscle) esophagus because it is composed of striated muscle to permit rapid emptying of the pharynx. Similarly, clear conceptions of the interrelationships of lower esophagus and stomach are an essential preliminary to any understanding of the normal control of gastric reflux.

The pharynx develops in the lateral walls and floor of the cranial part of the early foregut (1). Pharyngeal pouches first appear as grooves which resemble the gills of aquatic vertebrates. As these pouches develop they become modified and give rise to a number of diverse structures including the walls of the pharynx, the middle ear and the parathyroid, thymus and thyroid glands.

The esophagus arises in direct continuity with the developing pharynx and connects it to the dilated portion of the foregut which later becomes the stomach (Fig. 1.1). A small diverticulum, which buds off the anterior aspect of the proximal esophagus, increases in size and differentiates to form the lungs.

As the embryo grows, the esophagus rapidly lengthens and, with this lengthening, its lumen is first obliterated and later recannulates. During its early development the esophagus is lined by columnar epithelium, but later this undergoes metaplasia to form a stratified squamous epithelial lining. Disturbances in these embryologic developments give rise in later life to several disorders such as esophageal atresia, tracheosophageal fistula, the columnar-lined esophagus and esophageal reduplications.

The value of embryology to the physician can be illustrated by citing such clinical conditions as anomalous development of the esophagus and lung buds, which gives rise to a variety of congenital defects ranging from an isolated tracheoesophageal fistula to various combinations of fistula and esophageal atresia. Most of these defects present as emergencies in the newborn, but occasionally small fistulas may continue unrecognized into adult life. Sometimes isolated patches of columnar epithelium (which commonly represent embryologic rests) are seen in the esoph-

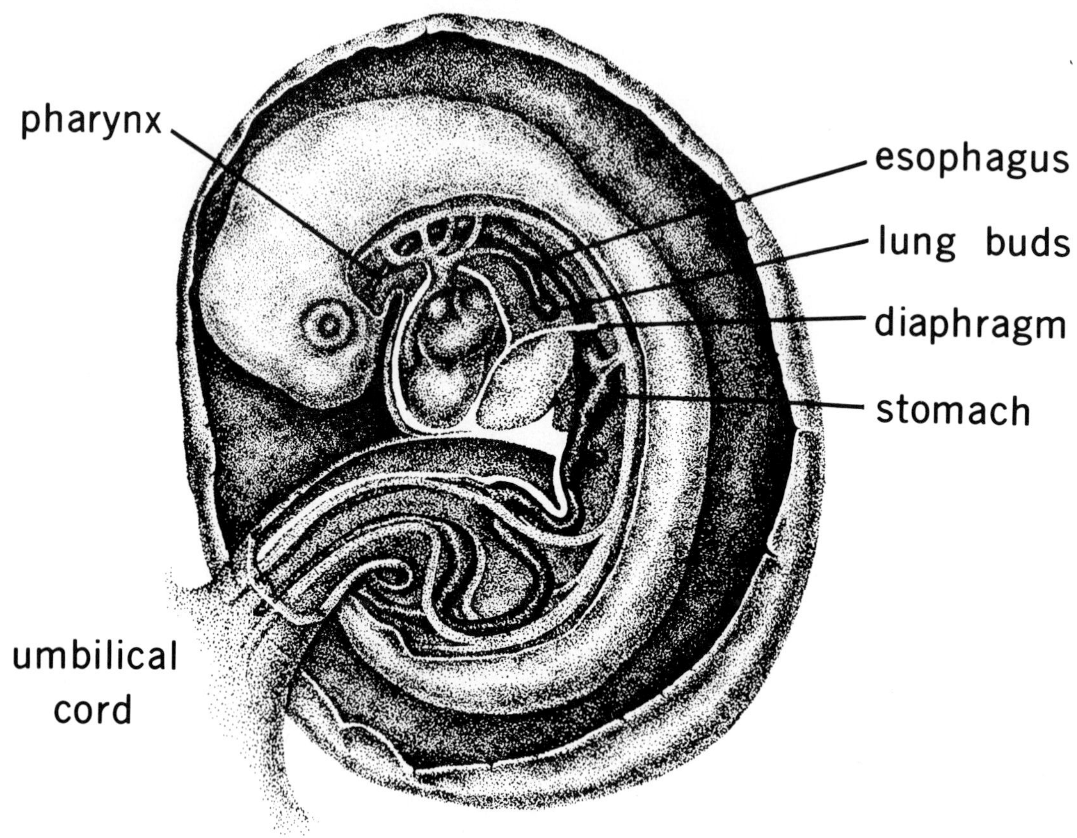

Figure 1.1
In the 5-mm embryo the esophagus connects the pharynx to the dilated foregut, which becomes the stomach. At this stage the diaphragm is already formed. Lung buds develop by growing forward from the primitive esophagus, then divide to form the bronchi of the developing lungs.

agus. The complete lining of the lower esophagus with columnar epithelium, which is rare, is usually first recognized in the adult. Reduplications develop during the stage of esophageal fusion and recannulation, and these may present clinically during either infancy or adult life.

Pharynx and Cricopharynx

The organization of pharyngeal musculature is totally different from that in the cricopharynx and body of the esophagus (2, 3). The fan-shaped pharyngeal muscles, which develop in the endodermal pouches, arise anterolaterally from the pterygoid process, hyoid bone and thyroid cartilage. As the superior, middle and inferior constrictors and the stylopharyngeus (Fig. 1.2), they sweep posteriorly and are inserted into a median raphe, which runs from the base of the skull to the level of the cricopharyngeus muscle. The outer surfaces of the pharyngeal muscles are covered by loose areolar tissue and the inner surfaces are lined by the pharyngobasilar fascia. This strong fibrous membrane is attached to the base of the skull, to the hyoid bone and to the skeleton of the larynx. The pharynx is lined by stratified squamous epithelium which is continuous with the mucosa of the nasopharynx, mouth, larynx and esophagus.

The pharynx can be divided into three compartments: the nasopharynx, oral pharynx and laryngeal pharynx. The passage between oral pharynx and nasopharynx is referred to as the pharyngeal isthmus (Fig. 1.3). Because of these communications with the larynx and nasal passage, disorders of the pharynx which interfere with the passage of

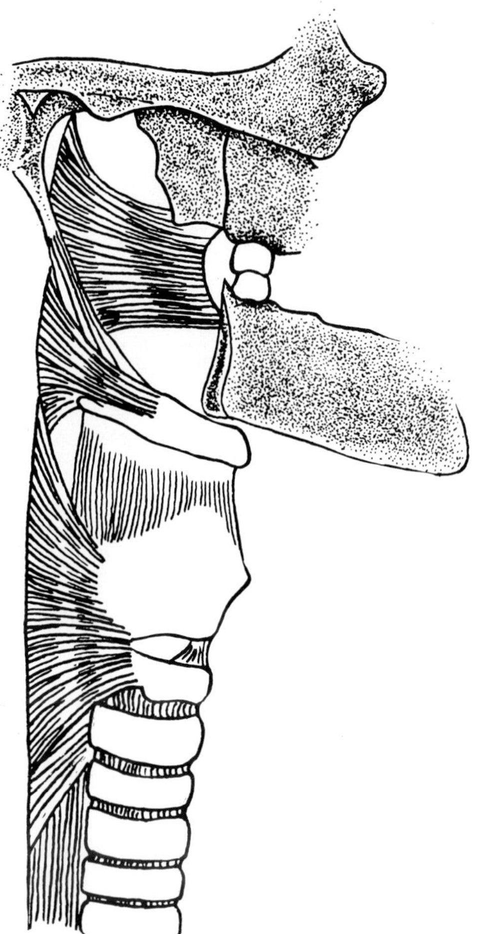

Figure 1.2
Four muscles form the pharyngeal wall—the superior, middle and inferior constrictors and the stylopharyngeus. The constrictors arise from the pterygoid process, hyoid bond and thyroid cartilage, and sweep posteriorly in a fan shape, to be inserted into a median posterior raphe.

food may provoke forward spillage with aspiration, or upward spillage and nasal regurgitation. During the normal swallow, muscular activity is coordinated to control the descending food bolus and force it through the cricopharynx.

The structures continuous with the pharynx are, posteriorly, the prevertebral fascia and cervical vertebrae and, laterally, the carotid sheaths which contain the carotid arteries and veins, and the vagus nerves.

Cricopharynx

The cricopharyngeus arises as a separate muscle from the posterior aspect of the cricoid cartilage (4). It has no posterior fibrous raphe, and this may assist in maintaining constant closure of the proximal esophagus except during deglutition. In 1907 Killian (5) described a weak area between the inferior pharyngeal constrictor and the upper margins of cricopharyngeus posteriorly, Killian's triangle, through which it is alleged pharyngeal diverticula make their way. In recent years, many workers have denied the existence of a triangular zone devoid of muscle. However, the pharyngeal and cricoid muscles anatomically are separate, and diverticula, when they do form, develop at this site.

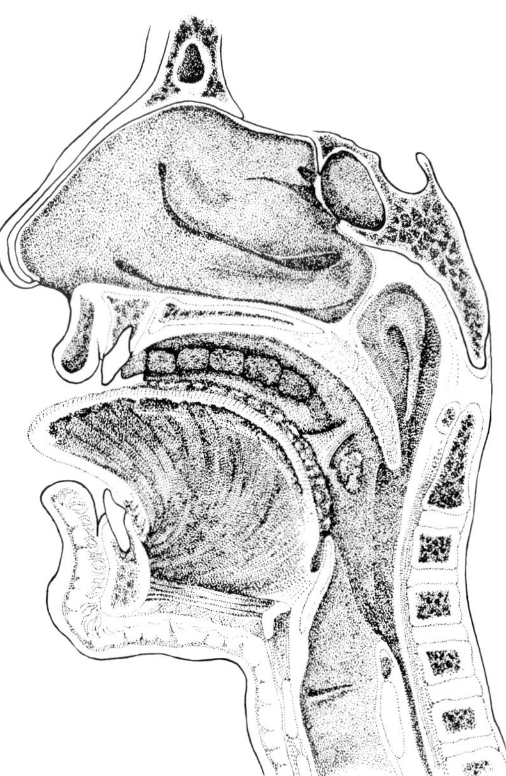

Figure 1.3
The pharynx can be divided into nasopharynx, oropharynx and laryngeal pharynx. The soft palate can close the nasopharynx during swallowing and the trachea is protected both by the epiglottis and by elevation of the larynx behind the tongue.

Pharynx and cricopharynx have both parasympathetic and sympathetic innervations. The former is through the vagus, the glossopharyngeal and the bulbar roots of the accessory nerve. The vagal fibers are distributed through its pharyngeal and laryngeal divisions. These structures are also innervated by the recurrent laryngeal branches of the vagus, but this is limited to the upper esophagus and cricopharyngeus. Sympathetic nerve supply is derived from branches of the cervical sympathetic ganglia (6, 7).

Because of the nerve supply of these muscles, the pharyngeal and cricopharyngeal motor functions may be altered by congenital disorders of the autonomic nervous system, by bulbar disorders, by injury to the neck, or through damage to the recurrent laryngeal nerves by intrathoracic disease (8). Although the nerve pathways are not fully understood, it is possible for neurogenic disorders to involve the pharynx or the cricopharyngeus independently.

The pharynx receives its arterial supply from many small vessels including some from the ascending pharyngeal, ascending palatine, the greater palatine, facial and maxillary arteries. Venous drainage is to the pharyngeal venous plexus, which communicates with both the pterygoid plexus and the internal jugular veins. Lymph drainage of the pharynx passes dominantly to the upper deep cervical lymph glands.

Esophagus

The esophagus extends from the lower margin of the cricopharyngeus (the level of the 6th cervical vertebra) to a point 2 cm below the diaphragm where it joins the stomach. It is a hollow muscular tube 24 cm long and 2.5 cm in its maximal diameter (Fig. 1.4). The esophagus, which in health and at rest is empty, apart from small quantities of mucus, is closed by the cricopharyngeus at its upper end and by the gastroesophageal high pressure zone at its lower end.

Seen in cross section, the outer surface of the esophagus is composed of loose areolar tissue without serosal covering. The outer layer of longitudinal muscle is continuous throughout its length and blends into the gastric musculature below. Immediately deep to this, the circular layer of muscle spirals around the organ and becomes continuous

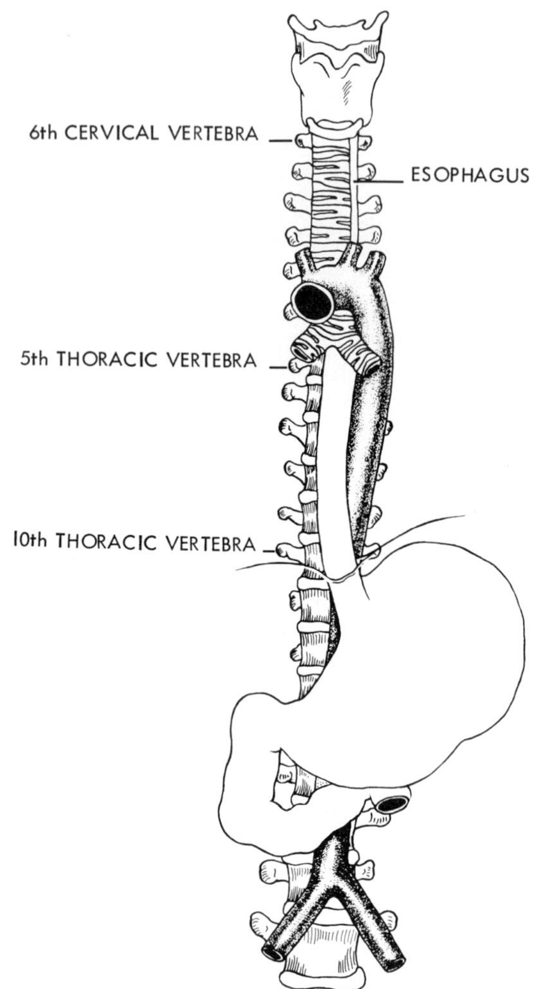

Figure 1.4
The esophagus begins at the level of the cricoid at the 6th cervical vertebra. It traverses the lower neck and thorax to end by joining the stomach in the upper abdomen. Its major relations to the spine, trachea, aorta and heart can be seen in this figure.

with the circular layer of gastric muscle. The muscle in the upper third of the esophagus is striated and in the lower two-thirds is smooth. Because of this difference in muscular arrangement, motor waves are conducted faster through the upper esophagus than through the lower esophagus. Also the presence of mixed types of muscle explains why myogenic disorders involve only one type of esophageal muscle and usually do not involve the whole esophagus.

The submucosa of the esophagus contains

racemose glands which secrete into the lumen and help to lubricate the food particles during their descent. Its stratified squamous lining is continuous above with the pharyngeal mucosa and ends below at a clearly delineated point near the lower end of the esophagus, where it meets the columnar gastric mucosa. In outline this squamocolumnar junction may be regular or serrated, and commonly the lower esophagus may contain small islands of gastric mucosa. Occasionally, the entire lower esophagus may be lined with columnar epithelium up to the level of the tracheal carina, but whether this is a congenital anomaly or a response to reflux and esophageal ulceration remains a matter of controversy (9).

The esophagus follows a slightly devious course from pharynx to stomach and curves toward the left in the base of the neck and upper mediastinum, where its lateral margin lies 4 to 6 mm to the left of the trachea. The esophagus returns to the midline at the level of the 6th thoracic vertebra and once again swings to the left at the level of the 7th thoracic vertebra, crossing the aortic arch at the level of the 8th vertebra and passing through the diaphragm at the level of the 10th thoracic vertebra to terminate approximately 2 cm below the diaphragmatic level at the proximal margin of the stomach (Fig. 1.4).

The anatomic relations of the esophagus vary at different levels. In the upper thorax it lies behind the trachea until it reaches the tracheal carina, then it passes behind the aortic arch to lie at the right lateral side of the aorta and behind the heart. The thoracic duct, in its course upward and toward the base of the neck, passes posteriorly to the esophagus. These relationships determine the sites of predilection for esophageal disease and explain why esophageal disease often involves contiguous organs.

Neurologic Control

The nerve supply to the esophagus consists of both vagal parasympathetic nerves and a sympathetic nerve supply from the cervical ganglia and from the lower thoracic ganglia (10). The vagal nerve supply is derived primarily from the body of the vagal nerve, but in addition the recurrent laryngeal nerve supplies the upper third of the esophagus and the cricopharyngeus muscle.

Blood Supply and Lymphatics

Blood supply is derived from numerous small vessels, the most important of which include the inferior thyroid artery, the aortic segmental branches, branches from the left gastric artery, short gastrics and the left phrenic artery.

Lymphatic drainage occurs both to the left gastric lymph nodes and celiac axis and also spreads proximally to nodes around the hilum of the left and right lungs, the subcarina, tracheobronchial angles and paratracheal lymph glands. Proximal drainage is to the scalene lymph nodes at the base of the neck on both the right and left sides.

Gastroesophageal Junction

The term, gastroesophageal junction, has been applied to the lower 4 cm of the esophagus where it passes from the thoracic cavity through the tunnel between the diaphragmatic crura for a distance of 2 cm into the upper abdominal cavity. The junction terminates at its point of union with the proximal stomach. This area has received various names, one of the most common being the cardia, a term used by Fabricius (1618), who attributed it to Galen (A.D. 130–200) (11). The name "cardia" was coined when physicians recognized that symptoms arising in the gastroesophageal junction were similar to those found in patients with cardiac disease.

In the normal subject no macroscopic transition can be recognized between the body of the esophagus and the gastroesophageal junction (12). In such disease states as diffuse spasm (primary disordered motor activity) and achalasia, the appearance of this junction is still normal but the esophagus proximal to it shows muscular hyperplasia, thus delineating clearly the muscular zone of the gastroesophageal junction (13, 14). Most workers who have described the anatomy of this region have not recognized any muscular sphincter mechanism, but Botha (11) has demonstrated that a zone of distinct muscle thickening can be recognized in most normal subjects when the esophageal mucosa has been stripped away. The muscular thickening he described arises from the circular muscle layer. More recent studies (12) have confirmed that a histologic sphincter is present at the gastroesophageal junction which corresponds to the high pressure zone (Fig. 1.5).

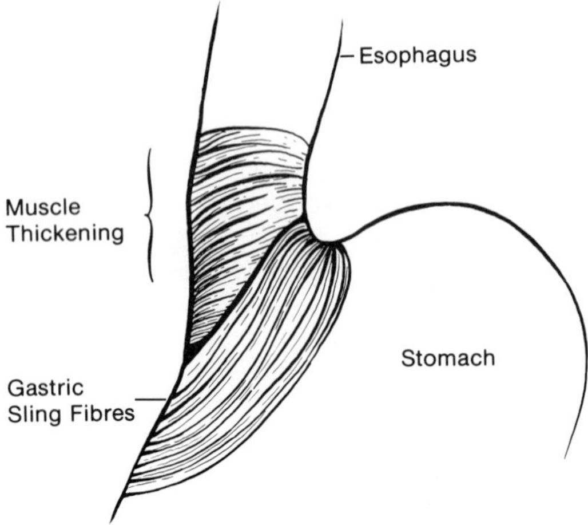

Figure 1.5. Muscular Anatomy of the Gastroesophageal Junction
Muscular thickening has been demonstrated histologically at the lower end of the esophagus and blending into the gastric sling fibers. This thickening corresponds to the approximate HPZ as demonstrated manometrically.

At the junction of the esophagus and stomach a muscular sling (the bundle of His) blends into the muscle fibers of the esophagus at its upper margin. This muscular sling runs from the lateral margin of the junction of stomach and esophagus down to the lesser curvature of the stomach. The term, mucosal rosette, describes the more prominent longitudinal folds of esophageal mucosa at the level of the gastroesophageal junction. The junction of squamous mucosa with the cardiac gastric mucosa is usually abrupt, but some subjects have islands of gastric mucosa which extend up into the lower esophagus. The racemose glands, described earlier, occur more frequently in the esophageal submucosa at this level. The angle of entry of esophagus to stomach varies between 70 and 180 degrees (Fig. 1.6) (11). The angle is formed when the esophagus enters the stomach on its lesser curvature and the fundus of stomach bulges laterally.

The esophagus is attached to the diaphragm by means of the phrenoesophageal ligament and the gastrophrenic ligament, both of which consist of folds of pleura and peritoneum supported by dense elastic tissue fibers.In the normal subject these ligaments are quite strong and effectively restrict esoph-

ageal movement at this level. The vessels and nerves pass deep to these ligaments on the muscular surface of the esophagus and accompany it in its course through the diaphragm. The right vagus nerve, which lies along the right margin of the distal esophagus as it passes through the diaphragmatic tunnel, then passes into the walls of the lesser sac and down the lesser curvature of the stomach. The left vagus nerve is accompanied by sheaths of small vessels that run on the greater curvature of the stomach as the short gastrics and supply a rich vascular network to the esophagogastric fat pad. The fat pad, which is situated on the anterior surface of the stomach and lower esophagus immediately below the attachments of the phrenoesophageal ligament, varies in size with the obesity of the patient.

The relationship of the peritoneum to the lower esophagus is of considerable clinical importance. On its anterior and lateral margins the peritoneum is mostly reflected off the esophagus by the phrenoesophageal ligament. Posteriorly the lesser sac may extend up as far as the esophagus but usually ends 2 to 3 cm below the esophagogastric junction; here it leaves a bare area of proximal stomach and esophagus that is in direct contact with the diaphragmatic crurae. Occasionally small bursal communications develop in which sacs of peritoneum extend from the lesser or greater peritoneal sac through the diaphragmatic hiatus and into the thorax for a distance of 3 to 4 cm.

Diaphragm

The relationships of the diaphragm to the esophagus may vary widely. Most commonly the right crus dominates in formation of the esophageal hiatus, and the left crus plays a lesser and more variable part in this muscular sling. These crura arise from the sides of the second, third and fourth lumbar vertebrae, pass upward and around the esophagus and aorta and are inserted into the central diaphragmatic tendon (Fig. 1.7). Fibers also arise from the median arcuate ligament which crosses the anterior surface of the aorta immediately above the celiac axis. Botha (11) and Collis have shown that there is considerable variability in the formation of the crura. The right crus dominates in 55.1 per

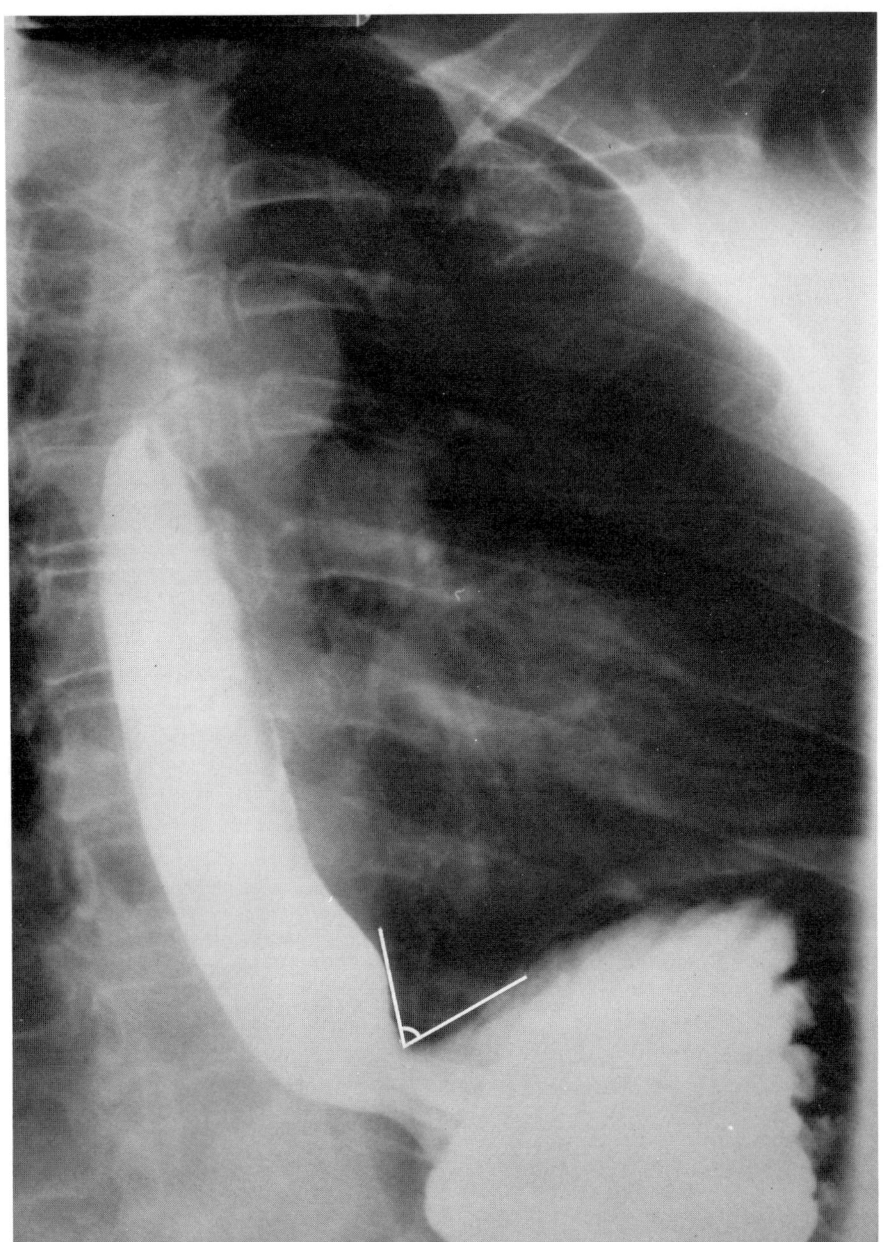

Figure 1.6
Radiologic study shows the angle of entry of esophagus to stomach. This film was taken specifically
to illustrate the cardiac angle, which in this particular patient measured 80 degrees.

cent, but there is some degree of shift to the
left in 34.8 per cent and a shift to the right in
10.1 per cent. Large transverse bands connect
the crural margins in 15.5 per cent and
smaller transverse bands in 17.9 per cent of
patients studied (15–18).

The diaphragm is innervated by the
phrenic nerve. The crural margins have their
own specific innervation: the right lateral
margin of the right crus is supplied from the
right phrenic nerve, and the left margin of
the right crus together with the left crus is
supplied by the left phrenic nerve.

This brief anatomical description may per-

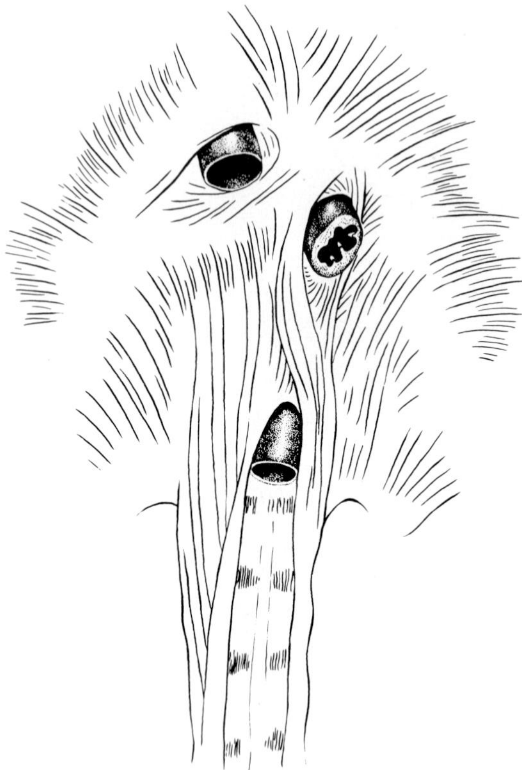

Figure 1.7
The esophagus passes through the diaphragm at the level of the 10th thoracic vertebra. At this point the right crus of diaphragm forms the major part of hiatal muscle—the left crus contributes only a small muscle bundle. This typical distribution is illustrated here.

mit the reader to discern the rudiments of esophageal function. In the mouth food is broken down before swallowing. Pharyngeal action propels the food bolus to the cricopharynx and esophagus, and supplies the muscular control which prevents spillage forward to the larynx or upward to the nasal passage. The cricopharynx, which is the narrowest part of the gastrointestinal tract, relaxes to allow the food to pass into the body of the esophagus. Gravity, coordinated motor function and lubrication combine to assist the descent of the food bolus; thus, seconds following the initiation of the swallow, food passes through the gastroesophageal junction

and into the stomach. Once food is in the stomach, the lower esophagus closes off and prevents reflux.

These simple concepts will now be expanded into a more detailed analysis of motor function and control before proceeding to a study of specific esophageal motor disorders.

References

1. Hamilton, W. J., Boyd, J. D., and Mossman, W. H.: *Human Embryology.* W. Heffer & Sons, Ltd., Cambridge, 1956.
2. Brash, J. C.: *Cunningham's Textbook of Anatomy.* Oxford University Press, London, 1951.
3. Grant, J. C. B.: *A Method of Anatomy*, Ed. 6. Williams & Wilkins, Baltimore, 1958.
4. Ellis, F. H., Jr.: Upper esophageal sphincter in health and disease. Surg. Clin. North Am., *51:* 553, 1971.
5. Killian, G.: The mouth of the esophagus. Laryngoscope, *17:* 421, 1907.
6. Hwang, K., and Grossman, M. I.: Note on the innervation of cervical portion of human esophagus. Gastroenterology, *25:* 375, 1953.
7. Hwang, K., Grossman, M. I., and Ivy, A. C.: Nervous control of the cervical portion of the esophagus. Am. J. Physiol., *154:* 343, 1948.
8. Henderson, R. D., Boszko, A., and vanNostrand, A. W. P.: Pharyngoesophageal dysphagia and recurrent laryngeal nerve palsy. J. Thorac. Cardiovasc. Surg., *68:* 507, 1974.
9. Smith, R. A., and Smith, R. E.: *Surgery of the Esophagus: The Coventry Conference.* Butterworths, London, 1972.
10. Valdes-Dapena, A. M., and Stein, G. N.: *Morphologic Pathology of the Alimentary Canal: Gross, Radiographic and Microscopic.* W. B. Saunders, Philadelphia, 1970.
11. Botha, G. S. M.: *The Gastro-Oesophageal Junction.* J. & A. Churchill Ltd., London, 1962.
12. Liebermann-Meffert, D., Allgower, M., Schmid, P., and Blum, A.L.: Muscular equivalent of the lower esophageal sphincter. Gastroenterology, *76:* 31, 1979.
13. Smith, B.: *The Neuropathology of the Alimentary Tract.* Williams & Wilkins, Baltimore, 1972.
14. Henderson, R. D., Ho, C. S., and Davidson, J. W.: Primary disordered motor activity of the esophagus (diffuse spasm); diagnosis and treatment. Ann. Thorac. Surg., *18:* 327, 1974.
15. Low, A.: A note on the crura of the diaphragm and the muscle of Treitz. J. Anat., *42:* 93, 1907.
16. Ellis, F. G., Kauntze, R., and Trounce, J. R.: The innervation of the cardia and lower oesophagus in man. Br. J. Surg., *47:* 466, 1960.
17. Collis, J. L., Kelly, T. D., and Wiley, A. M.: Anatomy of the crura of the diaphragm and the surgery of hiatus hernia. Thorax, *9:* 175, 1954.
18. Collis, J. L., Satchwell, L. M., and Abrams, L. D.: Nerve supply to the crura of the diaphragm. Thorax, *9:* 22, 1954.

CHAPTER 2

Normal Esophageal Motor Activity: Function and Control

Esophageal Function

The esophagus is the only nonabsorbing segment of the gastrointestinal tract (1). It runs from the cricopharyngeus muscle to the stomach as a musculomembranous structure, whose sole function is to transport oropharyngeal content to the stomach, or during vomiting to act as a route for gastric evacuation.

Following the development of the esophagoscope by Chevalier Jackson in 1890 (2), our understanding of esophageal disorders advanced rapidly. The early applications of contrast radiology further increased this accessibility, and since the early fifties extensive application of manometric techniques has provided detailed data concerning normal and disordered esophageal function. In the sixties and early seventies, the major advances came from increased sophistication in instrumentation, and from the more accurate correlation of available information. Thus, since Jackson's day each new development has produced more and better data so that the literature on the esophagus, once weak and fragmentary, has grown tremendously and shows no sign of slackening.

Since the major function of the esophagus is transport, most of the dysfunction in this organ is related to disorders of transport. Transport can be obstructed mechanically by the development of a fibrous or malignant stricture or functionally through some failure in the motor transport mechanism. The many and varied motor transport disorders are due either to disturbance or failure of myogenic or neurologic function, or the esophagus may respond to injury by muscle spasm. These motor transport problems are the principal subject of this book.

Mouth

For normal function, the human body requires the nourishment it obtains from food. The act of eating brings considerable pleasure. Most of this pleasure is derived from the taste of food products, but much of it is lost if, following chewing, the swallowed food particles become obstructed or produce pain during their passage into the stomach. For chewing, the mouth is equipped with powerful muscles of mastication, with teeth and with saliva to lubricate the food bolus and start early enzymatic breakdown. The food particles are broken down to a particular size acceptable to the esophagus and stomach. With mastication completed, the swallowing process begins. During swallowing, the mouth is closed and the food bolus forced backward by the tongue to the posterior pharynx (Fig. 2.1). From this site it can pass into the nasopharynx, the larynx or down through the cricopharyngeal sphincter to the esophagus. Under normal circumstances the nasopharynx is effectively closed off by the muscles of the soft palate and the larynx is pulled up underneath the tongue and partially protected by the epiglottis (3).

With this directional control, the food particles are then forced downward and through the cricopharyngeus sphincter into the esophagus. Swallowing can be initiated voluntarily or by reflex action in response to stimulation of sensory areas in the anterior and posterior pillars of the fauces and the sides and posterior walls of the pharynx (4). Once initiated, swallowing continues as a reflex action and

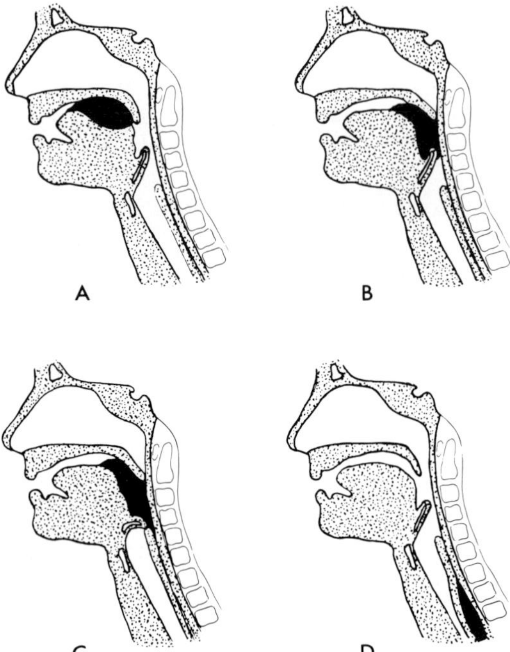

Figure 2.1. Sequence of Events during Swallowing

While the food bolus is in the mouth, nasal respiration continues (A); with swallowing, the nasopharynx is closed and the larynx is pulled forward and upward, closing off the larynx (B and C). The food is propelled through the cricopharynx to the body of the esophagus (D) by the combined action of the pharyngeal motor wave and the mechanical thrust of the tongue.

the bolus of food passes through the pharynx, cricopharynx and esophagus to the stomach.

Gravitational and Motor Propulsion

Two major components are responsible for transport of the food bolus: gravity and motor propulsion (4, 5). The relative effects of each of these depend to some extent on the consistency of the bolus. Solid food particles are aided by gravity, but their descent is considerably assisted by the forward propulsive force of the pharyngeal and esophageal motor waves. Liquid, by contrast, descends rapidly through the pharynx and esophagus by gravity, and motor contraction of the esophagus only clears away residual food fragments.

Gravitational descent is accelerated by the thrust of the tongue, which exerts on the upper pharynx a pressure of 10 to 20 cm of water (6, 7). The bolus rapidly descends through the pharynx, slowing slightly at the cricopharyngeus, then descending to the gastroesophageal junction where its forward motion is again reduced. Slowing at the cricopharyngeus may be due to the abrupt narrowing of the food passage at this level. At the level of the gastroesophageal junction, liquid which is descending by gravity is held up until the gastroesophageal junction relaxes. Solid food descends much more slowly, and usually the propulsive peristalsis of pharynx and esophagus carries it through the cricopharynx and the gastroesophageal junction.

Normal Esophageal Motor Function

For the purposes of description, esophageal motor function is divided into that of the pharynx, cricopharynx, body of the esophagus and gastroesophageal junction. Motor waves initiated in the pharynx pass through the entire length of the esophagus to the distal margin of the gastroesophageal junction. Although the motor waves so initiated vary in their amplitude, duration and velocity at each level, they remain coordinated and thus supply a continuous propulsive force. The esophagus itself is closed proximally by the cricopharyngeus and distally by the gastroesophageal junction high pressure zone (HPZ). Proximally the cricopharyngeus muscle acts as an anatomic sphincter, closing the esophagus and relaxing only in response to deglutition. Distally the HPZ closes the esophagus, relaxing to allow forward flow of food, but at all other times remains closed and acts as an important barrier to reflux of gastric content.

Pharyngoesophageal Junction

In this book, the pharynx, cricopharynx and upper esophagus are referred to as the pharyngoesophageal junction. The pharynx extends from the base of the tongue and posterior aspect of the soft palate to the upper margin of the cricopharyngeus muscle. The pharyngeal motor wave, which is of rapid velocity, 5 to 10 cm per second (Fig. 2.2), is usually described as a single motor wave (8), although some authors have described an initial low amplitude pressure rise preceding the major motor wave (9). This preliminary increase in pressure may be due to the propulsive force of the tongue, or may mark the entry of the food bolus into the pharynx.

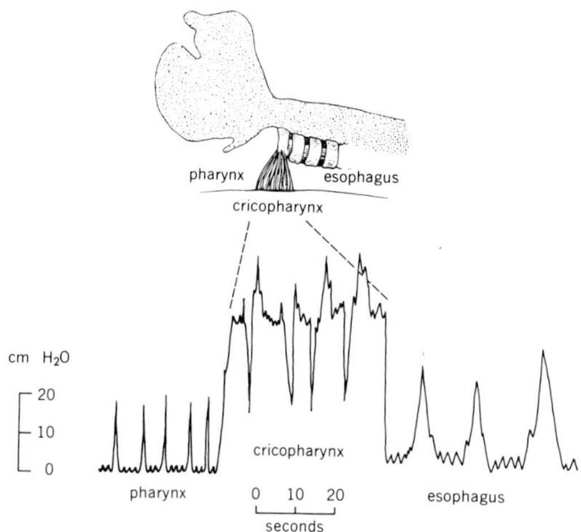

Figure 2.2. Motor Function of Cricopharynx
In this figure anatomic structure is correlated with motor changes. Pharyngeal motor activity is of high amplitude and short duration. The cricopharynx presents a constant pressure barrier which responds to deglutition by relaxation and then contraction. Relaxation of the cricopharyngeal sphincter is coordinated with the pharyngeal motor wave so that pharyngeal pressure reaches its peak at the instant of maximal cricopharyngeal relaxation. The pharyngeal and cricopharyngeal motor waves then sweep into the esophagus as the esophageal motor wave. It should be noted that the cricopharynx, by its constant tone, closes off the upper esophagus and it relaxes only in response to deglutition.

When pharyngeal pressures are recorded during the swallowing of a 1-cm marshmallow, this early pressure rise becomes more prominent, and may represent a direct response to the food bolus rather than contraction of the pharyngeal wall. The amplitude of the pharyngeal pressure wave varies from 15 to 80 cm of water and its duration is ½ second.

The cricopharyngeus muscle, which is approximately 2 cm in length, maintains a constant intraluminal pressure of from 10 to 60 cm of water. As the pharyngeal motor wave passes through the cricopharyngeus, it is preceded by local relaxation, which reduces cricopharyngeal pressure to the resting level in the upper esophagus. (This phase of relaxation is immediately preceded by a short pressure rise of 10 cm of water.) Pharyngeal contraction and cricopharyngeal relaxation

are so synchronized that the peak of pharyngeal contraction corresponds to the maximum relaxation in the cricopharyngeus. This coordination maintains a positive pressure gradient from pharynx through cricopharynx and into the upper esophagus. Following relaxation the cricopharynx contracts, then returns to basal tone, effectively closing off the sphincter and the upper end of the esophagus. Peristaltic contraction in the cricopharyngeus involves the entire length of the muscle and continues into the esophagus as the esophageal peristaltic wave (10).

The pressure in the body of the esophagus is directly related to intrapleural pressures, and hence will change with changes in intrapleural pressure and in response to alterations in body position and the distribution of blood of the lungs (11, 12).

Body of Esophagus

Esophageal peristalsis is a continuation of the motor wave from pharynx through cricopharynx. As noted earlier, the esophageal motor wave is preceded by a slight fall in basal esophageal pressure (13, 14), probably related to elevation of the larynx and alterations in the respiratory pattern during deglutition (Fig. 2.3). Following relaxation, esophageal pressure rises sharply, followed by a

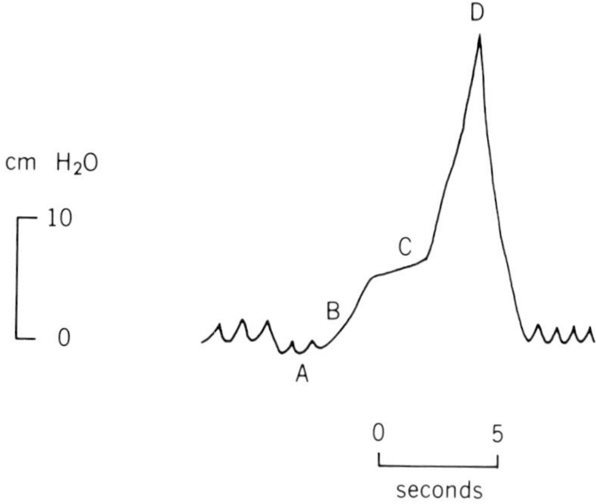

Figure 2.3. Esophageal Motor Wave
Components of the esophageal motor wave: (A) pressure fall preceding motor wave; (B) sharp increase in pressure stimulated by entry of food bolus to esophagus; (C) slowly rising plateau of pressure due to bolus descent; and (D) peristaltic esophageal motor wave.

gradually rising plateau of pressure, which terminates in the major peak of the peristaltic wave. The entry of the bolus into the esophagus provokes the initial sharp rise in pressure (15), the descent of the food bolus through the esophagus gives the gradually increasing plateau and the final motor contraction phase produces the coordinated peristaltic wave. Peristalsis moves rapidly through the upper esophagus but gradually slows until, at the lower esophagus, the motor wave advances only at a rate of 2.5 cm per second. In the upper esophagus, peristaltic waves tend to be of lower amplitude and shorter duration. These pressures and velocities probably differ because in the proximal esophagus most of the musculature is striated, whereas in the distal esophagus it is pure smooth muscle. (Striated, or skeletal, muscle is capable of faster contraction than is visceral smooth muscle.)

Disordered Motor Activity

Motor activity can become disordered in the normal as well as in the diseased esophagus and may manifest two types of waves—secondary and tertiary (16). Secondary motor waves arise within the body of the esophagus and progress distally, producing normal relaxation and contraction at the gastroesophageal junction (Fig. 2.4). Tertiary motor waves are localized zones of spasm and hence are not propagated (Fig. 2.5).

In the normal subject, 10 per cent of motor waves may be disordered and occasionally this percentage is even higher (10). Experimentally secondary peristalsis can be initiated by balloon distention in the lower esophagus but only rarely in the upper esophagus. Associated with distention and secondary disordered motor activity (DMA) the cricopharyngeal sphincteric tone also increases (17). Instillation of a liquid bolus into the esophagus also raises the cricopharyngeal pressure. The pressure response is more marked to 0.1 N hydrochloric acid than to saline. These pressure responses may act as a body defense mechanism to gastroesophageal reflux confining the refluxed bolus to the esophagus and protecting the lungs (18). In the aging esophagus, (DMA) becomes more marked (10, 19). Apart from its presence in the normal and ageing esophagus, DMA also develops in association with any form of esophageal irri-

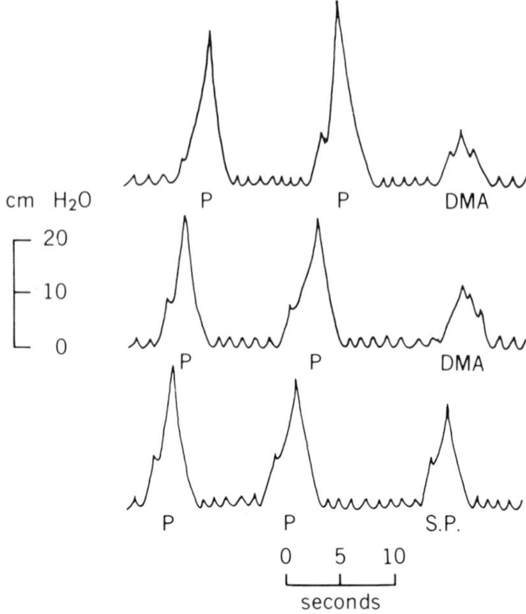

Figure 2.4. Secondary Disordered Motor Activity
Secondary disordered motor activity arises in the body of the esophagus and is propagated distally. In this figure, esophageal pressure is recorded at three levels 5 cm apart. Peristaltic motor waves (P) progress from one level to the next, whereas disordered motor waves (DMA) are simultaneous. Here a normally propagated peristaltic wave (P) is followed by a spastic disordered motor wave (DMA) which then is propagated distally as a secondary peristalsis (SP).

tation. Myogenic and neurogenic esophageal disorders also produce DMA; however, the form of the esophageal motor wave varies with the disease process (19–23).

Gastroesophageal Junction

The lower esophagus is demarcated by a physiologic HPZ, which separates the body of the esophagus from the stomach. This zone has been given several names, including gastroesophageal junction, high pressure zone and gastroesophageal sphincter, all of which are used synonymously and apply to the distal esophageal segment which, by maintaining an elevated pressure, acts as a barrier to reflux of gastric content into the esophagus. This zone has been demonstrated by esophageal manometric studies (Fig. 2.6), by radi-

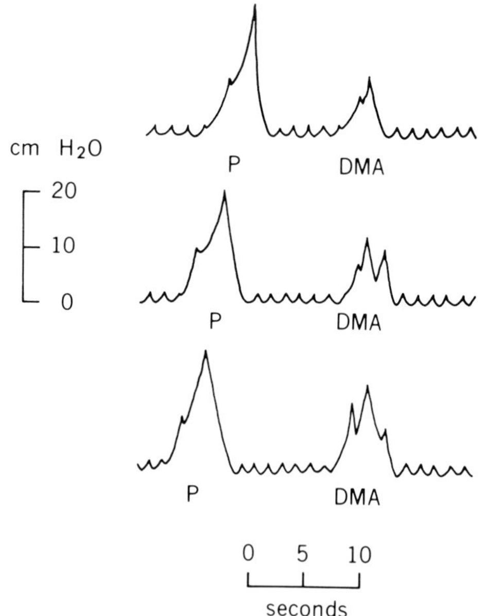

Figure 2.5. Tertiary Disordered Motor Activity Tertiary disordered motor activity arises in the body of the esophagus. In this figure a peristaltic motor wave (P) is followed by a nonpropagated disordered motor wave (DMA) of the tertiary type.

ologic studies (Fig. 2.7) and by endoscopy; the last shows an empty or closed segment of distal esophagus. This area is usually considered to be a physiologic zone without recognizable muscular thickening. However, Botha and more recently Liebermann-Meffert et al. have shown that an anatomic sphincter is present (24, 25). The mean pressure of the HPZ is 15 to 30 cm of water and the zone varies in length from 2 to 4 cm (26, 27) (Fig. 2.6). With deglutition, relaxation begins 1.5 to 2.5 seconds after the initiation of the swallow and continues for up to 10 seconds. This relaxation, which reduces the pressure in the HPZ, neutralizes the pressure barrier, and produces a pressure gradient from esophagus into stomach (28). Relaxation terminates with the arrival of the esophageal peristaltic motor wave. The wave continues through the HPZ as the postrelaxation contraction. At the distal end of the zone, coordinated esophageal activity ceases and is replaced by gastric motor activity. It should be noted that gastric and esophageal motor activity are independent of each other.

The relaxation seen in the HPZ is more prolonged than that in the cricopharyngeus. When a liquid bolus of barium descends by gravity through the esophagus, it slows at the gastroesophageal junction before it descends into the stomach during the period of relaxation. Solid fragments under the control of esophageal peristaltic activity are passed through and cleared by the coordinated esophageal and gastroesophageal junctional contraction. This coordinated contraction wave arrives at the gastroesophageal junction approximately 10 seconds after the initiation of deglutition, and, once it has passed through the junction, motor activity in the esophagus ceases until a new motor complex is initiated by deglutition.

Pressure Inversion Point— "Physiologic Diaphragm"

Esophageal manometric studies of the gastroesophageal junction show a point at which respiratory positive deflections in the abdomen become respiratory negative deflections in the intrathoracic esophagus (Fig. 2.7). This point of pressure change, "the pressure inversion point (PIP)," is important because it marks the point at which the balance of intraabdominal pressures causing the respiratory positive deflections is overcome by the correspondingly balanced pressures within the thorax. In the normal subject this point falls within the gastroesophageal HPZ. The pressure inversion point (29, 30) can be regarded as the physiologic diaphragm, separating the thorax from the abdomen. In the normal subject it lies close to the level of the diaphragm, whereas, in the individual with a hiatal hernia, the physiologic diaphragm may lie within the thoracic cavity or within the herniated gastric fundus, leaving the gastroesophageal junction entirely respiratory negative.

In hiatal hernias, variations in the site of the PIP are of diagnostic value because here the inversion point may become more proximal or more distal. If the PIP moves during manometric studies the HPZ will fluctuate, changing from respiratory positive to respiratory negative; this phenomenon is referred to as double respiratory reversal (DRR). When present, DRR indicates diminished competence of the junction and is regarded as a diagnostic feature of hiatal hernia (Fig. 2.8).

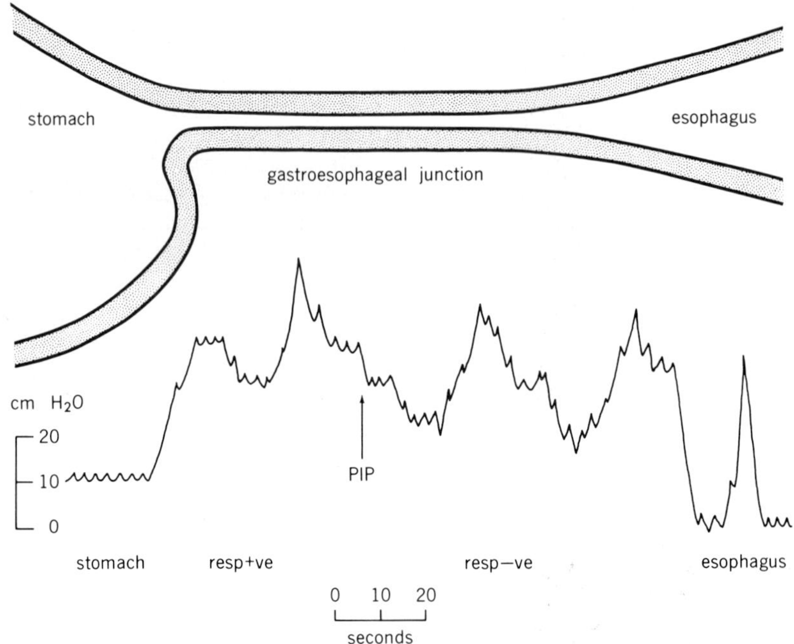

Figure 2.6. Gastroesophageal Junction
In the gastroesophageal junction, a high pressure zone (HPZ) maintains pressure as a barrier between esophagus and stomach. This zone demarcates the lower end of the esophagus. The pressure inversion point (PIP) is the point at which respiratory pressure changes (''inverts'') from positive in the abdomen to negative in the thorax. The gastroesophageal junction maintains a pressure barrier at rest and responds to deglutition by relaxation followed by contraction and resumption of the protective function.

Control of Motor Function

Neurogenic

The oral phase of swallowing is controlled by sensory fibers from the glossopharyngeal and superior laryngeal branch of the vagus nerve. This activity is relayed through the medulla and motor control exerted through fibers of C1, C2, and C3 (31). The medullary swallowing center can be initiated voluntarily or may be activated by afferent sensory stimulation from the oropharynx, hypopharynx, or esophageal body. Initiated activity from the esophagus may result in a complete swallow or may produce peristalsis only in the body of the esophagus (32). This type of deglutive response arising in the esophagus and propagating distally would be secondary DMA.

Peristalsis in the pharynx, cricopharynx and the esophagus is controlled by the vagus and by cervical and thoracic sympathetic fibers. The vagal fibers are distributed to the myenteric plexuses in the esophageal wall, and the postganglionic vagal fibers subserve coordinated esophageal function. The esophagus also appears to have β-adrenergic fibers which, when activated, lower the pressure in the high pressure zone during deglutition. Zfass and colleagues (33–37) have described α-adrenergic fibers which act to increase smooth muscle contractions.

Myogenic

The longitudinal muscle fibers in the lower esophagus assist in the coordination of esopageal function by conducting the motor wave (35–37). Evidence of such "myogenic" conduction has been gained chiefly from electromyographic studies of the lower esophagus in animals (38). This type of conduction appears to be a second and distinct method for coordinating esophageal motor function.

Gastric Reflexes

Gastroesophageal reflux is prevented in part through the responsiveness of the gastroesophageal junction to increases in intra-ab-

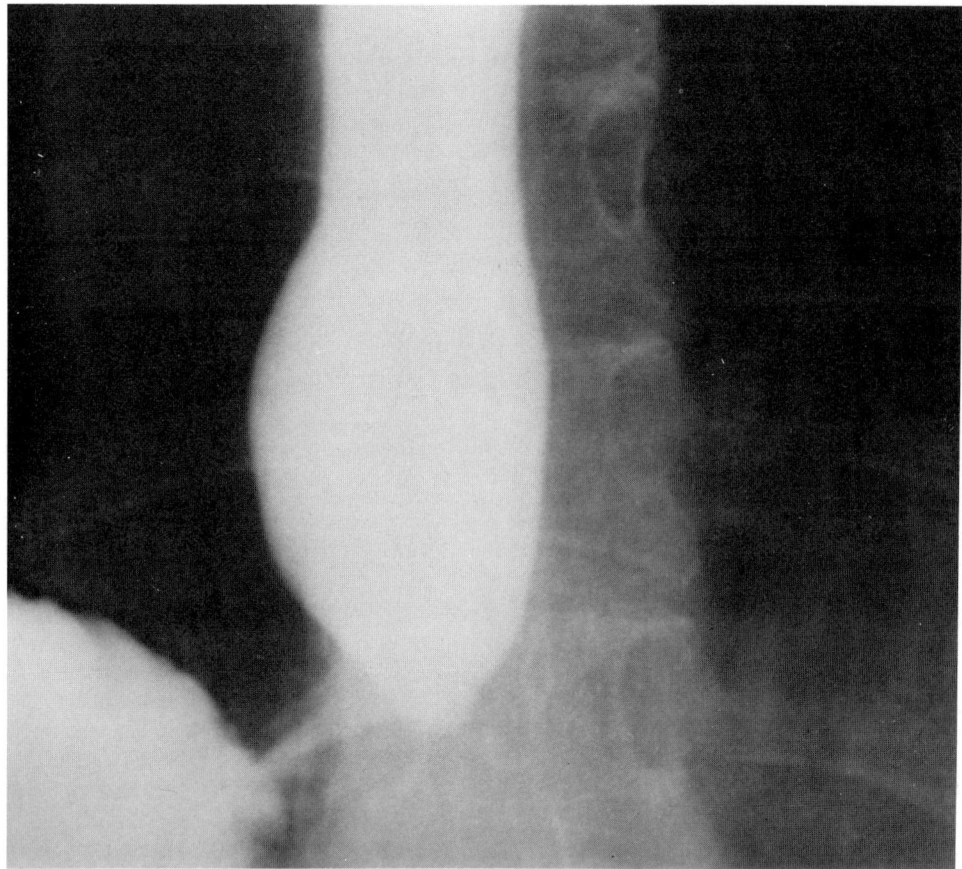

Figure 2.7. Normal Barium Swallow
The distal esophagus dilates to form the phrenic ampulla. Immediately distal to this is the gastroesophageal high pressure zone which relaxes in response to deglutition.

dominal pressure. Increased gastric pressure produces a corresponding increase in gastroesophageal junctional pressure and, in this way, maintains an effective pressure barrier (39–41). This phenomenon has been studied manometrically by recording the pressure in the HPZ when abdominal compression is applied and a Teflon ball is withdrawn simultaneously from the stomach into the esophagus. By these methods it has been shown that the pressure in the HPZ increases even more than the pressure in the adjacent stomach. This augmented increase in HPZ pressure indicates that the response to abdominal compression is neurogenic rather than a passive response to extrinsic elevation of peritoneal pressure. The response of the gastroesophageal junction to increased intra-abdominal pressure is reduced in the presence of a hiatal hernia. Pressures in the gastro-esophageal junction increase in response to gastric motor activity in experimental animals, but this finding has not yet been confirmed in humans (42).

Hormonal Control

Gastrointestinal hormones are polypeptides released from various parts of the intestine in response to ingested food. There are many such hormones, but not all have a proved physiologic role. Those most likely to involve the HPZ and esophageal function are gastrin, cholecystokinin (CCK), secretin and glucagon. Other described hormones may affect esophageal function; however, their roles have not been elucidated. These other hormones include vasoactive intestinal polypeptide (VIP), gastric inhibiting polypeptide (GIP), motilin and some of the prostaglandins (43–50).

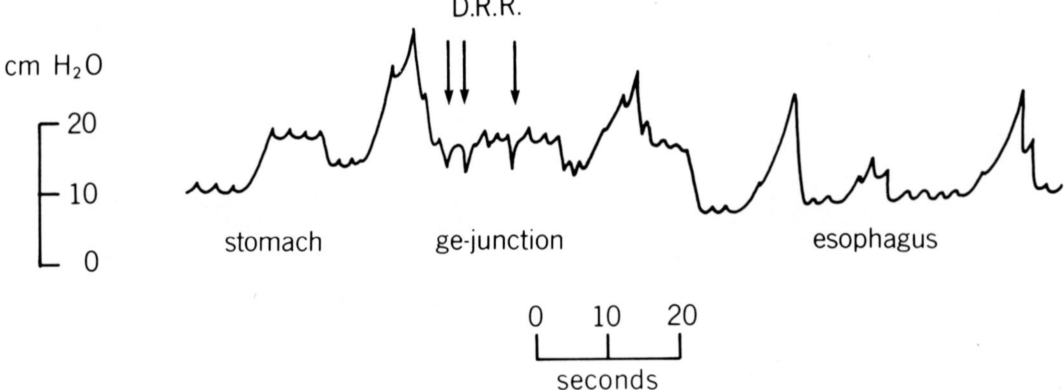

Figure 2.8. Double Respiratory Reversal in Hiatal Hernia
Double respiratory reversal is commonly seen in patients with a hiatal hernia. Instead of a sharp demarcation between respiratory positive and respiratory negative zones in the gastroesophageal junction, there are fluctuations from respiratory positive to respiratory negative. These fluctuations reflect the incompetence of the junction and its tendency to slip in and out of the thoracic cavity.

Gastrin

Gastrin is released from the antrum of the stomach in response to vagal stimulation and gastric alkalinization. Early studies suggested that it might be responsible for basal tone in the HPZ and an observed HPZ tone elevation following gastric alkalinization or a protein meal. The pressure changes which occur with alkalinization and to a protein meal do not correspond to elevations of serum gastrin and pressure elevations still occurred, although to a reduced degree, in patients with antrectomy. Serum gastrin levels vary in patients with vagotomy and pyloroplasty, Billroth I gastrectomy, Billroth II gastrectomy, Zollinger-Ellison syndrome and reflux; however, the HPZ tone cannot be correlated with these serum levels (51). Although the HPZ does respond to pharmacologic infusion of pentagastrin, it has not been possible to demonstrate a physiologic role although further study is clearly necessary (43–47, 52, 53).

Cholecystokinin (CCK)

This hormone is released from the proximal part of the small intestine and is primarily involved in regulating the function of the gallbladder and pancreas.

CCK endogenously and exogenously has been shown to reduce HPZ tone. A fatty meal is the major stimulus to CCK release and has been shown to be associated with a decrease in HPZ tone. Fat has also been shown to decrease the anticipated HPZ tone response to a protein meal (45, 54, 55).

Secretin

This hormone has a different polypeptide structure from gastrin and CCK. It is released from the proximal small intestine and stimulates pancreatic secretion.

While the hormone can not be shown to have a direct effect on the HPZ, it does antagonize the effects of gastrin and if gastrin has a role in the HPZ tone mechanism then it is likely that secretin also is active (45).

Glucagon

Glucagon is similar to secretin in structure and is released both from pancreas and small bowel. This hormone also antagonizes the effect of pentagastrin on the HPZ but has not yet been shown to have a physiologic role in control of the HPZ (45).

While the role of hormones in HPZ control has not been elucidated almost certainly, they do have a function and combined with neural control they aid in maintenance and regulation of tone.

Our knowledge of the various mechanisms which control the esophagus and gastroesophageal junction is becoming more complicated with each succeeding year (Fig. 2.9). In addition to the neurogenic, myogenic and hormonal controls, we must consider the ef-

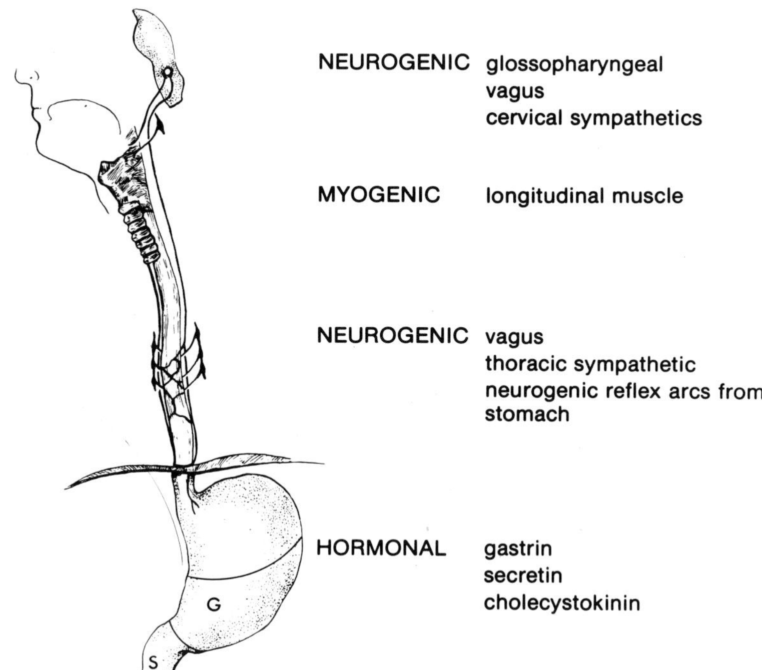

Figure 2.9. Esophageal Control Mechanisms
Esophageal motor function is coordinated through neurogenic, myogenic and hormonal mechanisms.

fects of endogenous dietary chemicals (56–58) on the control mechanism. For example, carminatives, nicotine (tobacco) and alcohol all may decrease esophageal motor activity and also reduce the tone of the gastroesophageal junction. Drug therapy (59) can affect the esophagus and alter motor function, particuarly drugs used to stimulate or block the autonomic nervous system. The complex interaction between these various control mechanisms moved Ingelfinger (60) to describe the gastroesophageal sphincter as a "sphinx."

References

1. Rosenow, E. C., III: Esophageal motility. Med. Clin. North Am., *54:* 863, 1970.
2. Jackson, C.: *The Life of Chevalier Jackson: An Autobiography.* Macmillan Co., New York, 1938.
3. Davenport, H. W.: *Physiology of the Digestive Tract, An Introductory Text.* Year Book Medical Publishers, Chicago, 1961.
4. Doty, R. W.: *Transactions of the Third Macy Conference on the Central Nervous System and Behavior.* Josiah Macy Jr. Foundation, New York, 1969.
5. Hightower, N. C.: Esophageal motility in health and disease. Dis. Chest, *28:* 150, 1955.
6. Negus, V. E.: Second stage of swallowing. Acta Otolaryngol. [Suppl.] *78:* 78, 1949.
7. Shedd, D. P., Kirchner, J. A., and Scatliff, J. A.: Oral and pharyngeal components of deglutition: A radiologic study in surgical patients. Arch. Surg., *82:* 373, 1961.
8. Kelley, M. L., Jr.: Esophageal motor function: Normal and pathological physiology as reflected by intraluminal manometric studies. Am. J. Dig. Dis., *9:* 553, 1964.
9. Atkinson, M., Kramer, P., Wyman, S. M., and Ingelfinger, F. J.: The dynamics of swallowing; 1. Normal pharyngeal mechanisms. J. Clin. Invest., *36:* 581, 1957.
10. Nagler, R., and Spiro, H. M.: Serial oesophageal motility studies in asymptomatic young subjects. Gastroenterology, *41:* 371, 1961.
11. Banchero, N., Schwartz, P. E., Tsakiris, A. G., and Wood, E. H.: Pleural and esophageal pressures in the upright body position. J. Appl. Physiol., *23:* 228, 1967.
12. Miller, A. D., Saunders, R. A., and Hopkin, L. E.: Relationship of intra-esophageal pressure to mouth pressure during the measurement of thoracic gas volume in the newborn. Biol. Neonate, *33:* 314, 1978.
13. Vantrappen, G., and Hellemans, J.: Studies on the normal deglutition complex. Am. J. Dig. Dis., *12:* 255, 1967.
14. Humphries, T. J., and Castell, D. O.: Pressure profile of esophageal peristalsis in normal humans as measured by direct intraesophageal transducers. Am. J. Dig. Dis., *22:* 641, 1977.
15. Dornhorst, A. C., Harrison, K., and Pierce, J. W.: Observations on the normal oseophagus and cardia. Lancet, *1:* 695, 1954.

16. Creamer, B., and Schlegel, J.: Motor responses of the esophagus to distension. J. Appl. Physiol., *10:* 498, 1957.

17. Enzmann, D. R., Harrell, G. S., and Zboralske, F. F.: Upper esophageal responses to intraluminal distension in man. Gastroenterology, *72:* 1292, 1977.

18. Gerhardt, D. C., Shuck, T. J., Bordeaux, R. A., and Winship, D. H.: Human upper esophageal sphincter; response to volume, osmotic and acid stimuli. Gastroenterology, *75:* 268, 1978.

19. Zboralske, F. F., Amberg, J. R., and Soergel, K. H.: Presbyesophagus; cineradiographic manifestations. Radiology, *82:* 463, 1964.

20. Fyke, F. E., Code, C. F., and Schlegel, J. F.; The gastroesophageal sphincter in healthy human beings. Gastroenterologia, *86:* 135, 1956.

21. Henderson, R. D., and Pearson, F. G.: Surgical management of esophageal scleroderma. J. Thorac. Cardiovasc. Surg., *66:* 686, 1973.

22. Henderson, R. D., Barichello, A. W., Pearson, F. G., Mugashe, F., and Szczepanski, M.: Diagnosis of achalasia. Can. J. Surg., *15:* 190, 1972.

23. Henderson, R. D., Ho., C. S., and Davidson, J. W.: Primary disordered motor activity of the esophagus (diffuse spasm). Ann. Thorac. Surg., *18:* 327, 1974.

24. Botha, G. S. M.: *The Gastro-Oesophageal Junction.* J. & A. Churchill Ltd., London, 1962.

25. Liebermann-Meffert, D., Allgower, M., Schmidt, P., and Blum, A. L.: Muscular equivalent of the lower esophageal sphincter. Gastroenterology, *76:* 31, 1979.

26. Cohen, S., and Harris, L. D.: Lower esophageal sphincter pressure as an index of lower esophageal sphincter strength. Gastroenterology, *58:* 157, 1970.

27. Davison, J. S.: Relaxation of the lower-oesophageal sphincter during swallowing. Digestion, *15:* 73, 1977.

28. Code, C. F., Creamer, B., Schlegel, J. F., Olsen, A. M., Donoghue, F. E., and Andersen, H. A.: *An Atlas of Esophageal Motility in Health and Disease.* Charles C Thomas, Springfield, Ill., 1958.

29. Harris, L. D., and Pope, C. E.: The pressure inversion point: its genesis and reliability. Gastroenterology, *51:* 641, 1966.

30. Atkinson, M., Edwards, D. A. W., Honour, A. J., and Rowlands, E. N.: The oesophagogastric sphincter in hiatus hernia. Lancet, *2:* 1138, 1957.

31. Doty, R. W., and Bosma, J. F.: An electromyographic analysis of reflex deglutition. J. Neurophysiol., *19:* 44, 1956.

32. Diamant, N. E., and El-Sharkawy, T. Y.: Neural control of esophageal peristalsis. Gastroenterology, *72:* 546, 1977.

33. Zfass, A. M., Prince, R., Allen, F. N., and Farrar, J. T.: Inhibitory beta adrenergic receptors in the human distal esophagus. Am. J. Dig. Dis., *15:* 303, 1970.

34. Daniel, E. E., and Chapman, K. M.: Electrical activity of the gastrointestinal tract as an indication of mechanical activity. Am. J. Dig. Dis., *8:* 54, 1963.

35. Snape, W. J., and Cohen, S.: Control of esophageal and lower esophageal sphincter function; neurohumoral and myogenic factors. Front. Gastrointest. Res., *3:* 76, 1978.

36. Stoddard, C. J.: Current concepts of gastrointestinal motility and electrical activity. Br. J. Hosp. Med., *20:* 426, 1978.

37. Christensen, J.: The innervation and motility of the esophagus. Front. Gastrointest. Res., *3:* 18, 1978.

38. Sarna, S. K., Daniel, E. E., and Waterfall, W. E.: Myogenic and neural control systems for esophageal motility. Gastroenterology, *73:* 1345, 1977.

39. Boesby, S.: Effects of changes in the intragastric milieu on competence of the gastro-oesophageal region. A study in normal subjects. Scand. J. Gastroenterol., *12:* 215, 1977.

40. Lind, J. F., Warrian, W. G., and Wankling, W. J.: Responses of the gastroesophageal junctional zone to increases in abdominal pressure. Can. J. Surg., *9:* 32, 1966.

41. Henderson, R. D., and Rodney, K.: Tone of the gastroesophageal junction; its response to abdominal compression and to swallowing. Can. J. Surg., *14:* 328, 1971.

42. Diamant, N. E., and Akin, A. N.: The effect of gastric contractions on the lower esophageal sphincter. Gastroenterology, *63:* 38, 1972.

43. Cohen, S., and Lipshutz, W.: Hormonal regulation of human lower esophageal sphincter competence; interaction of gastrin and secretion. J. Clin. Invest., *50:* 449, 1971.

44. Castell, D. O., and Harris, L. D.: Hormonal control of gastroesophageal-sphincter strength. N. Engl. J. Med., *282:* 886, 1970.

45. Snape, W. J., and Cohen, S.: Hormonal control of esophageal function. Arch. Intern. Med., *136:* 538, 1976.

46. McGuigan, J. E.: Serum gastrin in health and disease. Am. J. Dig. Dis., *22:* 712, 1977.

47. Henderson, J. M., Lidgard, G., Osborne, D. H., Carter, D. C., and Heading, R. C.: Lower oesophageal sphincter response to gastrin-pharmacological or physiological? Gut, *19:* 99, 1978.

48. Sinar, D. R., O'Dorisio, T. M., Mazzaferri, E. L., Mekhjian, M. D., Caldwell, J. H., and Thomas, F. B.: Effect of gastric inhibitory polypeptide on lower esophageal sphincter pressure in cats. Gastroenterology, *75:* 263, 1978.

49. Koelz, H. R., Lepsien, G., Hollinger, A. P., Säubreli, H., Largiader, F., Arnold, R., Blum, A. L., and Siewert, R.: Effect of intraduodenal peptone on the lower esophageal sphincter pressure in the dog. Gastroenterology, *75:* 283, 1978.

50. Meissner, A. J., Bowes, K. L., Zwick, R., and Daniel, E. E.: Effect of motilin on the lower oesophageal sphincter. Gut, *17:* 925, 1976.

51. McCallum, R. W., and Walsh, J. H.: Relationship between lower esophageal sphincter pressure and serum gastrin concentration in Zollinger-Ellison syndrome and other clinical settings. Gastroenterology, *76:* 76, 1979.

52. Windsor, C. W. O.: Gastroesophageal reflux after partial gastrectomy. Br. Med. J., *2:* 1233, 1964.

53. Henderson, R. D.: Gastroesophageal reflux following gastric operation. Ann. Thorac. Surg., *26:* 563, 1978.

54. Resin, H., Stern, D. H., Richard, A. L., Sturdevant, M. D., and Isenberg, J. I.: Effect of C-terminal octapeptide of cholecystokinin on lower esophageal sphincter pressure in man. Gastroenterology, *64:* 946, 1973.

55. Behar, J., and Biancani, P.: Effect of cholecystokinin-

octapeptide on lower esophageal sphincter. Gastroenterology, *73:* 57, 1977.

56. Dennish, G. W., and Castell, D. O.: Inhibitory effect of smoking on the lower esophageal sphincter. N. Engl. J. Med., *284:* 1136, 1971.

57. Sigmund, C. J., and McNally, E. F.: The action of a carminative on the lower esophageal sphincter. Gastroenterology, *56:* 13, 1969.

58. Mayer, E. M., Grabowski, C. J., and Fisher, R. S.: Effects of graded doses of alcohol upon esophageal motor function. Gastroenterology, *75:* 1133, 1978.

59. Smith, G., Dalling, R., and Williams, T. I. R.: Gastro-oesophageal pressure gradient changes produced by induction of anaesthesia and suxamethonium. Br. J. Anaesth., *50:* 1137, 1978.

60. Ingelfinger, F. J.: The sphincter that is a sphinx. N. Engl. J. Med., *284:* 1095, 1971.

CHAPTER 3

Disordered Motor Activity of the Esophagus: Primary and Secondary

Having considered the normal motor function of the esophagus, we can now explore further the motor response of the esophagus to disease. For a fuller understanding of this response it is necessary to divide the motor changes into primary disorders and secondary disorders where the esophagus responds to local injury (Tables 3.1 and 3.2) (1, 2). Further subdivision is necessary because of muscle structure and function. The upper esophagus, cricopharynx and pharynx have striated muscle which, in general, is involved by a different group of disease processes than the lower smooth muscle esophagus. Primary motor disorders can be defined as those in which the motor changes are related to neurogenic or myogenic esophageal abnormality. In some it is possible to be specific and state that the motor changes are either neurogenic or myogenic. In many others, further investigation is necessary to elucidate the precise pathophysiology. Achalasia is the best known of the primary disorders affecting the lower esophagus and is now recognized as being neurogenic (3). Myotonia is related to a primary disorder of skeletal muscle and affects the upper third of the esophagus, cricopharynx and pharynx (4). Other primary disorders are less well understood, but fall into the primary categorization because they are not related to exposure to a specific exogenous or endogenous esophageal irritant (5).

Secondary motor disorders are those related to exogenous and endogenous irritation. The irritation produces a secondary esophageal inflammation, and the motor changes found are secondary to this inflammatory change. The best example is the reflux of gastric content which produces esophagitis and is associated with a secondary motor change (6). Reflux affects both proximal and distal esophagus. Other causes of secondary disordered motor activity include the various chemical agents which may be ingested and which result in an esophageal burn. Secondary disorders also include esophageal inflammation from lodgment of foreign bodies or from an acute esophageal infection such as moniliasis.

This classification into primary and secondary disorders has greatly assisted categorization of disturbances of function and in so doing has increased our understanding of the various esophageal responses to these diseases.

Primary Motor Disorders

These need not be examined in depth here because each will be considered later at the time of fuller discussion of the disease. However, it may be helpful at this stage to review briefly the principal changes in some of the more important motor disorders to illustrate the wide variety of motor responses.

Achalasia

Achalasia is a neurogenic esophageal disorder (7) in which the motor changes affect both the gastroesophageal junction and the body of the esophagus. The junction fails to relax and in some patients the tone of the gastroesophageal junction is elevated (8). The body of the esophagus shows a total disorder of motor activity, and the motor waves are of low amplitude and prolonged duration (Fig. 3.1). The cricopharynx and pharynx exhibit normal motor function. A knowledge of the motor defect in achalasia permits a fuller understanding of the clinical and radiologic appearances, namely, how failure of relaxation in the junction and the presence of inef-

Table 3.1

Disordered Motor Activity—Lower Smooth Muscle Esophagus*

Primary	
Neurogenic	
Congenital	Hereditary spastic ataxia
	Riley-Day syndrome
Acquired	Achalasia
	Diffuse esophageal spasm
	Parkinsonism
	Alcoholism
	Diabetes
	Chagas' disease
Myogenic	Myotonia
	Thyrotoxicosis
Idiopathic	Scleroderma
Secondary	
Infections	Monilia
	Viral
	Secondary bacterial
Endogenous	Gastroesophageal reflux
Exogenous	Caustic
	Foreign body
Malignancy	Esophageal infiltration
	Obstruction

* Primary disorders are defined as those due to the diseases of the esophageal muscle or nerve supply. Secondary disorders are due to esophageal irritation or infiltration.

fectual low amplitude disordered motor waves in the esophagus leaves a constant pressure barrier, which prevents passage of food into the stomach. Obstruction is relieved only when food retained in the esophagus creates sufficient hydrostatic pressure to overcome the resistance in the junctional tone and allow emptying by gravity. This defect in motor function is believed to be neurogenic because in animal experiments various forms of esophageal denervation have produced motor changes similar to those seen in human achalasia (9, 10). The motor changes which develop in humans following esophageal denervation have not been described because there are no therapeutic indications for this type of denervation.

One patient in my own experience had proved esophageal denervation and she developed motor changes similar to those seen in achalasia.

Case 1. Mrs. L., age 70, developed voice changes and dysphagia simultaneously. Food obstruction at the midesophageal level was severe and occurred with each meal. She complained also of frequent regurgitation of food-tasting esophageal content. On examination she was shown to have an idiopathic right recurrent laryngeal nerve palsy. A Hollander test meal showed no gastric response to insulin stimulation. Radiologically she had a 10-cm hiatal hernia, and the body of the esophagus

Table 3.2

Disordered Motor Activity—Upper Esophagus, Cricopharynx and Pharynx*

I. Primary	
A. Neurogenic	
1. Congenital	Riley-Day syndrome
2. Acquired central	Stroke
	Bulbar polio
	Parkinsonism
3. Acquired peripheral	Recurrent laryngeal nerve injury or neuritis
B. Myoneurogenic	Myasthenia gravis
C. Myogenic	Myotonia dystrophia
	Thyrotoxicosis
II. Secondary	
A. Exogenous	Caustic burn
B. Endogenous	Gastroesophageal reflux
III. Idiopathic	
A. Cricopharyngeal bar	
B. Cricopharyngeal pouch	

* Primary and secondry disorders are classified in the same manner as for the lower esophagus. Cricopharyngeal bars and pouches are probably secondary to gastroesophageal reflux.

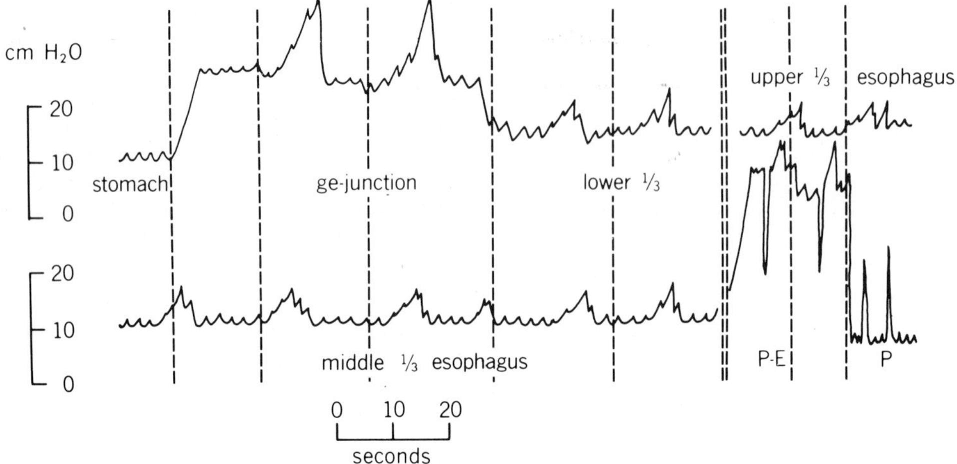

Figure 3.1. Manometric Tracing in Achalasia
This representation of manometric data is used to illustrate the actual motor traces obtained from patients. The pressure scale indicates pressure in centimeters of water (cm H₂O), and the time scale shows duration of motor waves in seconds. Single vertical lines indicate a 1-cm proximal move of motility catheters, and the double vertical line indicates a major move into the proximal esophagus. In achalasia the gastroesophageal junction (ge) is of normal or high normal tone and does not show relaxation in response to deglutition. Disordered motor activity in the body of the esophagus is total and of a low amplitude type. The pharyngoesophageal junction (P-E) and the pharynx (P) are normal.

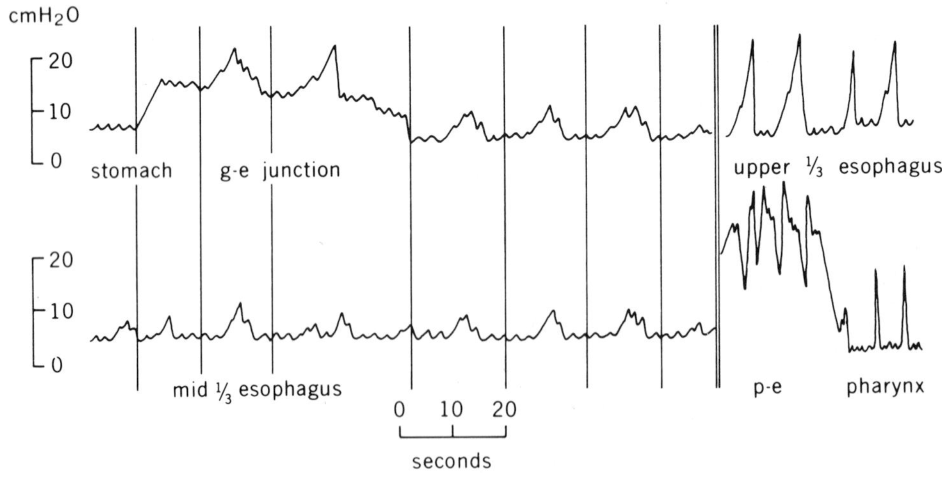

Figure 3.2. Neurogenic Esophagus
The patient (Mrs. L.) has a normal tone on the gastroesophageal (g-e) junction and contraction, but no relaxation in response to deglutition. The lower two-thirds of the esophagus is totally disordered with motor waves of low amplitude and prolonged duration. Peristalsis in the proximal esophagus is normal; the cricopharynx and pharynx are also normal. p-e, pharyngoesophageal junction.

showed no evidence of coordinated motor activity. Manometrically the gastroesophageal junction was of normal tone and did not show any relaxation in response to deglutition (Fig. 3.2). The lower two-thirds of the esophagus was totally disordered with low amplitude motor waves of prolonged duration. The proximal third of the esophagus showed normal peristalsis, and the cricopharyngeus and pharynx functioned normally.

This patient provided good evidence of at least partial denervation of the esophagus,

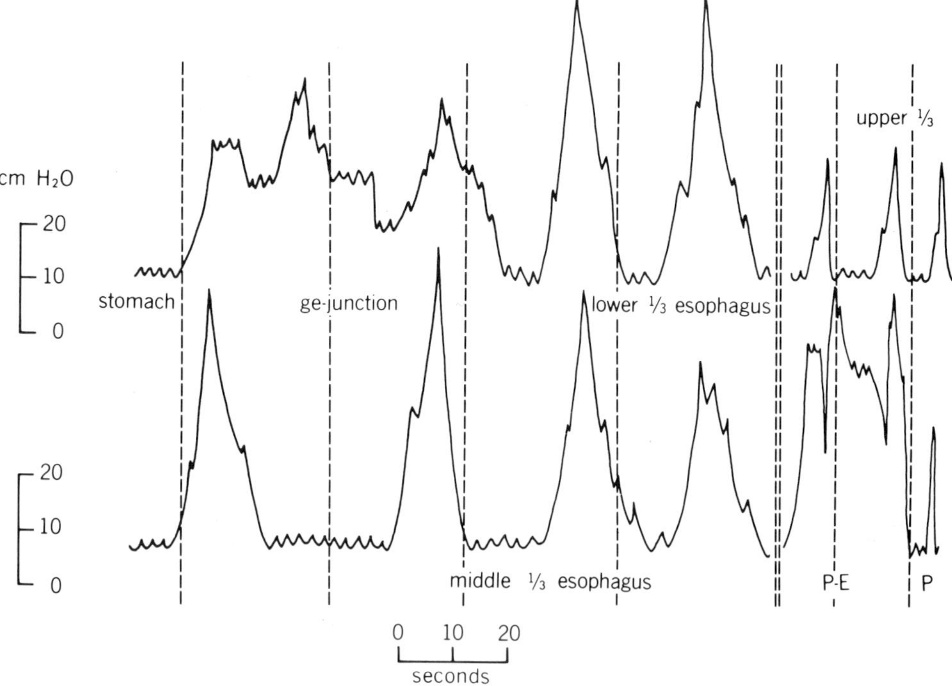

Figure 3.3. Diffuse Esophageal Spasm
In diffuse spasm (DES) the gastroesophageal (ge) junction is normal. In the lower two-thirds of esophagus disordered motor activity is severe and is usually of high amplitude and prolonged duration. The upper one-third of the esophagus, cricopharynx (P-E) and pharynx (P) are normal.

and the motor changes produced in the lower two-thirds of her esophagus were indistinguishable from achalasia.

Diffuse Spasm (DES)

Less is known about the etiology of diffuse spasm (DES) than about achalasia; however, investigation suggests that it too is a neurogenic disorder (11). Motor changes in DES are very different from those found in achalasia. The gastroesophageal junction is normal and relaxes and contracts well in response to deglutition (Fig. 3.3). The lower two-thirds of the body of the esophagus is involved in a severe disorder of motor activity and here the motor waves are of high amplitude and prolonged duration (12). In the proximal esophagus, cricopharyngeus and pharynx, the motor activity is normal. It should be noted that the motor response in the lower two-thirds, being of high amplitude, is very different from the secondary (low amplitude) disordered motor activity characteristic of esophageal injury.

Collagen Disorders

Scleroderma is the most frequent collagen disorder to involve the esophagus (13). It affects the lower two-thirds of the esophagus, that is, the smooth muscle portion, and produces a marked loss of esophageal contractility. The lower esophagus becomes adynamic (Fig. 3.4). Gastroesophageal tone is markedly reduced or totally absent. It has not yet been determined whether the changes are secondary to myogenic or neurogenic damage, and indeed both may be simultaneously involved (14).

Myotonia

This disorder is due to striated muscle degeneration (15) and as such is limited to the upper one-third of the esophagus, cricopharynx and pharynx. Motor activity in this segment is markedly reduced (Fig. 3.5).

Myasthenia Gravis

Esophageal involvement in myasthenia is similar to that in myotonia, and again the

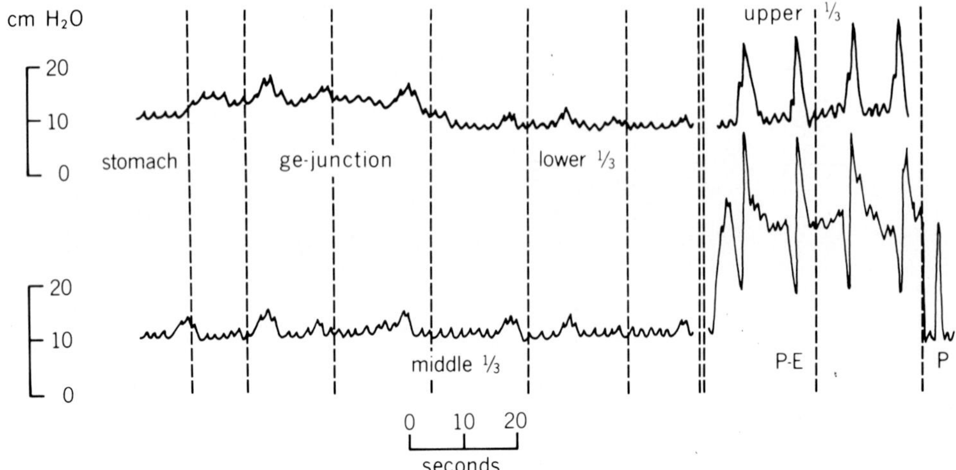

Figure 3.4. **Adynamic Esophagus (Scleroderma)**
In scleroderma (collagen disease), tone is lost in the gastroesophageal junction (ge) and distal two-thirds of esophagus, and the motor disorder is of low amplitude. The proximal one-third of esophagus and pharyngoesophageal junction (P-E) are usually normal. P, pharynx.

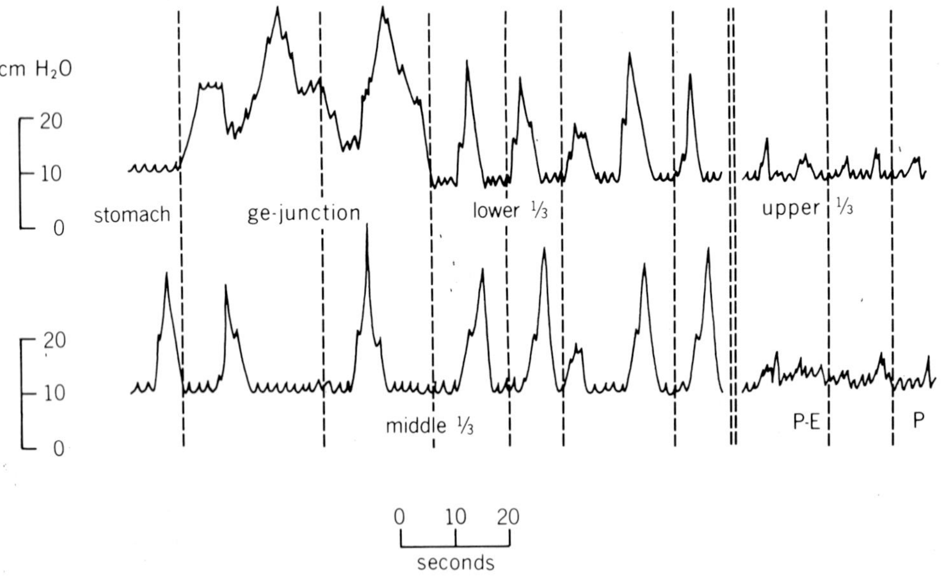

Figure 3.5. **Myotonia**
In myotonia the gastroesophageal (ge) junction and lower two-thirds of the esophagus are unaffected. The disease involves the proximal one-third of esophagus, pharyngoesophageal junction (P-E) and pharynx (P) and produces a marked loss of tone in these zones.

striated esophagus and pharynx are involved (16). There is a marked diminution in motor function in these areas. The myasthenia is due to a failure in chemical transmission at the myoneural junction.

The clinical presentations and motor ab-normalities in these esophageal diseases are varied, but they have one factor in common, namely, they involve one of the esophageal components necessary for normal esophageal function. This common denominator allows us to categorize them as primary esophageal disorders and to distinguish them from diseases giving rise to secondary disorders of esophageal motor activity.

Secondary Disordered Motor Activity

Secondary disordered motor activity (SDMA) is the response of the esophagus to injury, such as infection, ingestion of a foreign body or a chemical irritant, but the most common injury is due to reflux of gastric content into the esophagus. The response of the inflamed esophagus tends to be similar regardless of the factors producing the inflammation. Variation in esophageal response depends on the severity of the inflammation and upon its specific location. Hiatal hernia is associated with other motor changes which result from the new position of the gastroesophageal junction within the thoracic cavity.

In SDMA the motor changes seen in the body of the esophagus are categorized in terms of the percentage of secondary and tertiary disordered motor waves. Usually the motor waves are reduced in amplitude although they may be prolonged in duration. To a large degree the extent of the disorder varies with the severity of the inflammation which produced the disordered activity.

Secondary Disordered Motor Activity and Gastroesophageal Reflux

The motor changes seen in patients with hiatal hernias or with gastroesophageal reflux are related in part to the presence of the gastroesophageal junction within the thoracic cavity, and in part to the effects of refluxed gastric content upon the lower esophagus (17). Gastroesophageal junctional displacement gives rise to a high pressure zone that is dominantly respiratory negative or shows variations in its negative and positive response to respiration, described as "double respiratory reversal." The intrathoracic location may also alter the shape of the gastroesophageal junction. As defined manometrically, the record may show some high and peaked respiratory waves at its lower end corresponding to the position of the diaphragm; this will be followed by a plateau of relative inactivity and then pressure changes from the more active gastroesophageal junction during its typical response to deglutition (Fig. 3.6). Other motor changes seen in the area of the gastroesophageal junction may be partly related to the intrathoracic position, but most of the response is related to reflux and reflects the effects of mucosal damage at the junctional level.

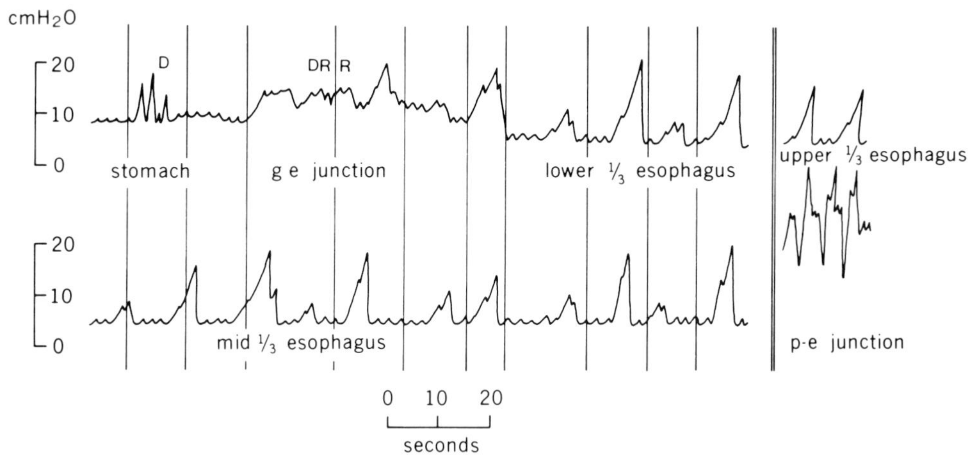

Figure 3.6. Manometric Pattern in Hiatal Hernia
Patients with gastroesophageal reflux and a hiatal hernia may show characteristic motor changes. This tracing illustrates high spiked respiratory waves at the level of the diaphragm (D), followed by a plateau of pressure in the segment of stomach above the diaphragm. The gastroesophageal junction (ge), which is totally respiratory negative, shows a poor deglutition response and a double respiratory reversal (DRR). This patient has a moderate degree of low amplitude disordered motor activity in the body of the esophagus. p-e, pharyngoesophageal.

Animal experimentation has been of great value in clarifying the motor changes associated with hiatal hernia and gastroesophageal reflux. The experimental creation of hiatal hernia produces very little motor defect but, if gastric acidity is raised concurrently by histamine stimulation, esophagitis (18) develops and the severity of the motor defect so produced is proportional to the stage of the esophagitis. The motor defect thus produced consists of increased secondary disordered motor activity in the body of the esophagus and reduction in the tone of the gastroesophageal junction. This experimental model, although helpful in demonstrating the development of secondary disordered motor activity, goes too far because it combines the effects of surgical manipulation of the esophagus, the creation of hiatal hernia and the effects of reflux and gastric acid stimulation.

Isolated esophagitis can be produced and its effects can be studied in the absence of hiatal hernia. Henderson and colleagues (19–21) produced experimental esophagitis by perfusing the esophagus with decinormal hydrochloric acid, bile, bile salts and a mixture of acid and bile or bile salts. In this experiment each dog was perfused with a specific mixture 4 hours daily for 21 days. Esophagitis developed and was assessed endoscopically and by biopsy at 3-day intervals. Manometry was performed also at 3-day intervals and these manometric studies were compared with others made before perfusion. Under these conditions esophagitis develops, the tone of the gastroesophageal junction declines and the secondary disordered motor activity increases sharply in the body of the esophagus. The severity of the motor disorder in these experimental animals is directly proportional to the stage of esophagitis noted endoscopically. When the perfusion is stopped, the esophagitis progressively resolves over a period of 5 to 6 days, the motor defect abates and esophageal motor function eventually returns to normal (Fig. 3.7). This type of study clearly demonstrates that secondary disordered motor activity can be produced by esophageal irritation alone without an associated hiatal hernia.

Many studies in humans with reflux esophagitis have attempted to correlate the degree of esophagitis with the degree of esophageal motor change (22). This correlation is very clear in patients with extensive ulcerative

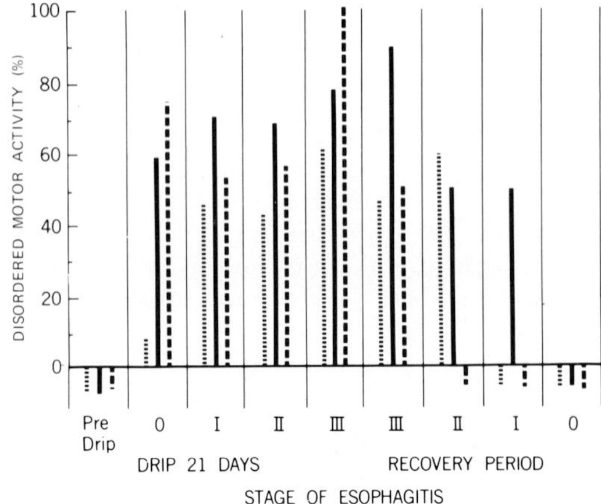

Figure 3.7. Role of Bile and Acid in Esophagitis
When esophagitis was induced by infusion of bile and acid, esophagitis developed and the percentage of disordered motor activity progressively increased. When the infusion was stopped, esophagitis resolved and disordered motor activity disappeared. Disordered motor activity is shown as a percentage from 0 to 100 and esophagitis is staged from 0 to III. The infusion was run for 21 days until Stage III esophagitis developed, then the dogs were studied for 21 days during resolution of the esophagitis.

esophagitis or with a peptic stricture. However, many patients who have no evidence of esophageal ulceration endoscopically have a severe associated motor defect. It is this group of patients who have no ulceration but have major motor changes who require careful evaluation to determine, if at all possible, the origin of these motor abnormalities.

In experimental animals there is a clear relationship between esophageal ulceration and the severity of the concurrent motor defect, and in the human ulcerative esophagitis is clearly associated with severely disordered esophageal motor activity. However, the reader should mark the differences between the acute animal experiment and the human disease. In the human the severity of reflux may alter from time to time and ulceration within the lumen of the esophagus may heal. As this process continues, repeated cycles of ulceration and healing may produce extensive inflammatory changes within the wall of the esophagus and as the inflammation spreads, the wall of the esophagus becomes thickened by a deposition of scar tissue. If the patient is evaluated clinically when he is in a stage of healing, the only recognizable endoscopic changes will be those of mucosal thickening and mucosal pallor. However, in such patients it is now possible to correlate at the time of operation the extent of motor disorder with the presence of esophageal wall thickening. This thickening, which is clear evidence of established esophageal disease, provides a much better indication of the extent of disordered motor activity than any other parameter of esophageal investigation.

I have studied the association between esophageal wall changes and the severity of disordered motor activity in the esophagus in 104 patients (23) before operative correction of gastroesophageal reflux. Each patient was studied preoperatively by manometry, radiology and endoscopy. At the time of thoracotomy the esophageal wall was carefully mobilized to the aortic arch level and palpated before being categorized as being thickened or normal. We considered thickening to be present only when the change was clearly detectable and when, in association with thickening, the wall was firm and of a woody consistency. These changes are characteristic and, when he looks for them, the operating surgeon will recognize them readily.

As noted above, the esophageal motor change in these patients was studied by preoperative manometric evaluation. The tone of the gastroesophageal junction was recorded and, in addition, motor waves in the lower half of the esophagus were categorized either as "peristaltic" or "disordered." Disordered motor waves were then expressed as a percentage of all motor waves present within the lower esophagus. Similarly, we evaluated the motor waves in the proximal esophagus and calculated the percentage of disordered motor activity. At thoracotomy 37 of the 104 patients had a thickened esophageal wall and 35 of the 37 had more than 40 per cent disordered motor activity in their lower esophagus. Of 67 patients who had a normal esophageal wall, 51 had less than 40 per cent disordered motor activity (Fig. 3.8). This correlation is important because it shows clearly that, as panmural esophagitis develops and the wall thickens, the percentage of disordered motor activity also increases. In the proximal esophagus, no association was found between panmural esophagitis, wall

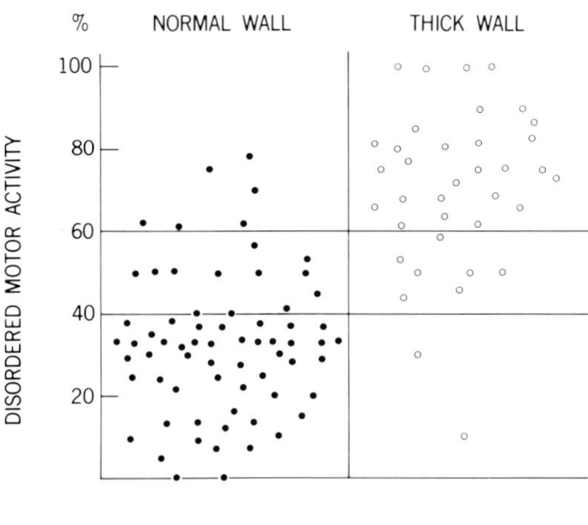

Figure 3.8
Correlation of esophageal wall thickness as judged at thoracotomy and distal disordered motor activity (DMA). The severity of DMA in the distal half of the esophagus is a good predictor of esophageal wall thickening and shortening. Most patients with a thick wall had more than 60 per cent DMA, and most of those with a normal wall had less than 40 per cent DMA.

thickening and disordered motor activity. Thus, we have concluded that the changes of reflux esophagitis are confined almost entirely to the esophagus below the aortic arch level and that only in advanced disease would we expect to find panmural esophagitis in the upper esophagus. Although reduced in those patients with severe esophagitis, the tone of the gastroesophageal junction did not correlate closely with the presence of panmural esophagitis and wall thickening.

Separation of primary and secondary esophageal disorders is of great help in evaluating esophageal disease. The primary disorder is associated with a primary defect of neurogenic or myogenic function within the esophagus. A wide variety of these disorders has been described and fortunately each one tends to have a characteristic motor pattern. Secondary disorders are nonspecific responses which the esophagus makes to injury, and hence the motor pattern in any one is likely to be indistinguishable from another. Specific changes do occur at the gastroesophageal junction in the presence of an anatomic hiatal hernia, and these are valuable in distinguishing this specific secondary disorder from other secondary disorders related to injury only. However, it should be noted that the motor changes specific to hiatal hernia are confined to the gastroesophageal junction and consist of variations in the junction that are directly related to its intrathoracic position. A full understanding of these distinctions is essential to the clinical recognition of esophageal motor disorders, and this subject will be pursued further in chapters on the individual disease processes.

Investigation of Primary and Secondary Motor Disorders

History, radiology, manometry, acid perfusion, reflux testing and endoscopy are all important in the diagnosis and evaluation of esophageal motor disorders.

History

History is essential in the diagnosis of esophageal disease. A carefully taken history will allow localization of the disease to the esophagus in the majority of patients and often will be specific in allowing a diagnosis of the motor defect.

Reflux and secondary disordered motor activity (DMA) is the commonest disorder. In most patients a characteristic history of food-induced and posturally related pain with antacid relief is strong evidence of the disorder. If recognizable reflux to the throat is present or excessive eructation, hiccoughing, nausea, vomiting or dysphagia are present, the diagnosis can be made by history alone and further investigation is confirmatory and to evaluate esophageal reflux damage.

Most other motor disorders can be localized to the esophagus by history but require investigation to differentiate them from gastroesophageal reflux. Esophageal pain and dysphagia are the two most common presenting symptoms. In specific instances the presence of systemic disease will be of diagnostic value. This is more likely to be present in primary cricopharyngeal disorders; for example, voice change and dysphagia would indicate recurrent laryngeal nerve palsy and systemic myotonia or myasthenia gravis would indicate the appropriate cricopharyngeal motor disorders. In the lower esophagus scleroderma is associated with Raynaud's phenomena or diabetic and alcoholic

neuropathy may be associated with esophageal symptoms.

Radiology

Pain and dysphagia are the most common presenting symptoms of esophageal motor disorders. When these present as new symptoms, or become more severe, radiology is usually the first investigation and the most readily obtained. When dysphagia is a new and presenting symptom, radiology is essential to exclude malignancy.

Radiology has diagnostic limitations (24) in esophageal motor disorders. For accuracy it is necessary that the study be done with great care and that the radiologist is aware of the potential diagnostic problems.

Fluoroscopy is essential and may be combined with full plate and 70 or 90 mm exposures. Cinefluoroscopy allows repeat viewing and careful assessment of motor function; however, it is not always readily available. Cine studies are of most value in cricopharyngeal disorders as the rapid rate of transit makes conventional radiology less accurate.

My preference in radiology is to combine a liquid barium examination with a barium sandwich particularly when dysphagia is the dominant symptom. The use of solids more closely approximates a normal meal and is more likely to produce recognizable obstruction. This maneuver has frequently been of diagnostic value where other investigations were normal.

Case 2. Mrs. A., age 45. This patient was treated surgically for severe reflux symptoms by transabdominal Nissen hiatal hernia repair 3 years before her evaluation. Dysphagia was a dominant residual symptom unresponsive to repeated dilatation up to #60 Fr. She had been previously evaluated manometrically, endoscopically and radiologically and considered normal.

Because of persistent symptoms and a weight loss of 30 pounds, she was referred for further studies. At that time she was reduced to a liquid and semisolid diet.

The most specific investigative finding was radiology. The liquid barium study was considered normal, with no evidence of hernia recurrence or reflux. When solids were swallowed they obstructed at the gastroesophageal junction and were regurgitated. (Fig. 3.9). Endoscopically there was no obstruction and a #60 bougie could be passed without recognizable resistance. Manometrically

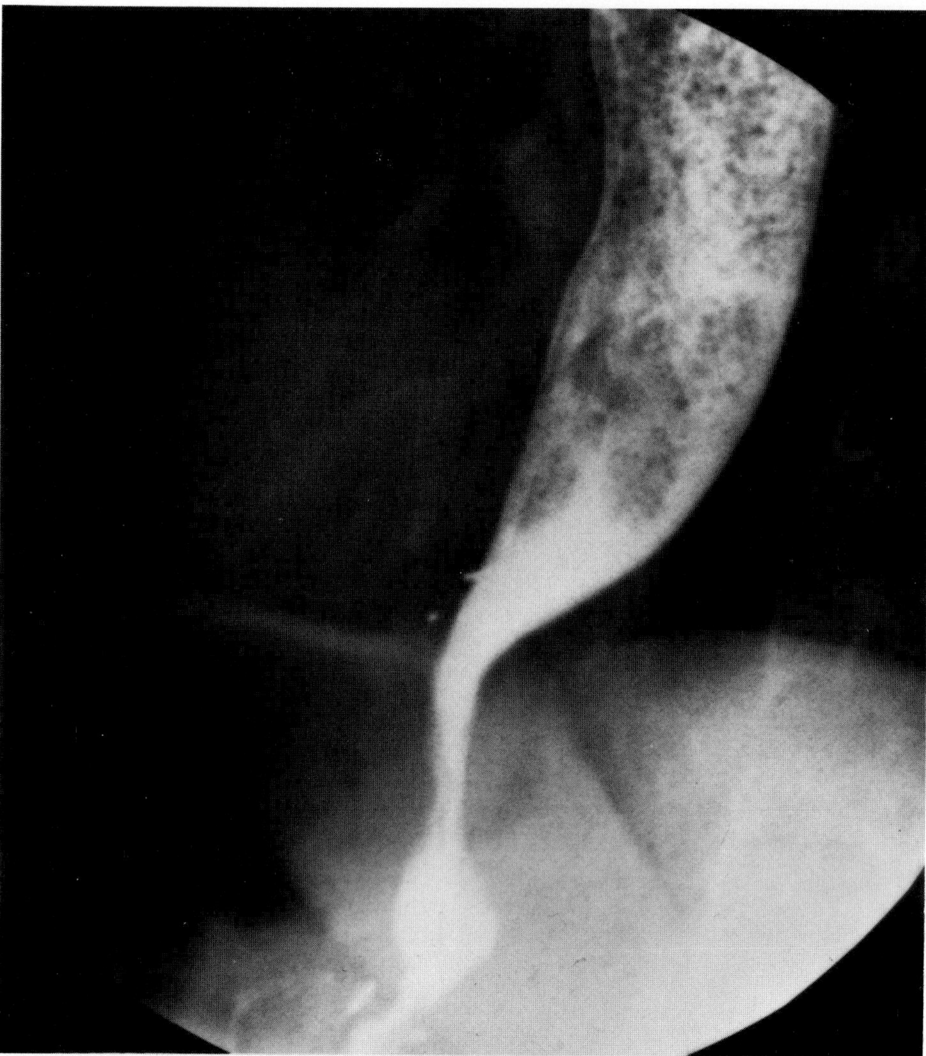

Figure 3.9
Mrs. A., Case 2, was reported as having normal radiologic studies. When a barium beef sandwich
was added food obstruction was clearly demonstrated. The obstruction was not apparent endoscopically and a #60 Fr. bougie could be passed. This motor obstruction produced severe symptoms
and restricted her diet.

the only abnormality was a high tone gastroesophageal junction.

A clinical diagnosis of a tight fundoplication
repair was made and confirmed surgically. Repeat
hernia repair has given effective symptom relief,
and the patient has returned to a normal weight.

In this instance the use of solids with radiology was of critical diagnostic importance.
Had this investigation been carried out earlier

the patient could have been spared considerable distress.

Esophageal wall thickening (12) may be of
importance in recognizing the presence of
diffuse spasm. This radiologic finding is only
possible if the patient is rotated so that spot
films show the esophagus clear of the thoracic
spine.

Motor function can be demonstrated radiologically; however, it is not as reliable a

method as esophageal manometry. Severe DMA will give a characteristic corkscrew pattern (Fig. 3.10) and may demonstrate obstruction to liquids or solids. Liquid swallows in a head down position are useful in assessing loss of motor function in patients with scleroderma. An adynamic esophagus is more difficult to recognize with the patient vertical as liquid barium will fall under the effects of gravity. Occasionally in scleroderma (25) and frequently in achalasia or diffuse spasm an air-filled esophagus will be present, and this is of diagnostic importance.

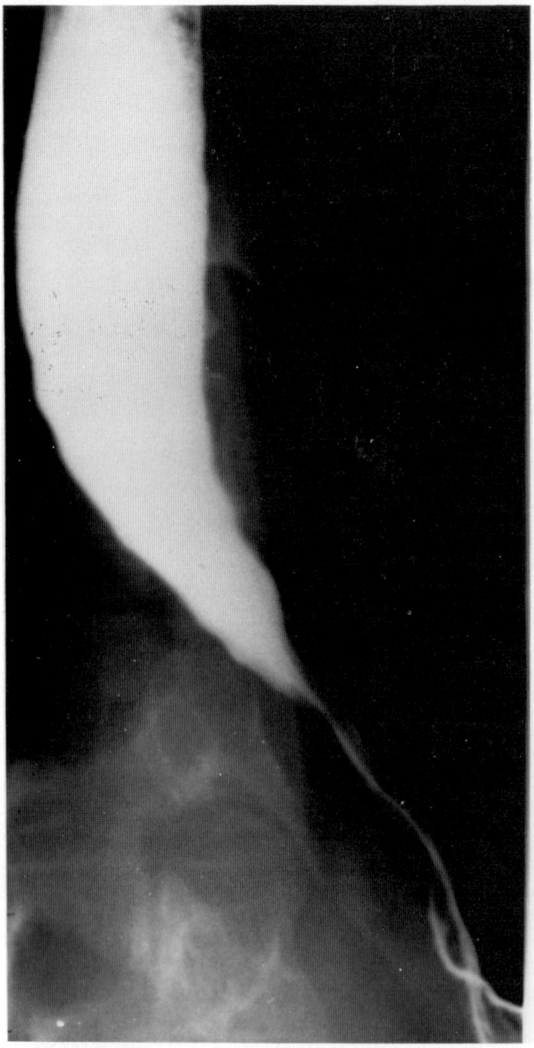

Even with careful radiology, a specific diagnosis cannot always be made; however, the study is important in excluding stricture and in recognizing carcinoma, a hiatal hernia or reflux.

Esophageal Manometry

Methods of Recording

Three basic methods of recording esophageal pressures have been described. In 1899 Meltzer (26, 27) used a small balloon as the pressure sensor and recorded the first esophageal pressure waves. Interest in recording esophageal pressures again increased in the 1950's and balloon measurements together with water-filled, noninfused tubes were used. The addition of constant water infusion made it possible to record more accurate pressures and to quantitate the tone of the gastroesophageal junction and the amplitude of esophageal motor waves. Infusion systems have persisted with various modifications up to the present (28–32).

Miniaturized pressure transducers have been introduced. One of the earliest was the Millhon-Crites transducer (33). Various modifications of these transducers have resulted in a stable system capable of recording esophageal pressures (34, 35) (Sensotec EMP3) (Fig. 3.11).

Water-perfused systems require a constant forward flow of water from a pump, and pressure recordings are produced by esophageal contraction impeding the water flow. Strain gauges record back pressure, and the effects can be documented using a pen-writing or ultraviolet light recorder.

The constant infusion catheter system is very simple to construct and produces reliable data. Since pressure recordings are dampened by the viscosity of water flow and the resistance of the tubing, this system is slow in its response to pressure change. In the lower smooth muscle esophagus, slow response rates are of no importance as motor changes are correspondingly slow. In the cricopharynx and pharynx cycles of contraction and relaxation may be complete within 0.5 to 1 second, and some of the peaks of pressure

Figure 3.10
The radiologic features of DES vary; however, recognizable features include spasm and a thickened esophageal wall. In this x-ray study there was increased motor activity and wall thickening was 7 mm. Manometry excluded achalasia and confirmed the presence of diffuse spasm of the PRV (peristalsis: relaxation: vigorous) type.

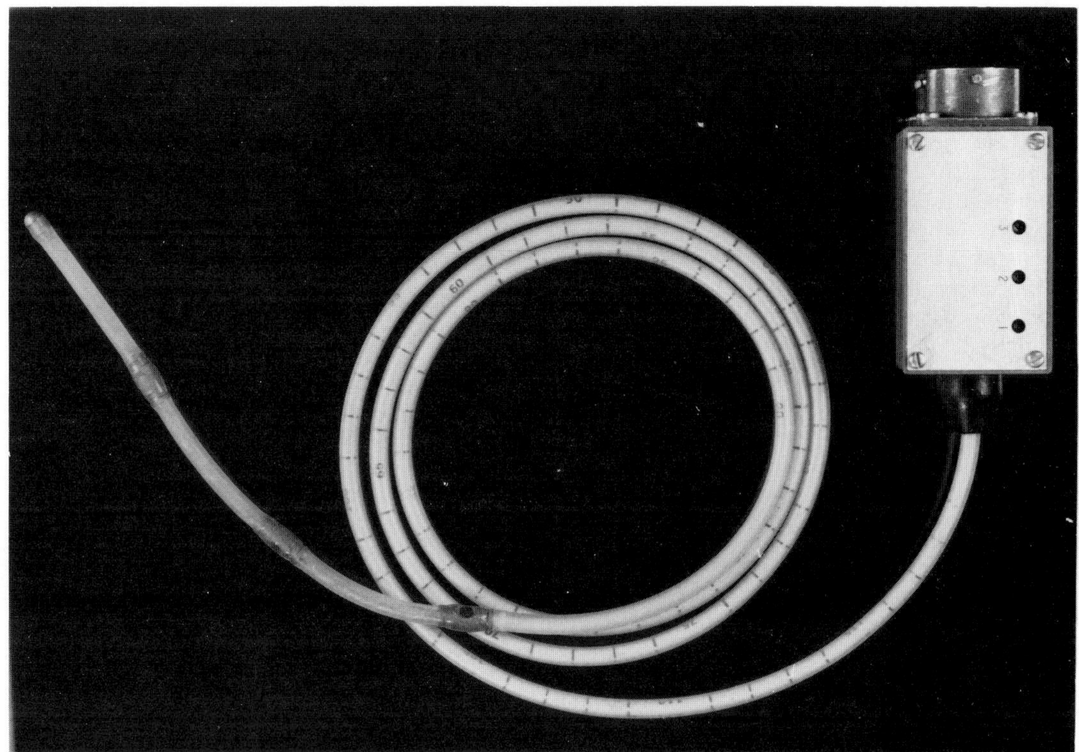

Figure 3.11
The solid state catheter has an end transducer and eliminates the frictional resistance present in the water-perfused systems. Because of its construction, it is capable of recording rapid pressure changes, and it is particularly valuable in the study of the cricopharyngeus.

change are missed by this recording system. In the lower esophagus when pressures rise too high they tend to stop forward flow of water, and the peak is mechanically cut off. If water flow is fast enough, this pressure cutoff is of less importance as water pressure is sufficient.

Using the miniaturized pressure transducer, the water pump system is no longer necessary and impulses from the transducers are directly recorded. Because of absent frictional resistance rapid frequency pressure changes in the cricopharynx and pharynx are more accurately recorded. In the lower esophagus pressure changes also are recorded without difficulty. There are as yet unsolved problems with the miniaturized transducer system. The most common difficulty is electric interference from cardiac contraction and interference from external electrical sources. This interference adds considerably to the difficulty of interpretation. More important is the

difference in pressure recorded by these two systems. Water-perfused catheters in general record lower pressures than the transducer system (36). Comparative studies with multiple recordings on the same patients have shown much more variability in the recordings using the miniaturized system than with the water-perfused system.

Hay et al. in 1979 (37) compared the two systems with multiple recordings in a group of 17 healthy volunteers. With the water-perfused system the high pressure zone (HPZ) tone was statistically similar both with multiple recordings on one day and also when the recordings were repeated several days later. Using the miniaturized transducer same day recordings were statistically similar but not as close as with the water infusion system. With the transducer recordings at several day intervals no statistical correlation was achieved between the recorded HPZ tones.

These findings suggest that the water-perfused system is more accurate as a method of documenting esophageal motor change.

Clinical Application

Manometric studies are the most accurate method of defining motor disorders in the esophagus and as such should be used in all patients where an accurate diagnosis cannot be established by history and radiology alone. Manometry is of particular value in cricopharyngeal abnormalities, but in this location high speed tracings are necessary for clearer definition of motor change. In the lower esophagus primary motor abnormalities are very difficult to diagnose without manometry.

Case 3. Mrs. M., age 42 years, was originally investigated for problems of dysphagia. Based on history and radiology only she was diagnosed as achalasia and treated by transabdominal Heller myotomy. Postoperatively she developed severe reflux symptoms with continued dysphagia, nausea and vomiting.

When seen for evaluation this patient had an ulcerative esophagitis secondary to gastroesophageal reflux. Radiology confirmed the presence of reflux and endoscopy with biopsy excluded malignancy. Manometry demonstrated peristaltic motor activity in the body of the esophagus. The HPZ had been myotomized and was not manometrically recognizable; however, the presence of peristalsis excluded achalasia.

Surgical correction of reflux has given effective symptomatic relief. Misdiagnosis originally was based on questionable radiologic esophageal dilatation considered to be an early achalasia. While radiology is usually accurate in Stage II and Stage III achalasia (38), it is not accurate and must never be used as grounds for surgical intervention in Stage I achalasia.

Practical Approach to Manometry

In my practice, manometry is used routinely in the investigation of patients with

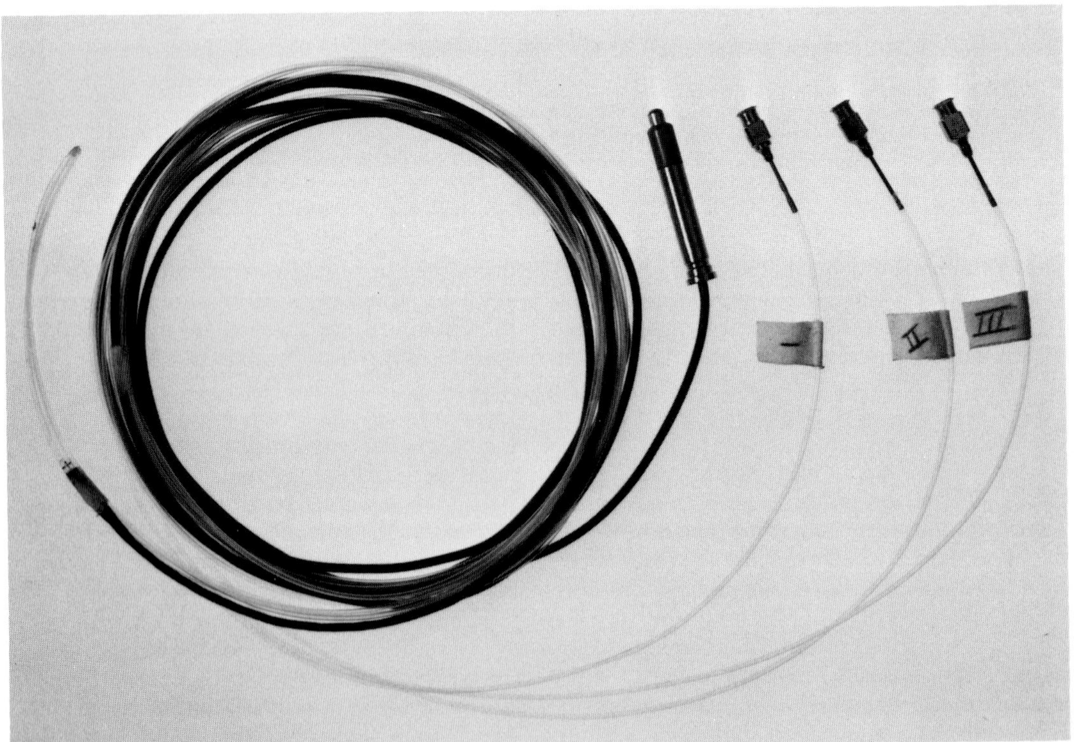

Figure 3.12
The water-perfused system is reliable and has been tested over years of clinical and experimental use. The catheters we use are polyethylene tubes (PE 190) with an internal diameter of 0.047 inch and an outer diameter of 0.067 inch. Three catheters are fused together and have distal side openings. A pH lead can be attached to the catheter assembly.

significant esophageal disorders. The patient is fasted overnight or 4 hours before testing. Catheters are passed by mouth and usually swallowed without difficulty. The manometric catheters are three polyethylene tubes (PE 190) with distal side openings 2.5 and 5 cm apart. Included with the tubes is a Beckman pH probe. For pH recording, the patient's finger is placed with an external electrode in a concentrated potassium chloride solution (Figs. 3.12 and 3.13).

With the tubes in the stomach perfusion is started using a 2202 modified Harvard pump with 100 cc Teflon-lined syringes. Water infusion is at 6.8 cc per tube per minute. Gastric pH is recorded by the probe. The tubes are then slowly withdrawn at 1-cm intervals using continuous recording with a 1508 ultraviolet Honeywell visicorder and Statham P23 De strain gauges.

Good recordings must be obtained at each level before withdrawal is continued. When the tubes lie 5 cm above the gastroesophageal junction, the patient is tested for reflux using leg raising or abdominal compression. Continuous pH recording allows recognition of reflux at any level. Gastric acidification is carried out if the gastric pH is high at the commencement of the study.

When indicated, 0.1 N hydrochloric acid perfusion is carried out through the proximal catheter at a level 5 cm above the gastroesophageal junction. This is continued for a minimum of 20 minutes unless it causes the patient too much distress.

Catheter withdrawal is then completed to the cricopharyngeal level. At this point, paper speed is increased from 1 mm per second to 1 cm per second. Recording at this level is difficult due to patient intolerance; however, with care a good recording is almost always possible.

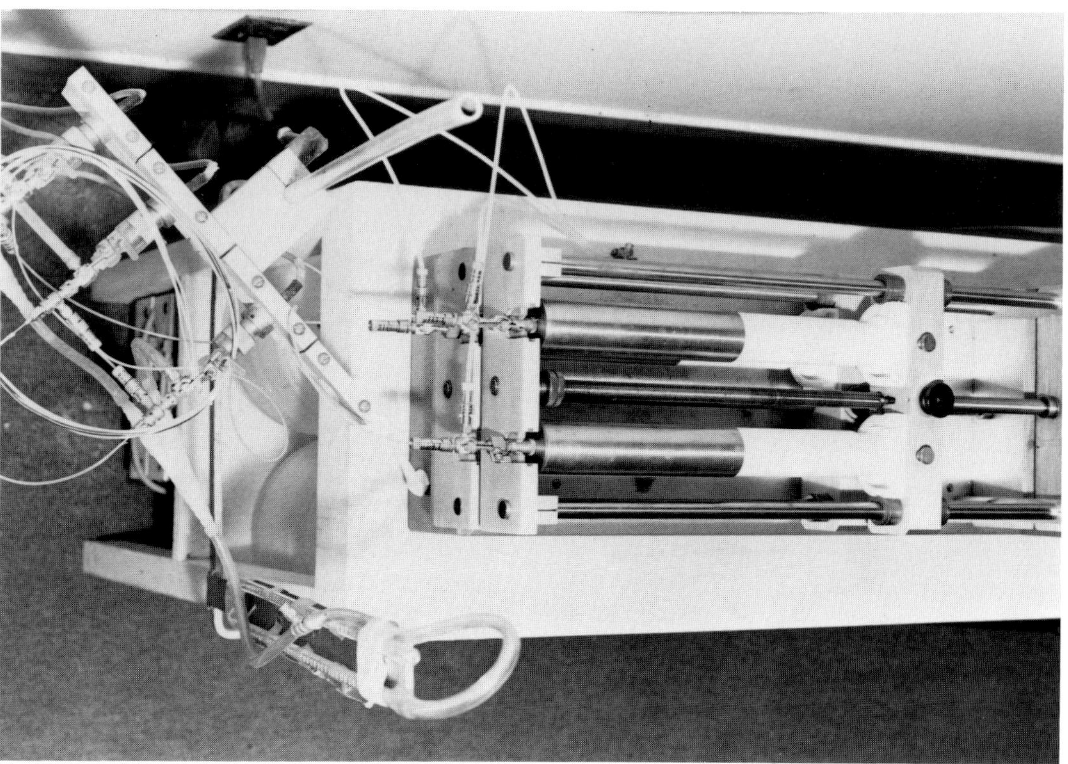

Figure 3.13
Using a water-perfused system pressure changes are measured by Stathem P23 De strain gauges and the pressures are recorded using an ultraviolet recorder. Constant water flow is maintained by a Harvard pump. In our pump assembly viewed from above we use 100 cc metal syringes with Teflon-coated barrels. The strain gauges are attached to the outflow and to the water-perfused catheters.

The entire study can be completed in 1 hour with good patient tolerance, and a reproducable quality of record is almost always achieved.

Recording of pH is important in patients with reflux as their major problem. This can be done as an isolated study or combined with manometry. Twelve- and 24-hour pH monitoring is becoming a popular method of study and will be discussed in detail in Chapter 6 when the evaluation of patients with hiatal hernia and reflux is considered.

Endoscopy

Endoscopy is reserved for patients with more major disease and with particular diagnostic problems. If malignancy is suspected, endoscopy is mandatory. In my practice, any patient being considered for esophageal surgery will have endoscopy performed for the purpose of documenting esophageal pathology, excluding malignancy and recognizing distal pathology in stomach or duodenum.

Rigid endoscopy is less frequently used for diagnostic purposes; however, it is clearly better for assessing esophageal malignancy and allows better biopsy material to be obtained. Many endoscopists are not skilled in the use of the rigid esophagoscope, and it is my clinical impression that malignancies are being missed because of this.

Fiberoptic flexible esophagogastroduodenoscopy is a major advance and allows accurate assessment of esophagus, stomach and duodenum. Distal pathology must be excluded as malignancy can simulate achalasia and duodenal ulceration can aggravate reflux.

When ulceration or stricture is present in the esophagus I always brush and biopsy to exclude malignancy. Without tissue for pathologic examinations an in situ or early invasive malignancy can be missed. In the past, routine biopsy of the esophagus was performed; however, I have found this to be of little value and on two occasions had significant bleeding which required transfusion.

Case 4. Mr. E., age 66. This patient presented with a long history of intractable heartburn. Radiologically a hiatal hernia was present with a small polypoid mass in the midesophagus. Initial fiberoptic endoscopy visualized a 1-cm polyp in the midesophagus at the upper margin of a Barrett

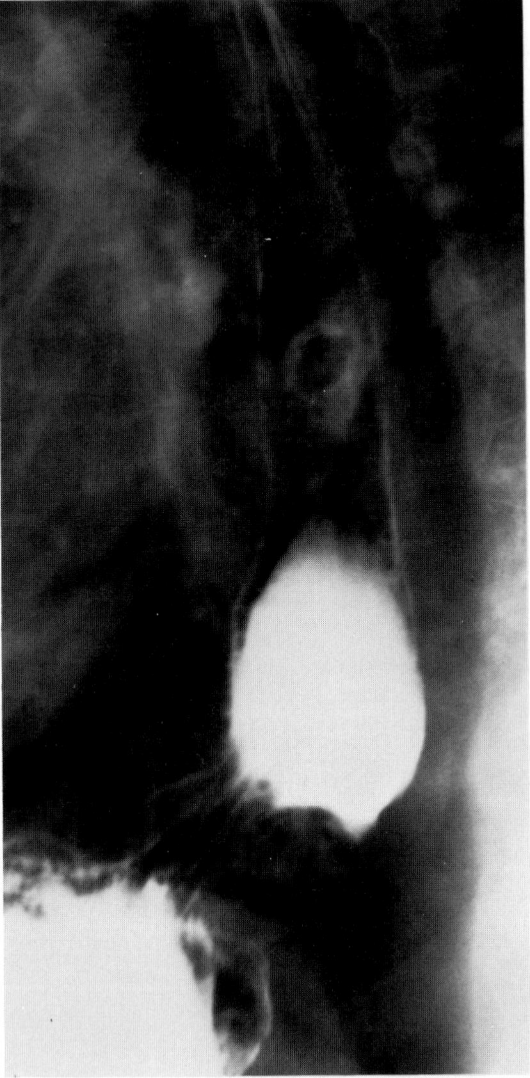

Figure 3.14
Mr. E., Case 4, was noted radiologically to have a hiatal hernia with reflux and an esophageal polyp. Flexible fiberoptic endoscopy with multiple small biopsies did not show malignancy; however, rigid esophagoscopy and biopsy confirmed the presence of a small adenocarcinoma in the polyp.

esophagus (Fig. 3.14). Four biopsies were obtained and all were benign.

He was electively admitted for surgical reflux correction 6 weeks later, and endoscopy was repeated using the rigid esophagoscope. With a larger biopsy specimen a tissue diagnosis of adenocarcinoma was established. At surgical resection a 1-cm malignant lesion was present without nodal involvement and muscular invasion. Use of the rigid esophagoscope allowed a more adequate biopsy and proved essential in the management of this patient. These basic investigative techniques are all necessary in the evaluation of patients with primary and secondary motor disorders of the esophagus. In the following chapters more specific investigative detail will be outlined for each disease entity.

References

1. Palmer, E. D.: The hiatus hernia-esophagitis-esophageal stricture complex. Am. J. Med., *44:* 566, 1968.
2. Nelson, P. G.: Observations on dysphagia. Med. J. Aust., *2:* 924, 1970.
3. Silber, W.: Achalasia. Lancet, *2:* 1289, 1975.
4. Schotland, D. L., and Rowland, L. P.: Muscular dystrophy: features of ocular myopathy, distal myopathy and myotonic dystrophy. Arch. Neurol., *10:* 433, 1964.
5. Tatelman, M., and Keech, M. K.: Esophageal motility in systemic lupus erythematosus, rheumatoid arthritis and scleroderma. Radiology, *86:* 1041, 1966.
6. Siegel, H. A.: The radiology corner; esophageal moniliasis. Am. J. Gastroenterol., *59:* 454, 1973.
7. Cassella, R. R., Ellis, F. H., Jr., and Brown, A. L., Jr.: Fine-structure changes in achalasia of esophagus; 1. Vagus nerves. Am. J. Pathol., *46:* 279, 1965.
8. Henderson, R. D., Barichello, A. W., Pearson, F. G., Mugashe, F., and Szczepanski, M.: Diagnosis of achalasia. Can. J. Surg., *15:* 190, 1972.
9. Higgs, B., Kerr, F. W. L., and Ellis, F. H.: The experimental production of esophageal achalasia by electrolytic lesions in the medulla. J. Thorac. Cardiovasc. Surg., *50:* 613, 1965.
10. Carveth, S. W., Schlegel, J. F., Code, C. F., and Ellis, F. H.: Esophageal motility after vagotomy, phrenecotomy, myotomy and myomectomy in dogs. Surg. Gynecol Obstet., *114:* 31, 1962.
11. Gillies, M., Nicks, R., and Skyring, A.: Clinical, manometric and pathological studies in diffuse oesophageal spasm. Br. Med. J., *2:* 527, 1967.
12. Henderson, R. D., Ho, C. S., and Davidson, J. W.: Primary disordered motor activity of the esophagus (diffuse spasm). Ann. Thorac. Surg., *18:* 327, 1974.
13. Henderson, R. D., and Pearson, F. G.: Surgical management of esophageal scleroderma. J. Thorac. Cardiovasc. Surg., *66:* 686, 1973.
14. Cohen, S., Fisher, F., Lipshutz, W., Turner R., Myers, A., and Schumacher, R.: The pathogenesis of esophageal dysfunction in scleroderma and Raynaud's disease. J. Clin. Invest., *51:* 2663, 1972.
15. Fischer, R. A., Ellison, G. W., Thayer, W. R., Spiro, H. M., and Glaser, G. H.: Esophageal motility in neuromuscular disorders. Ann. Intern. Med., *63:* 229, 1965.
16. Schwab, R. S., and Viets, H. R.: Roentgenoscopy of the pharynx in myasthenia gravis before and after prostigmine injection. A.J.R., *45:* 357, 1941.
17. Atkinson, M., Edwards, D. A. W., Honour, A. J., and Rowlands, E. N.: The oesophagogastric sphincter in hiatus hernia. Lancet, *2:* 1138, 1957.
18. Baue, A. E., and Hoffer, R. E.: The effects of experimental hiatus hernia and histamine stimulation on the intrinsic esophageal sphincter. Surg. Gynecol. Obstet., *125:* 791, 1967.
19. Henderson, R. D., Mugashe, F. L., Jeejeebhoy, K. N., Szczepanski, M. M., Cullen, J., Marryatt, G., and Boszko, A.: Synergism of acid and bile salts in the production of experimental esophagitis. Can. J. Surg., *16:* 12, 1973.
20. Henderson, R. D., Mugashe, F., Jeejeebhoy, K. N., Cullen, J., Boszko, A., Szczepanski, M., and Marryatt, G.: The motor defect of esophagitis. Can. J. Surg., *17:* 112, 1974.
21. Henderson, R. D., Mugashe, F., Jeejeebhoy, K. N., Cullen, J., Szczepanski, M., Boszko, A., and Marryatt, G.: The role of bile and acid in the production of esophagitis and the motor defect of esophagitis. Ann. Thorac. Surg., *14:* 465, 1972.
22. Affolter, H.: Pressure characteristics of reflux esophagitis. Helv. Med. Acta, *33:* 395, 1967.
23. Henderson, R. D.: Correlation of esophageal wall changes and disordered motor activity. Unpublished data, 1976.
24. Steiner, G. M.: Gastro-oesophageal reflux, hiatus hernia and the radiologist, with special reference to children. Br. J. Radiol., *50:* 164, 1977.
25. Henderson, R. D., and Pearson, F. G.: Surgical management of esophageal scleroderma. J. Thorac. Cardiovasc. Surg., *66:* 686, 1973.
26. Code, C. F., and Schlegel, J. F.: The pressure profile of the gastro-esophageal sphincter in man; an improved method of detection. Mayo Clin. Proc., *33:* 406, 1958.
27. Meltzer, S. J.: On the causes of the orderly progress of peristaltic movements in the oesophagus. Am. J. Physiol., *2:* 266, 1899.
28. Dodds, W. J., Hogan, W. J., Arndorfer, R. C., and Dent, J.: Efficient manometric technic for accurate regional measurement of esophageal body motor activity. Am. J. Gastroenterol., *70:* 21, 1978.
29. Boesby, S., Söndergaard, E. Y., and Madsen, T.: Oesophageal peristalsis. A simple system for the recording of oesophageal peristalsis, and the influence of bolus volume on peak peristaltic pressure amplitude. Scand. J. Gastroenterol., *13:* 149, 1978.
30. Sundström, G., and Ulmsten, U.: Lateral-hole catheters compared with shielded-hole catheter systems in oesophageal manometry. Scand. J. Clin. Lab. Invest., *37:* 661, 1977.
31. Dent, J., Culross, J., and Morris, J. M.: A pneumatically driven pump for constant perfusion manometry. Aust. J. Exp. Biol. Med. Sci., *55:* 293, 1977.
32. Arndorfer, R. C., Stef, J. J., Dodds, W. J., Linehan, J. H., and Hogan, W. J.: Inproved infusion system for intraluminal esophageal manometry. Gastroenterology, *73:* 23, 1977.
33. Millhon, W. A., Hoffman, D. E., Jarvis, P., Cross, J., Millhon, U. S., and Crites, N. A.: Preliminary report on Millhon-Crites intraesophageal motility probe. Am. J. Dig. Dis., *13:* 929, 1968.
34. Wallin, L., Boesby, S., and Madsen, T.: Comparative pressure measurements in the oesophagus by means of in situ tip-transducers and external transducer ssystems. Scand. J. Clin. Lab. Invest., *38:* 375, 1978.
35. Kaye, M. D., Showalter, J. P., Rock, K. C., and Johnson, E.: A circumferentially-sensitive miniature pressure sensor for study of human esophageal motility. Med. Res. Eng., *12:* 10, 1977.

36. Earlam, R.: *Clinical Tests of Oesophageal Function*, pp. 1–21. Crosby Lockwood Staples, London, 1975.
37. Hay, D. J., Goodall, R. J. R., and Temple, J. G.: The reproducibility of the station pullthough technique for measuring lower oesophageal sphincter pressure. Br. J. Surg., *66:* 93, 1979.
38. Henderson, R. D., Barichello, A. W., Pearson, F. G., Mugashe, F., and Szczepanski, M.: Diagnosis of achalasia. Can. J. Surg., *15:* 190, 1972.

CHAPTER 4

Physiologic Control of Reflux

Gastroesophageal reflux is the most common cause of esophageal symptoms (1). At one time reflux was considered to be the universal accompaniment of hiatal hernia; e.g., in 1962 Botha (2) said "I have not yet seen free reflux without herniation, and am convinced that such a condition does not exist." However, many patients have been recognized who have symptomatic reflux but do not have a radiologically demonstrable hernia (3). Although this controversy—namely, whether hiatal hernia is required for reflux—is the central issue in current discussions of physiologic methods of reflux control, its importance must not be exaggerated, because all agree that the reflux, not the hernia, is the source of the patient's symptoms. Hiatal hernia is chiefly a radiologic diagnosis, whereas gastroesophageal reflux is recognized from the symptomatology, or from the findings on endoscopy, radiology or pH reflux testing in the body of the esophagus. A hernia that is demonstrable radiologically may be associated with reflux, but this will be confirmed by one or usually more than one of these diagnostic maneuvers. If a hiatal hernia is not seen on radiologic examination but there is good evidence of reflux, this is often termed "reflux without hernia," but the investigation cannot be allowed to end there because further radiologic evaluation may demonstrate a hiatal hernia. In my own review of 93 consecutive patients who required operation for gastroesophageal reflux, 16 did not have a radiologically demonstrable hernia and 9 of 16 did not have radiologic reflux. All patients had clinical, manometric or endoscopic evidence of reflux, and in all 93 patients a surgical procedure designed to control reflux corrected their symptoms.

The difficulties in precise radiologic diagnosis of a hernia (3, 4) and the tendency of subsequent radiologic studies to show a hernia make it unwise to take a rigid position as Botha did, namely, that there could be no reflux without herniation. Rather it seems reasonable to say that the majority of patients with reflux have a hiatal hernia; however, some patients have reflux without a radiologically demonstrable hernia.

Having counseled caution in this controversy, it is now desirable to evaluate the various control mechanisms which are believed to operate in the prevention of reflux.

Control Mechanisms

In the normal subject, gastroesophageal reflux is prevented by anatomic, neurogenic and hormonal mechanisms (Table 4.1). Anatomically, the diaphragm, phrenoesophageal ligament, mucosal rosette, gastric muscular sling, angle of entry of esophagus to stomach, the intra-abdominal segment of esophagus and the gastroesophageal high pressure zone (HPZ) have all been considered to make some contribution to control. Neurologically, the parasympathetic and sympathetic neurologic control of esophageal motor activity is assisted by vagal reflex mechanisms from the stomach. The hormones, gastrin, secretin, cholesystokinin and glucagon were considered to be important in reflux control; however, recent evidence suggests that their role is less important.

Anatomic Reflux Control

Diaphragm

The diaphragm separates the abdominal and thoracic cavities and, in addition, through its attachments to the esophagus, maintains that organ in its normal position (Fig. 4.1). Radiologically the diaphragm indents the esophagus during respiration (5);

Table 4.1
Control of Gastroesophageal Reflux

1. Anatomic:
   a. Intra-abdominal segment of esophagus
   b. Gastroesophageal junctional tone
   c. Mucosal rosette
   d. Gastric sling
   e. Angle of entry to stomach
   f. Phrenoesophageal ligament
   g. Diaphragm
2. Neurogenic:
   a. Autonomic nerve activity
   b. Gastric reflexes
3. Hormonal:
   a. Gastrin
   b. Secretin
   c. Cholecystokinin
   d. Glucagon

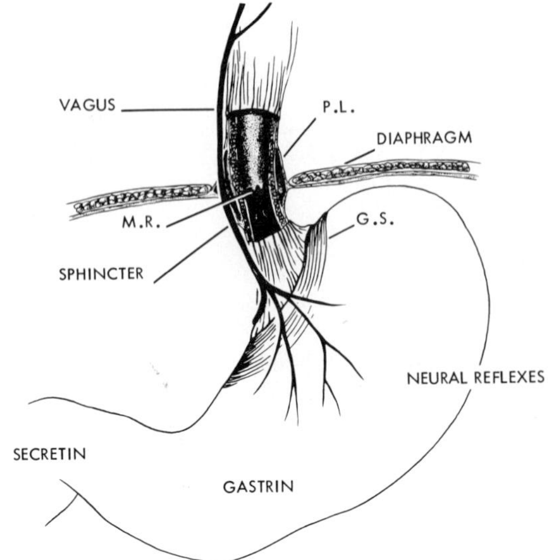

Figure 4.1.   Physiologic Control of Reflux
Anatomic, neurologic and humoral mechanisms of reflux control are illustrated. The principal anatomic controls are the diaphragm, phrenoesophageal ligaments, mucosal rosette, gastric sling fibers, angle of esophageal entry, the intra-abdominal segment of esophagus and the gastroesophageal sphincter mechanism. P.L., phrenoesophageal ligament; M.R., mucosal rosette; G.S., gastric sling fibers, sphincter-gastroesophageal high pressure zone.

however, this pressure effect usually cannot be recognized on the manometer and does not appear to be important in preventing reflux. Paralysis of the diaphragm does not produce reflux and, experimentally, excision of the diaphragm with preservation of the phrenoesophageal ligament does not produce reflux. Pressure studies within the esophageal lumen occasionally show high spiking respiratory waves at the precise point where the esophagus passes through the diaphragm. These changes, although valuable in recognizing the location of the diaphragm, do not raise basal esophageal pressure and do not appear to play a part in the control of reflux (6).

Despite the evidence that the role of the diaphragm in preventing reflux is minor, I have noted a high incidence of reflux symptoms in patients following pneumonectomy, particularly on the left side. This may be related to elevation of the diaphragm or may be secondary to distortion of the esophagus from mediastinal shift.

Phrenoesophageal Ligament

The phrenoesophageal ligament, which attaches the esophagus to the diaphragm, consists of pleural and peritoneal reflections separated by areolar tissue (7, 8). In the normal individual, this ligament acts as an anchor but, when a hiatal hernia develops, the ligament becomes attenuated and can no longer hold the gastroesophageal junction at the level of the diaphragm.

Bombeck and colleagues (7) have suggested that, in the patient with hiatal hernia, the stretched phrenoesophageal ligament pulls the gastroesophageal junction laterally and by so doing reduces sphincteric tone (9). In experimental animals it has been shown that shortening the phrenoesophageal ligament reduces the tone of the gastroesophageal junction; however, this experimental model is so crude that it probably should not be applied to the human situation. In humans with hiatal hernia the ligament is so thinned out and of such poor quality that it can hardly exercise any control function. It is, to say the least, doubtful that this ligament is a major factor in reducing the tone of the gastroesophageal junction in these patients.

Mucosal Rosette

In humans the mucosal rosette (Fig. 4.2) is seen radiologically and endoscopically. In most patients the folds of esophageal mucosa can be seen to interlock; however, they do not appear to have any valvular action. Experimentally the esophageal mucosa can be excised without producing reflux (10).

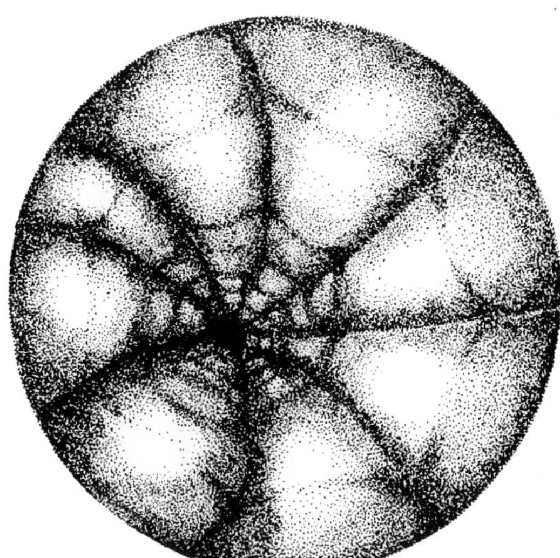

Figure 4.2
Mucosal folds are puckered together at the gastroesophageal junction. These folds do close the junction but do not exert any valvular action which could maintain gastroesophageal competence.

Endoscopically, under local anesthesia, I have frequently noted gastric mucosal prolapse through the HPZ when patients retch. This prolapse may be significant in stretching the esophagus and lowering HPZ tone. Retching and vomiting are common symptoms in patients with reflux.

Gastric Muscular Sling

In the normal subject, the gastric musculature contains a muscular sling, which runs from the esophagogastric angle down toward the lesser curvature of the stomach. The sling can only be recognized after the gastric serosa has been stripped off. We have no evidence that the sling interposes any pressure barrier and, indeed, in experimental animals this sling can be divided without producing reflux (10). However, recent anatomic studies (11) of the human esophagus show the HPZ to lie in the distal esophagus with its muscular fibers blending into the gastric muscular sling. Because of this anatomic relationship it is entirely possible that the sling fibers and the HPZ act in unison as a pressure barrier.

Angle of Entry of Esophagus to Stomach

The angle of entry—that made when the esophagus joins the stomach—is between 70 and 110 degrees in the human subject (Fig. 4.3) (2). No one has demonstrated that this angle is important in preventing reflux, and indeed its removal during proximal gastrectomy does not produce reflux (10).

In various fundoplication procedures done in the course of hiatal hernia repair (Fig. 4.4), the angle of entry is greatly exaggerated (12–14). This exaggerated angle may be important in preventing reflux following surgical correction; however, the angle created surgically bears no resemblance to that seen in the normal subject. It is difficult to see how the stomach could exert any effective extrinsic pressure in the normal subject without more direct contact with the esophagus.

The Intra-abdominal Segment and the HPZ

It is generally agreed that reflux control depends upon the tone of the HPZ. Controversy remains as to the relative importance of the intra-abdominal segment of the esophagus and the HPZ (15). Before proceeding further it is important to define the term "hiatal hernia" and it is necessary to document the properties of the HPZ and to look at the potential value of an intra-abdominal segment of esophagus.

What is a Hiatal Hernia?

Hiatal hernia is a radiologic diagnosis. It was recognizably present in 77 of 93 consecutive patients treated surgically for reflux. Endoscopically in the 16 patients without a radiologic hernia it was possible to show incompetence of the HPZ: manometrically it was possible to show a low tone HPZ and pH reflux tests were positive. Although the manometric and endoscopic findings indicated reflux they did not indicate the presence of a hiatal hernia. At the time of surgery a small hiatal hernia cannot be differentiated from lax diaphragmatic crura. The only examination we have which defines the presence of a hernia is radiology, and in this group of 93 patients 16 did not have a radiologic hernia.

Radiologists vary in what they define as a hernia. The definite hernia with absent peristalsis and mucosal folds visible above the diaphragm is obvious. A small hiatal hernia has not been clearly defined radiologically. Normal radiologic studies on one examination do not exclude the finding of a hiatal hernia in subsequent examinations. Because

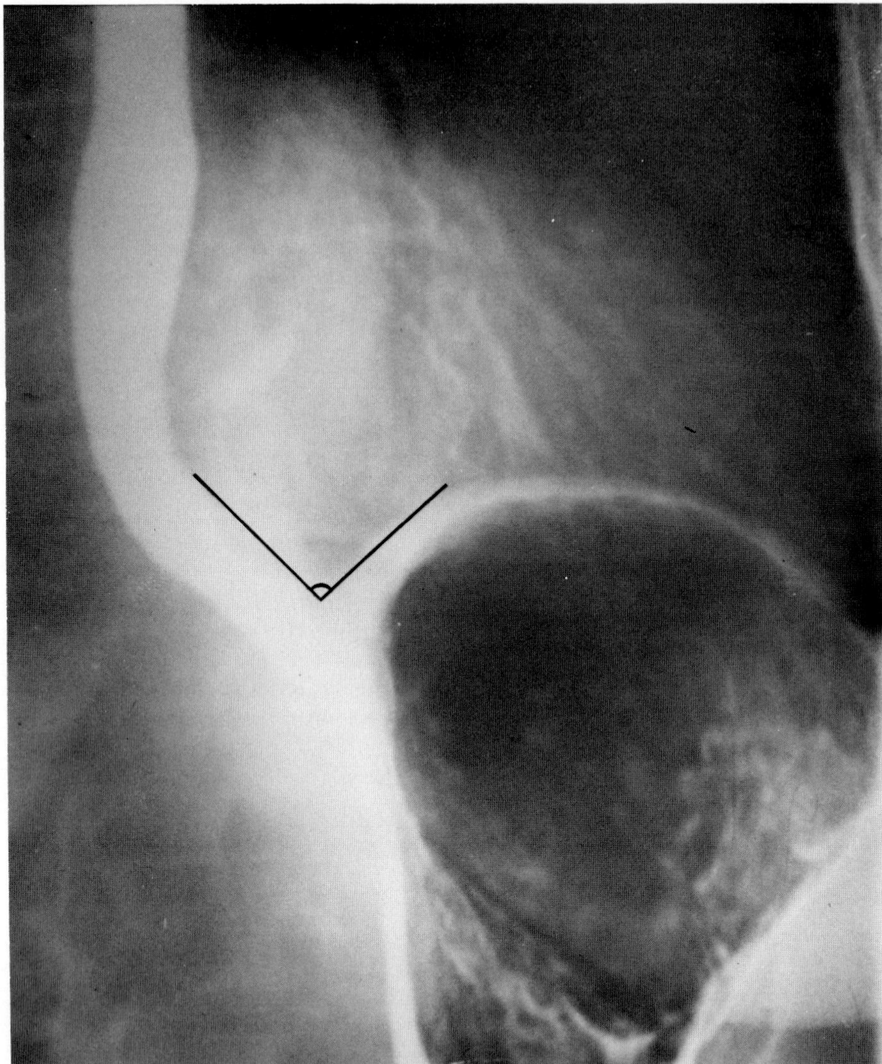

Figure 4.3
Angle of entry of esophagus to stomach varies from 70 to 110 degrees. The angle on this radiograph, which was taken specifically to demonstrate this angle, is 95 degrees.

of the variables discussed it is not possible to use reported radiologic data to state definitely that a hernia is absent (16). As a corollary to this statement it is not possible to say whether these 16 patients did or did not have an effective intra-abdominal segment to their esophagus.

Properties of the HPZ

The HPZ is situated at the lower end of the esophagus. Manometrically its mean tone is 15 to 20 cm H_2O using a water-perfused manometric system. It is known that the tone of the HPZ can vary from one examination to another (17) and that it will vary in response to various injested foods, alcohol, carminatives and tobacco (18–21). There is evidence that the HPZ (22, 23) tone will decrease when the stomach is acidified.

Increased gastric pressure causes an augmented tone increase in the HPZ (24–27), and this can be shown to be reduced following truncal vagotomy (28) suggesting that vagal reflexes from the fundus of stomach are important in maintaining tone.

Hormonal control is not clearly estab-

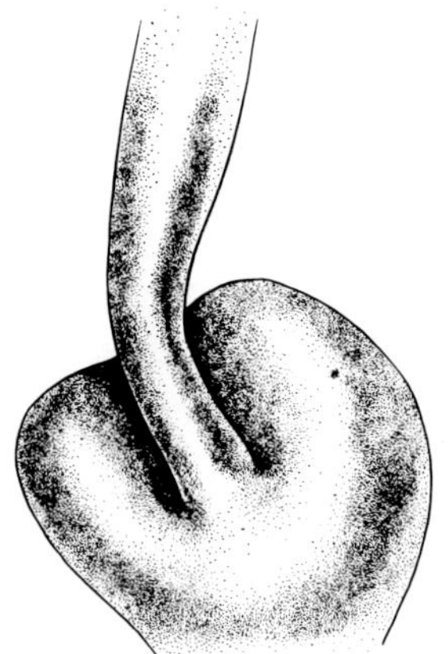

Figure 4.4
Following fundoplication, the stomach is wrapped around the distal esophagus for a distance of 5 cm. This creates a very acute angle of entry of esophagus to stomach and close contact of gastric and esophageal walls. This situation is totally different from that seen in the normal subject (Fig. 4.3).

lished. As originally conceived, gastrin, secretin and cholecystokinin were all potentially involved in reflux control (29–31). When food was swallowed the alkalinized stomach released gastrin and gastrin increased HPZ tone. Secretin was released with gastric emptying and caused a decrease in HPZ tone. The cholecystokinin mechanism was activated by fatty foods with a decrease in HPZ tone. More recent studies with endogenous gastrin release (32–34) have failed to correlate HPZ tone with gastrin levels. Despite the lack of evidence of a gastrin-HPZ tone relationship, it has been shown that infusion of acid into the stomach increases the tendency to reflux (23). The cholecystokinin mechanism lowering HPZ tone probably accounts for reflux following a fatty meal.

Properties of an Intra-abdominal Segment

Theoretically when an intra-abdominal segment is present it will act to prevent reflux by exposing the HPZ to surrounding intraperitoneal pressure. Mechanically this would be a significant advantage in preventing reflux; however, its necessity has not been established.

There are available laboratory studies (Fig. 4.5) in which the HPZ of dogs has been excised and replaced by an end-to-end anastomosis with tubed segments of stomach or colonic interpositions (35). Using this laboratory approach it is possible to show that 2 to 3 cm of tubed stomach, below the diaphragm, are sufficient to prevent reflux and 10 cm of colon interposition will prevent reflux. The stomach tube had a higher tone than the colon segment. In both instances when the tubes were myotomized and tone reduced to 0 cm H_2O, reflux occurred. These are animal studies; however, they are of value in demonstrating the antireflux properties of an intra-abdominal tubed segment.

DeMeester et al. (36) have constructed an in vitro model which has shown that the competence of an intra-abdominal toneless segment of esophagus is directly related to its length and that this competence is increased by the presence of intrinsic tone. This model illustrates the objectives to be accomplished by surgical correction of reflux. The length of esophagus necessary to prevent reflux in this in vitro model was 3 cm, which is similar to the length of tubed stomach required to produce competence in the experimental animal.

These various investigations indicate the potential value of an intra-abdominal segment and explain why surgical procedures which produce an intra-abdominal segment can effectively control reflux. Despite this factual information, it is not possible to say that an intra-abdominal segment is essential.

Reflux Control by HPZ and Intra-abdominal Esophagus

Patients with a hiatal hernia may be asymptomatic. Under these circumstances sphincter alone appears capable of controlling reflux. It is known that normal subjects who are tested for reflux with the pH probe may have reflux following a meal (37). The amount of reflux which occurs in the normal patient is less than in those with heartburn.

Clearly an argument can be made on both sides. Botha in 1962 stated that a hiatal hernia was always present with reflux (2). Cohen and Snape in 1978 state, "Recent understanding of the pathogenesis of gastroesophageal reflux disease as owing to LES incompetence has led to improvement in both the diagnosis and treatment of this disorder" (38). Edwards in 1978 states, "A common view is that the lower esophageal sphincter is the sole component of the antireflux mechanism. Other methods of investigation especially radiology

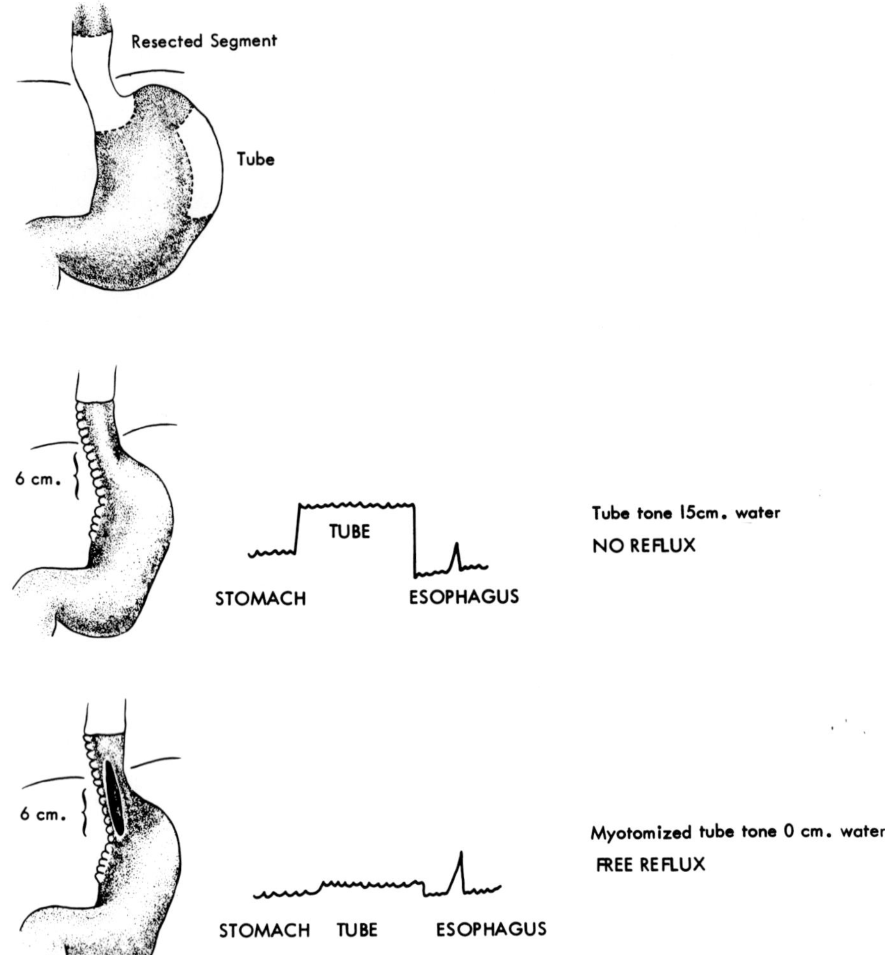

Figure 4.5.   Gastric Tube Replacement of Lower Esophagus
(Top) The resected zone of esophagus includes the gastroesophageal junction. The tube is taken from the greater curve of stomach and anastomosed to the esophagus. (Center) With the tube 6 cm below the diaphragm, the tube prevents reflux by virtue of its tone and its intra-abdominal position. (Bottom) When the intra-abdominal segment is myotomized, free reflux recurs.

and the effects of surgery suggest that the position of the sphincter and the size and shape of the hiatus are at least as important as the sphincter in the control of reflux" (39).

Who is correct in this argument? How important is the sphincter in reflux control? Certainly a simplistic concept of a low tone sphincter giving reflux and a high tone sphincter preventing reflux is no longer tenable as many patients with severe reflux symptoms have a high or normal tone sphincter. Experimentally it is possible to reduce the tone of the HPZ by inducing esophagitis (40–42) with a bile and acid drip technique. This study suggests that esophagitis reduces sphincter tone and indeed may be the cause of the low tone sphincter encountered in patients with severe reflux. Once sphincter tone is reduced then the reflux potential is increased. Studies in 359 patients with intractable reflux symptoms treated surgically by total fundoplication gastroplasty (TFG (43, 44): Nissen gastroplasty) are interesting and help support the concept of reflux damage producing a low tone sphincter rather than the primary disorder being a low tone sphincter which then allows reflux.

Of the 359 patients treated surgically, 353

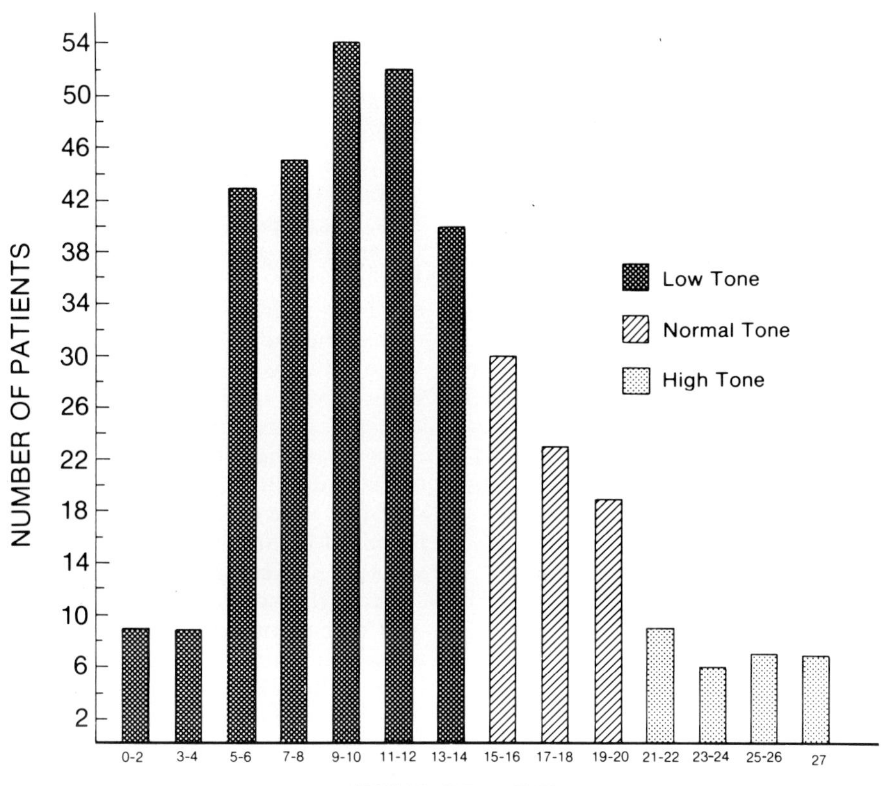

Figure 4.6.　HPZ Tone in 353 Patients with Reflux
Manometric evaluation of 353 patients with severe reflux symptoms requiring surgery shows a low tone HPZ in 71.4 per cent, normal tone in 20.4 per cent and a high tone in 8.2 per cent.

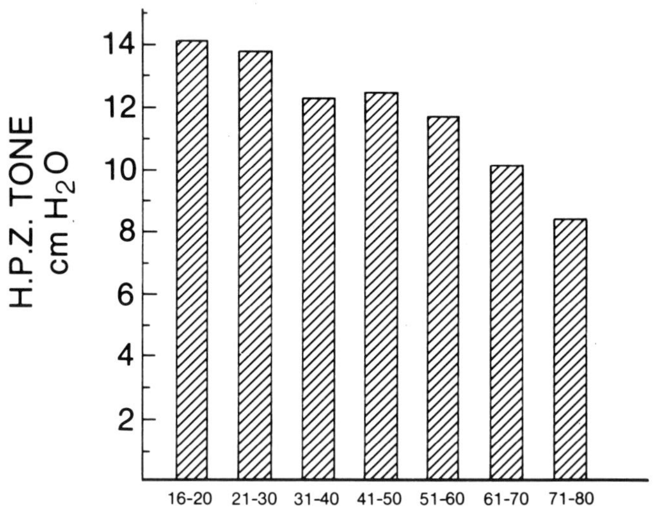

AVERAGE AGE 353 PATIENTS WITH REFLUX

Figure 4.7.　Comparison of HPZ Tone with Age in 353 Patients with Reflux
The HPZ tone in the 353 patients studied showed a slight, but definite, decrease with increasing age.

had preoperative esophageal manometry and 240 had follow-up manometry 3 to 12 months following surgery. The normal tone of the HPZ using this particular water-perfused system is 15 to 20 cm H_2O. In the present study of 353 patients with reflux 71.4 per cent had a low tone HPZ, 20.4 per cent a normal tone and 8.2 per cent a high tone HPZ (Fig. 4.6).

If HPZ damage develops and the tone falls after reflux has occurred, then one would expect to find a higher tone HPZ in young patients and also a fall in HPZ tone with duration of symptoms. In the age group under 20 years the average tone of the HPZ was 14.1 cm of H_2O, and this fell to 10.5 cm H_2O in the age group over 70 years (Fig. 4.7). Comparing HPZ tone with duration of symp-toms, when symptoms had been present for less than 1 year the average tone was 13.7 cm H_2O and when symptoms had been present for 6 to 30 years the average HPZ tone was 11.0 cm H_2O (Fig. 4.8).

Following TFG 240 patients had follow-up manometric studies to evaluate the effectiveness of surgical repair. The tone of the sphincter rose from a preoperative level of 12.04 cm H_2O average to a postoperative level of 18.35 cm H_2O average (an increase of 52.41 per cent). The increased tone is most marked in those with a very low tone sphincter and least in those with a high tone sphincter, suggesting that the measurable tone is true sphincter recovery rather than pressure generated by the surrounding fundoplication. If the pressure rise were due to the fundoplication then it should be an equal increment of pressure, additive to the preoperative tone (Table 4.2).

From this study it can be seen that 28.6 per cent of patients, despite severe reflux symptoms had a normal or high tone HPZ. The tone of the HPZ was higher in younger than in older patients and was higher in those with short duration disease than in those with long duration disease. Recovery of HPZ tone was most marked in those with a very low tone HPZ before surgery.

The only known effect of surgery in these patients was reflux control by fundoplication and by creating an intra-abdominal segment of esophagus. The findings suggest that reflux damages the HPZ over a period of years and that when reflux is controlled, the HPZ pressure returns to normal.

Based on this analysis, the tone of the HPZ is reduced because of reflux damage and is not primarily the cause of the reflux. However, as the HPZ tone decreases, reflux is likely to increase as an important mechanism of control is damaged.

Accepting that our knowledge of reflux

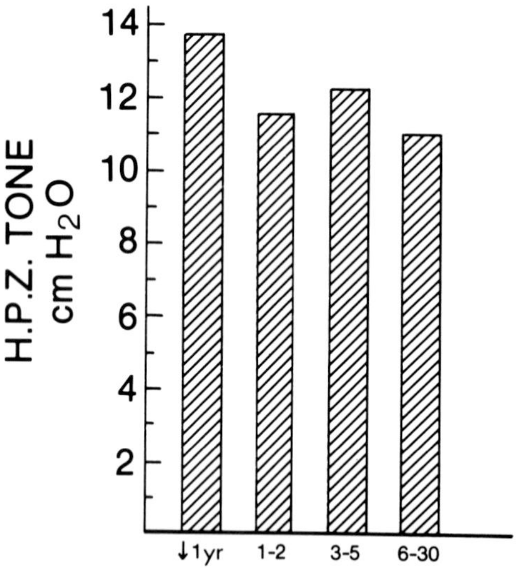

DURATION OF SYMPTOMS

Figure 4.8.   Comparison of HPZ Tone and Duration of Reflux Symptoms
Duration of symptoms in the 353 patients was also associated with a slight, but definite, decrease in HPZ tone.

Table 4.2
Reflux Control by TFG—Effect on HPZ Tone (240 Patients)*

No. of Patients	Preoperative Tone Range	Average Preoperative Tone	Average Postoperative Tone	Actual Tone Increase	Tone Increase
	cm H_2O	cm H_2O	cm H_2O	cm H_2O	%
13	0–4	2.62	12.92	10.3	393.1
69	5–9	7.13	17.16	10.03	140.67
88	10–14	11.59	18.28	6.69	57.72
44	15–19	16.96	19.48	2.52	14.86
26	20–27	23.54	20.46	−3.08	−13.08

* Following reflux control manometric evaluation in 240 patients showed an increase in HPZ tone which was greater in patients with a low tone HPZ and progressively decreased in those with higher HPZ tones.

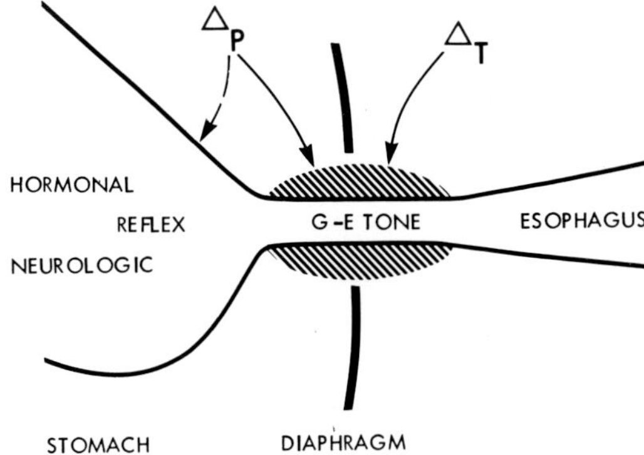

Figure 4.9. Normal Subject—Reflux Control
Δ_p is intraperitoneal pressure and Δ_T intrathoracic pressure. Under normal circumstances, reflux is prevented by hormonal and neurologic reflexes, together with the tone of the gastroesophageal junction (G-E tone) and its intraabdominal position. When Δ_T is increased, it acts on both stomach and gastroesophageal junction, and hence this pressure increase is counterbalanced and neutralized.

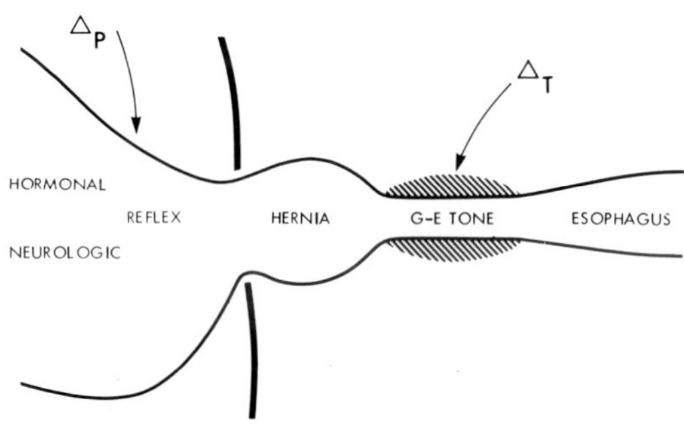

Figure 4.10. Hiatal Hernia Subject—Reflux
In a patient with a hiatal hernia, the intra-abdominal segment is lost, the neurologic reflexes are less effective and gastroesophageal (G-E) tone is the major barrier to reflux. Reflux, when it occurs, produces esophagitis which increases disordered motor activity (DMA) and decreases gastroesophageal junctional tone. Increased DMA delays esophageal emptying and increases the exposure of the esophagus to the refluxed bolus. Decreased junctional tone increases the potential to reflux and further accelerates esophageal damage.

control is still inadequate, I would support Edwards' concept that the HPZ is of prime importance in controlling intragastric pressure rises and the intra-abdominal segment and diaphragmatic hiatal opening are of major importance in resisting intraperitoneal pressure increases.

Coordination of Reflux Control

The diaphragm and phrenoesophageal ligaments are important in maintaining the esophagus in its correct position 2½ cm below the diaphragm. It is unlikely that the angle of entry of esophagus to stomach or the mucosal rosette is of much importance in preventing reflux (45).

Dominant in reflux control are the tone of the HPZ and the intra-abdominal segment of esophagus. The HPZ is a complex physiologic mechanism capable of responding to changes in gastric pressure, pH and gastric content. In the normal subject only minor and asymptomatic reflux occurs.

Two forces can act to produce reflux. One effect is an increase in peritoneal pressure such as that which occurs with obesity, lifting or ascites. This force acts also on stomach and directly compresses the intra-abdominal esophagus, counterbalancing any increase in gastric pressure (Fig. 4.9)

The second reflux-producing force is increased gastric pressure. This will occur fol-

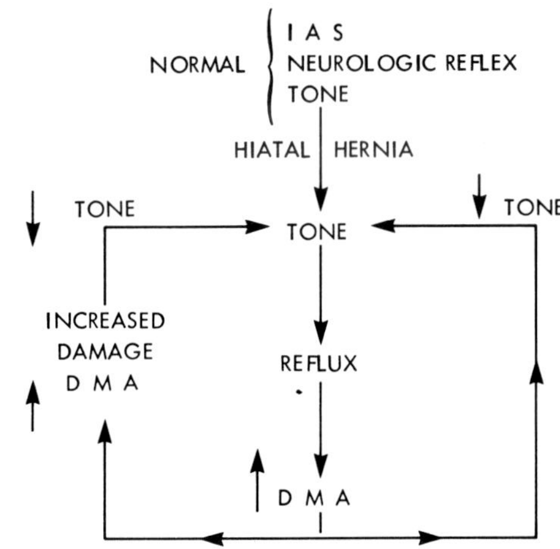

Figure 4.11
In the presence of a hiatal hernia, the intra-abdominal segment (IAS) is lost, the neurologic reflexes decrease and gastroesophageal tone is the major barrier to reflux. Reflux, when it occurs, produces esophagitis which increases disordered motor activity (DMA) and decreases gastroesophageal junctional tone. Increased DMA delays esophageal emptying and increases esophageal exposure to the refluxed bolus. Decreased junctional tone increases the potential to reflux and to further esophageal damage.

lowing a meal and will be exacerbated by overindulgence or by any change which delays gastric emptying. Gastric pressures act intraluminally and are counterbalanced by HPZ augmented tone increases which are neurogenic in origin. The gastrin mechanism, previously considered important, is unlikely to be responsible for acute HPZ tone changes following eating.

In the presence of a hiatal hernia the intra-abdominal segment of esophagus is lost, and acute increases in peritoneal pressure will increase gastric pressure without exerting a counterbalancing esophageal compression (Fig. 4.10). Reflux may occur under these circumstances. While it is only speculation, it is conceivable that a reflux produced by this type of extrinsic pressure may be the early reflux which will produce damage to the HPZ and reduce its tone. Once the tone is reduced, reflux will occur more readily and, indeed, when a hernia is present, there is evidence to suggest that the augmented HPZ pressure response to abdominal compression is reduced or absent.

Once reflux is established there are secondary changes of importance in increasing its damaging effect. Esophageal motor activity becomes disordered (46), and the esophageal clearance of the refluxed bolus is decreased (47) (Fig. 4.11). Recent studies have shown that secondary disordered motor activity results from lower esophageal distention and the cricopharyngeus may also increase its tone as a further method of containing the refluxed material (48).

With prolonged esophageal clearance and lowered HPZ tone, reflux is more likely to occur and is more damaging to the esophageal mucosa.

The next chapter will review the symptoms produced by gastroesophageal reflux and the clinical problems which may develop in patients with severe reflux.

References

1. Tuttle, S. G., Bettarello, A., and Grossman, M. L.: Esophageal acid perfusion test and a gastroesophageal reflux test in patients with esophagitis. Gastroenterology, *38:* 861, 1960.
2. Botha, G. S. M.: *The Gastro-Oesophageal Junction,* p. 204. J. & A. Churchill, Ltd., London, 1962.
3. Wolf, B. S., Brahms, S. A., and Khilnani, M. T.: The incidence of hiatus hernia in routine barium meal examinations. Mt. Sinai J. Med. N.Y., *26:* 598, 1959.
4. Berridge, F. R.: The mechanism at the cardia. III. Radiological aspects. Br. J. Radiol., *34:* 487, 1961.
5. Dornhorst, A. C., Harrison, K., and Pierce, J. W.: Observations on normal esophagus and cardia. Lancet, *1:* 695, 1954.
6. Allison, P. R.: Reflux esophagitis, sliding hiatal hernia, and the anatomy of repair. Surg. Gynecol. Obstet., *92:* 419, 1951.
7. Bombeck, C. T., Dillard, D. H., and Nyhus, L. M.: Muscular anatomy of the gastroesophageal junction and role of phrenoesophageal ligament; autopsy study of sphincter mechanism. Ann. Surg., *164:* 643, 1966.
8. Michelson, E., and Siegel, C. I.: The role of the phrenico-esophageal ligament in the lower esophageal sphincter. Surg. Gynecol. Obstet., *118:* 1291, 1964.
9. Hoag, E. W., Kiriluk, L. B., and Merendino, K. A.: Experiences with upper gastrectomy, its relationship to esophagitis with special reference to esophagogastric junction and diaphragm; a study in the dog. Am. J. Surg., *88:* 44, 1954.
10. Carveth, S. W., Schlegel, J. F., Code, C. F., and Ellis, F. H.: Esophageal motility after vagotomy, phrenecotomy, myotomy and myomectomy in dogs. Surg. Gynecol. Obstet., *114:* 31, 1962.
11. Liebermann-Meffert, D., Allgower, M., Schmid, P., and Blum, A. L.: Muscular equivalent of the lower esophageal sphincter. Gastroenterology, *76:* 31, 1979.
12. Belsey, R.: Functional disease of the esophagus. J. Thorac. Cardiovasc. Surg., *52:* 164, 1966.
13. Nissen, R., and Rossetti, M.: Surgery of hiatal and other diaphragmatic hernias. J. Int. Coll. Surg., *43:* 663, 1965.
14. Wolf, B. S., Heitmann, P., and Cohen, B. R.: The inferior esophageal sphincter, and manometric high pressure zone and hiatal incompetence. A.J.R., *103:* 251, 1968.
15. Field, P., and Stalker, M. J. B.: Incompetence of the cardiac sphincter without radiologic demonstration of hiatus hernia. Can. J. Surg., *11:* 412, 1968.
16. Steiner, G. M.: Gastro-oesophageal reflux, hiatus hernia and the radiologist, with special reference to children. Br. J. Radiol., *50:* 164, 1977.
17. Perez-Avila, C., and Irvin, T. T.: Interpretation of lower oesophageal pressure movements. Br. J. Surg., *62:* 663, 1975.
18. Nebel, O. T., and Castell, D. O.: Lower esophageal sphincter pressure changes after food ingestion. Gastroenterology, *63:* 778, 1972.
19. Dennish, G. W., and Castell, D. O.: Inhibitory effect of smoking on the lower esophageal sphincter. N. Engl. J. Med., *284:* 1136, 1971.
20. Chernow, B., and Castell, D. O.: Diet and heartburn. J.A.M.A., *241:* 2307, 1979.
21. Mayer, E. M., Grabowski, C. J., and Fisher, R. S.: Effects of graded doses of alcohol upon esophageal motor function. Gastroenterology, *75:* 1133, 1978.
22. Kaye, M. D.: On the relationship between gastric pH and pressure in the normal human lower oesophageal sphincter. Gut, *20:* 59, 1979.
23. Boesby, S.: Effect of changes in the intragastric milieu on competence of the gastro-oesophageal region. A study in normal subjects. Scand. J. Gastroenterol., *12:* 215, 1977.
24. Nagler, R., and Spiro, H. M.: Segmental response of the inferior esophageal sphincter to elevated intragastric pressure. Gastroenterology, *40:* 405, 1961.
25. Pope, C. E., II: A dynamic test of sphincter strength;

its application to the lower esophageal sphincter. Gastroenterology, *52:* 779, 1967.

26. Henderson, R. D., and Rodney, K.: Tone of the gastroesophageal junction; its response to abdominal compression and to swallowing. Can. J. Surg., *14:* 328, 1971.

27. Lind, J. F., Burns, C. M., and MacDougall, J. T.: "Physiological" repair for hiatus hernia—manometric study. Arch. Surg., *91:* 233, 1965.

28. Angorn, I. B., Dimopoulos, G., Hegarty, M. M., and Moshal, M. G.: The effect of vagotomy on the lower esophageal sphincter; a manometric study. Br. J. Surg., *64:* 466, 1977.

29. Sanders, M. G., and Schimmel, E. M.: Gastrin. Am. J. Med., *49:* 380, 1970.

30. Castell, D. O., and Harris, L. D.: Hormonal control of gastroesophageal-sphincter strength. N. Engl. J. Med., *282:* 886, 1970.

31. Cohen, S., and Lipshutz, W.: Hormonal regulation of human lower esophageal sphincter competence; interaction of gastrin and secretion. J. Clin. Invest., *50:* 449, 1971.

32. McGuigan, J. E.: Serum gastrin in health and disease. Am. J. Dig. Dis., *22:* 712, 1977.

33. Henderson, J. M., Lidgard, G., Osborne, D. H., Carter, D. C., and Heading, R. C.: Lower oesophageal sphincter response to gastrin—pharmacological or physiological? Gut, *19:* 99, 1978.

34. Goyal, R. K., and Rattan, S.: Neurohumoral, hormonal and drug receptors for the lower esophageal sphincter. Gastroenterology, *74:* 598, 1978.

35. Henderson, R. D., Boszko, A., Mugashe, F., Szczepanski, M. M., and Marryatt, G.: Oesophageal replacement by a gastric tube; an experimental study of the properties of the gastric tube. Br. J. Surg., *61:* 533, 1974.

36. DeMeester, T. R., Wernly, J. A., Bryant, G. H., Little, A. G., and Skinner, D. B.: Clinical and in vitro analysis of determinants of gastroesophageal competence. A study of the principles of antireflux surgery. Am. J. Surg., *137:* 39, 1979.

37. Kaye, M. D.: Postprandial gastro-oesophageal reflux in healthy people. Gut, *18:* 709, 1977.

38. Cohen, S., and Snape, W. J.: The pathophysiology and treatment of gastroesophageal reflux disease. New concepts. Arch. Intern. Med., *138:* 1398, 1978.

39. Edwards, D. A.: Reminiscences on the antireflux mechanism. South. Med. J., *71:* Suppl. 1, 1, 1978.

40. Henderson, R. D., Mugashe, F., Jeejeebhoy, K. N., Cullen, J., Szczepanski, M., Boszko, A., and Marryatt, G.: The role of bile and acid in the production of esophagitis and the motor defect of esophagitis. Ann. Thorac. Surg., *14:* 465, 1972.

41. Olsen, A. M., and Schlegel, J. F.: Motility disturbances caused by esophagitis. J. Thorac. Cardiovasc. Surg., *50:* 607, 1965.

42. Ramirez, J., Guarner, V., and Pazmino, F.: Alterations in motility of the esophagus in peptic esophagitis. Am. J. Proctol., *19:* 67, 1968.

43. Henderson, R. D.: The gastroplasty tube as a method of reflux control. Can. J. Surg., *21:* 264, 1978.

44. Henderson, R. D.: Reflux control following gastroplasty. Ann. Thorac. Surg., *24:* 206, 1977.

45. Henderson, R. D.: Gastroesophageal junction in hiatus hernia. Can. J. Surg., *15:* 63, 1972.

46. Kelley, M. L., Jr.: Esophageal motility studies in evaluation of hiatal hernia. N.Y. State J. Med., *66:* 595, 1966.

47. Booth, D. J., Kemmerer, W. T., and Skinner, D. B.: Acid clearing from the distal esophagus. Arch. Surg., *96:* 731, 1968.

48. Enzmann, D. R., Harell, G. S., and Zboralske, F. F.: Upper esophageal responses to intraluminal distension in man. Gastroenterology, *72:* 1292, 1977.

SECTION II

Hiatal Hernia

CHAPTER 5

Symptoms of Hiatal Hernia and Gastroesophageal Reflux

Patients with a hiatal hernia and/or gastroesophageal reflux develop a variety of symptoms that are related to reflux and represent the by-product of esophageal irritation. Pain as a significant complaint was first described by Fabricus (1648) and attributed to Galen (A.D. 130–200) (1). The first recognition of reflux as a cause of esophagitis is attributed to Quincke (1879) (2). Tileston (1906) (3) described 44 cases of reflux and for the first time outlined typical symptoms. Hamperl (1934) (4, 5) introduced the term peptic esophagitis.

The dominant symptoms are those of pain, the acidic taste of the refluxed bolus in the pharynx and dysphagia. Some patients also complain of burping, hiccoughing, "waterbrash," nausea or vomiting. In the typical patient, pain is the dominant symptom, but another component of the complex may occasionally predominate. Because this variability invites confusion and misdiagnosis, an esophageal history is a vital part of the physician's evaluation. If he takes it carefully, the history will be of cardinal importance, will often determine future investigation and from the outset may indicate the type of therapy.

The value of history is well illustrated by the following case.

Case 1. Mrs. M., age 40, had had symptoms of dysphagia for 5 years. Her complaints became progressively more severe and on radiologic evaluation she was shown to have a solitary gallstone. Cholecystectomy, which was performed 1 year before she was referred to me, had no effect on her clinical course. The information obtained on history alone established that her symptoms arose from her esophagus and permitted a precise diagnosis. (If such a history had been elicited earlier, she could have been offered treatment at the outset.)

This woman described her pain as right upper quadrant, epigastric and retrosternal. It occurred 5 minutes after each meal, lasted 30 to 60 minutes and was relieved by antacids. She was intolerant of fried foods, and felt full with only a small meal. She described reflux of gastric content into the throat once per week and a marked feature of her pain was excess salivation—"waterbrash." In addition she described definite gastroesophageal dysphagia occurring 3 to 4 times each week.

In review, several obvious features of this history suggest gastroesophageal reflux, but in particular the presence of reflux to the throat, waterbrash and dysphagia is so strongly suggestive of gastroesophageal reflux that it is difficult to accept that this woman was fully investigated before she was submitted to cholecystectomy. Further evaluation, namely radiology, manometry and acid perfusion, confirmed the presence of a hiatal hernia and gastroesophageal reflux. She was treated conservatively with antacids, bed elevation and dietary restriction and obtained marked improvement.

In evaluating pain, it is necessary first to chart carefully its predominant locations and distribution. The total duration of pain, frequency of episodes and the average duration of each episode must be elicited and recorded. The factors which precipitate the pain and the methods by which the patient achieves relief help to determine the type of pain and to distinguish esophageal pain from that arising in a related or contiguous organ.

In considering hiatal hernia and reflux, it should be recalled that the refluxed bolus, when it passes into the pharynx, induces a specific bitter, burning or sour taste. It is important to recognize this symptom, to determine its frequency and to inquire about any association between this and the coughing and choking of night aspiration. As noted earlier, other symptoms such as burping, hiccoughing, waterbrash, nausea and vomiting may predominate in the occasional patient. Dysphagia is a characteristic feature of many types of esophageal disease, and for full appreciation of this symptom a careful record is required of its frequency and duration; the types of food that stick, and its constancy or variability. If a patient regurgitates or aspirates during swallowing, his dysphagia is probably severe.

Anatomic Types of Hiatal Hernias

Hiatal hernias are of three anatomical types (6, 7). In Type I (Fig. 5.1) a sliding pouch of stomach passes up and into the chest; in Type II the gastric fundus rolls up beside the esophagus but the esophagogastric junction remains in its normal position beneath the diaphragm; Type III combines components of Type I and Type II. Reflux is the predominant symptom in Type I, but the symptoms in Type II are related to distension of the gastric fundal pouch. Type III hernia tends to combine the symptoms of Types I and II.

Type I Hiatal Hernia

Type I, the most common hiatal hernia (8, 9), accounts for at least 92 per cent of those recognized. In this type of hernia the dominant cause of symptoms is reflux and reflects the incompetence of the gastroesophageal junction (10, 11), which allows gastric content to flow into the body of the esophagus. The obvious questions "Why does reflux develop?" and "Can reflux develop in the absence of a hiatal hernia?" as yet have no simple answer. Reflux has been described in patients without a recognizable radiologic hiatal hernia (12, 13), and in any event anatomic "proof" of a Type I hiatal hernia almost always depends on its radiologic demonstration. How accurate is the radiologic diagnosis of a hiatal hernia? Reviewing radiologic data in a personal series of 428 patients treated surgically for reflux, a diagnosis of hiatal hernia was made in 297 (69.4 per cent), reflux only in 54 (12.6 per cent) and 77 (18 per cent) patients were considered entirely normal. The original diagnosis of reflux in these 428 patients was based on a combination of history, endoscopy, radiology and manometry, and in all, symptoms of reflux disappeared after operative repair. Clinically, it is common to observe that the patient in whom a hernia is not demonstrated may show a hernia on further radiologic studies. Since this is so, one cannot state that because a hernia is not demonstrated radiologically, a hernia will not appear later (14, 15). From radiologic studies, the reported incidence of hernias in the normal population ranges from 1.3 per cent (16) to 45 per cent (17), and this wide variability suggests the fallibility of radiologic techniques in such diagnoses. Since

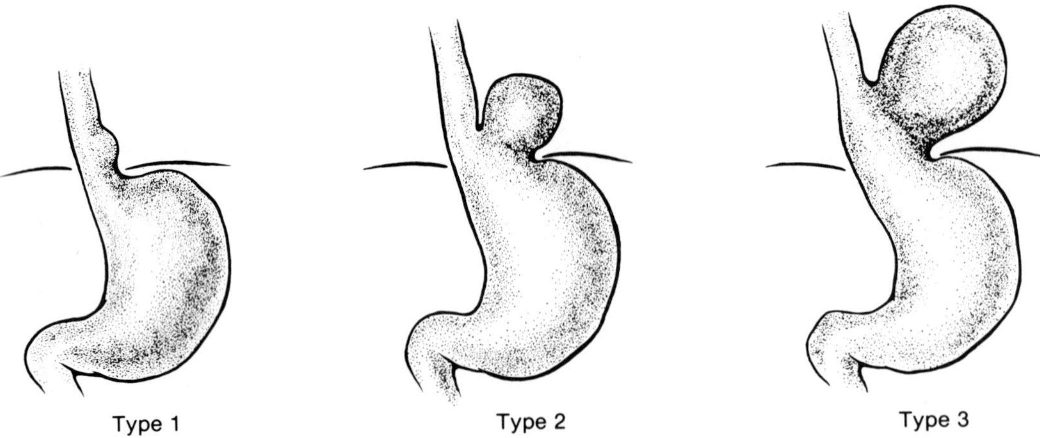

Figure 5.1. Types of Hiatal Hernia
Type I hiatal hernias are sliding hernias where stomach passes into the thorax through the esophageal hiatus. In the Type II hernia, the fundus of stomach rolls up beside the esophagus, usually through the esophageal hiatus. The gastroesophageal junction remains in its normal position. Type III hernias combine the Type I and Type II hernia.

the diagnosis of hiatal hernia is based chiefly on the radiologic examination and since these techniques are demonstrably inaccurate, we have not yet developed the criteria necessary to definitively answer the question "Can reflux develop in the absence of a hiatal hernia?" Regardless of whether one believes that a hernia is a prerequisite to reflux, it is generally accepted that reflux is responsible for most of the symptoms encountered (13).

Reflux

Irritation of esophageal mucosa by the refluxed gastric bolus produces most of the symptoms in hiatal hernia (18). The irritated mucosa becomes even more sensitive to further reflux, hence the peculiar and highly distressing "heartburn" typical of esophageal disease. Disordered motor activity (DMA) is a secondary and most important consequence of this irritation and is associated with esophageal food sticking in some patients. When it passes upward through the cricopharyngeal muscle into the pharynx, the presence of the refluxed bolus is signaled by its characteristic taste. Gastric content, when it is refluxed into the pharynx at night, may be aspirated into the tracheobronchial tree.

A careful history may make the diagnosis in up to 80 per cent of patients with hiatal hernias (19). A review of esophageal symptoms and their relative frequency is particularly helpful when the examiner assigns a "value" to each symptom in the light of their established diagnostic value (Table 5.1) (7, 10, 20). In this connection, we have reviewed the symptoms of 300 patients who had a demonstrable hiatal hernia. The frequency of the major symptoms was determined from the replies these patients made to specific questions. The following discussion of the symptomatology of hiatal hernia is based on the results of this study.

Esophageal Pain

The major complaint in most patients with a symptomatic hiatal hernia is pain, which may be produced by reflux, esophageal spasm or distention of the herniated stomach. The most frequent cause is esophageal irritation; here the pain varies with the character of the refluxed gastric content and the sensitivity of the mucosa. As the patient clearly describes

Table 5.1

Hiatal Hernia Symptoms: Comparison in Published Series*

Symptoms	Series (No. of Cases)			
	Hender-son (300)	Urschel and Paul-son (10) (636)	Skinner and Bel-sey (7) (1030)	Davis (20) (294)
	%	%	%	%
Heartburn	96.6	83	86	78
Reflux to throat	71.5	—	—	74
Reflux and aspiration	27.6	—	8	—
Waterbrash	30	—	—	—
Nausea and vomiting	46.3	21	—	—
Dysphagia total	78	40	54	44
Mechanical dys-phagia	8.3	—	19	—
Motor dys-phagia	69.7	—	35	—
Bleeding	2	11	15	6

* Considerable variations in the percentage of reported symptoms are evident in the published series. Much of this variation must depend on the care with which the patient's symptoms are elicited and recorded. When each symptom is carefully elicited it can be seen that major symptoms such as aspiration and dysphagia are very common.

it, this type of pain follows meals or comes with postural changes that produce gravitational reflux. Another source of pain is esophageal motor spasm, which can be detected radiologically in some patients. The spasm can also be demonstrated manometrically during acid perfusion which may produce both pain and spasm. A third source of esophageal pain is hernia distention. The abrupt distention of the hernia by an injected air bolus may produce pain in some patients. Removal of the air by suction gives rapid relief (Fig. 5.2). The relative importance of these various mechanisms remains speculative; however, all three play a part in the production of pain, probably in combination.

In its most typical distribution, the pain is epigastric and retrosternal, frequently going through to the back (Fig. 5.3). It may be referred to the neck, ears and jaw, and can be referred into the shoulders and down the arms as far as the elbows. Rarely this pain is

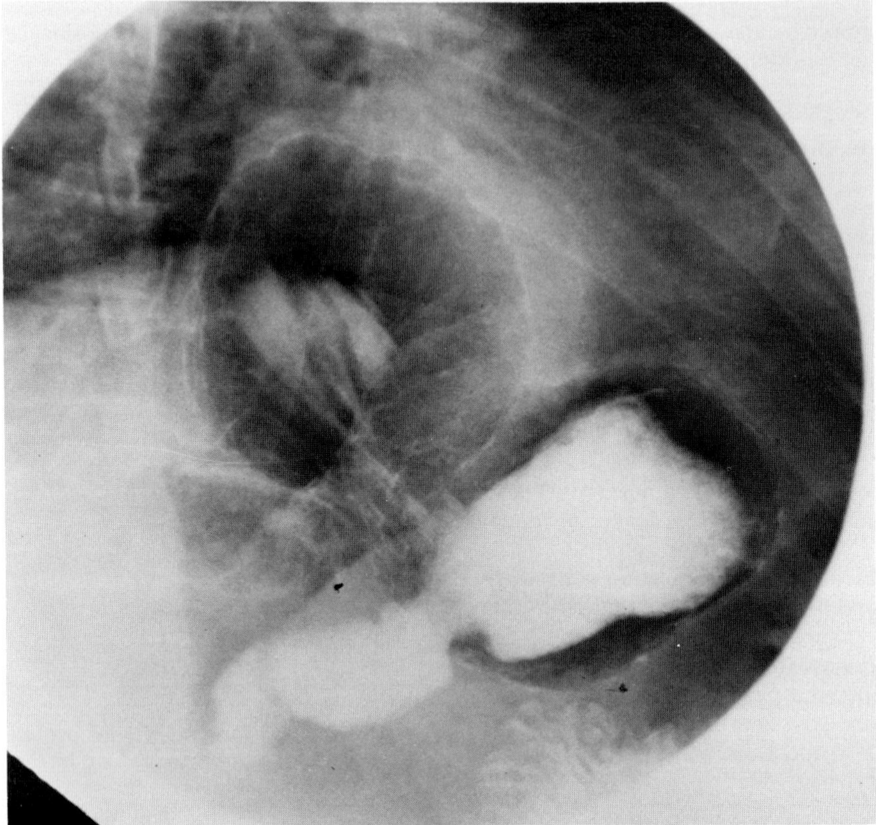

Figure 5.2. Large Type III Hiatal Hernia
The patient (Mrs. C.) had a large Type III hiatal hernia. She complained of chest pain with exercise, but this pain could be reproduced by distending her hernia with an air bolus. This radiograph shows the hernia distended by air; at the same time the patient's pain was reproduced.

described as radiating as far as the fingers. Such atypical esophageal pain is difficult to differentiate from that due to myocardial ischemia. Although it most often is described as "burning," the pain may be referred to as "knifelike" or "gripping."

Careful attention to factors which precipitate or relieve the symptom helps to determine whether the pain is due to esophageal disease. Typically, esophageal pain develops during the meal or within 5 to 10 minutes of its completion. Often the patient is most comfortable when he is hungry. Both the quality and quantity of food eaten are important. Tea, coffee, alcohol, carbonated beverages and spicy or fried food may produce symptoms or make the pain worse, and many patients seem to be sensitive to specific foods such as salmon, raw vegetables or acidic fruit (21). Typically patients with hiatal hernias consciously reduce the size of their meal because distention is the major aggravating factor. Postural change also produces pain. Commonly these patients cannot lie down following a meal, and exertion such as lifting or getting down to clean floors aggravates the pain. General exercise such as walking or climbing stairs usually does not reproduce their discomfort; however, pain produced by these maneuvers causes confusion with cardiac disease in some patients (22–25). Finally, esophageal pain may begin spontaneously and be unrelated to dietary or postural change.

The patient often discovers that he can reduce discomfort or avoid pain by not eating irritating foods and by eating small meals. When pain has developed, antacids may relieve it in many patients. Unlike the pain of cardiac disease, rest is rarely beneficial. Ni-

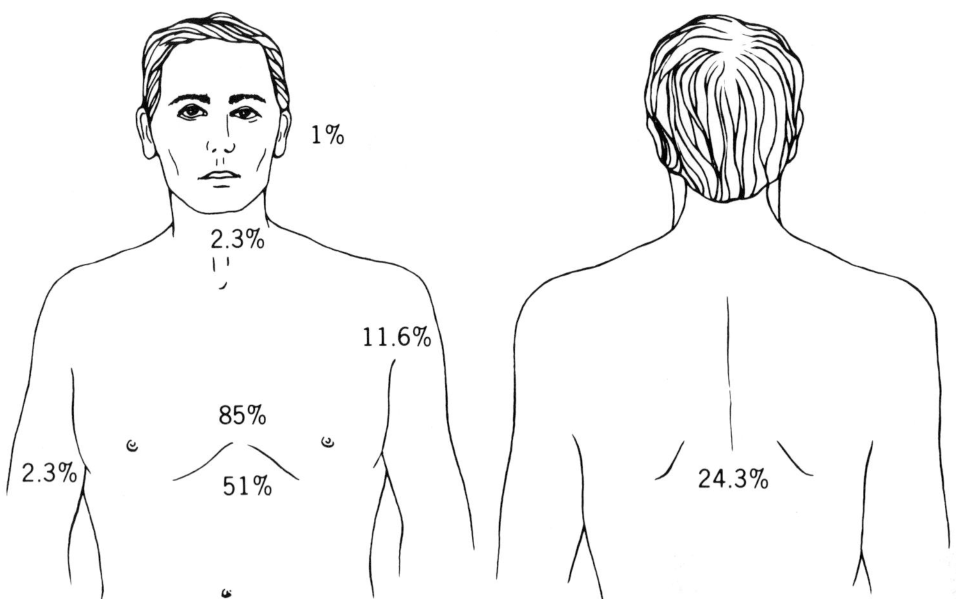

Figure 5.3. Pain Distribution with Hiatal Hernias (300 Patients)
Pain distribution was documented by history in 300 consecutive patients with a hiatal hernia. The dominant pains were epigastric, retrosternal and to the back, but a small proportion of patients had pain referred to the arms, jaw and ears. In 11.6 per cent of cases the pain was distributed to the left arm and in 2.3 per cent to the right arm.

troglycerin can relieve esophageal motor spasm, but the improvement usually does not come rapidly. With angina, relief comes within 3 minutes, whereas with esophageal pain it takes longer, and sometimes the patient, describes relief as taking up to 15 minutes.

Experience with 105 patients who presented with atypical chest pain illustrates the challenge posed by the differential diagnosis of esophageal pain (26, 27). In these patients the pain was sufficiently atypical to require a coronary angiogram or exercise cardiogram and each had radiologic, manometric and esophageal acid perfusion studies. After investigation we concluded that 43 of these 105 patients had "pure" esophageal dysfunction secondary to a hiatal hernia, and 12 had "pure coronary artery disease. Of the 43 atypical hiatal hernia patients, a high percentage had pain that was distributed to the arms and jaw (Table 5.2). In addition, the factors which precipitated and relieved the pain were much different from those in patients with more typical hiatal hernia symptoms. A comparison of the distribution of this pain and of precipitating and relieving factors (Table 5.3)

Table 5.2
Atypical Chest Pain of Esophageal Origin: Comparison with 300 Patients with Hiatal Hernias*

Origin of Pain	Atypical Chest Pain of Esophageal Origin (43 Patients)		Standard Hiatal Hernia Patients (300 Patients)	
	No.	% Distribution	No.	% Distribution
Epigastric	23	53.4	153	51
Retrosternal	40	93	255	85
Back	14	32.5	73	24.3
Left arm	23	53.4	35	11.6
Right arm	1	2.3	7	2.3
Both arms	2	4.6	0	0
Jaw	1	2.3	7	2.3
Ears	0	0	3	1

* The epigastric, retrosternal and back pain is similar in both the standard and atypical groups. In the atypical patients the distribution of pain to the arms is much more frequent. Distribution to one or both arms suggests cardiac pain and is a common reason for considering esophageal pain as atypical.

shows that it may be difficult to distinguish the symptoms of atypical esophageal disease from those of cardiac disease (23–30).

The following case illustrates the difficulties of pain differentiation.

Table 5.3
Atypical Chest Pain in 55 Patients*

Chest Pain	Esophageal (43)	Cardiac (12)
	%	%
Precipitating factors:		
Food	67	25
Posture	39	16
Exercise	55	41
Relief:		
Antacids	18	8
Nitroglycerin	20	33
Rest	18	33

* Chest pain is categorized as atypical when its distribution, precipitating or relieving factors differ significantly from those commonly encountered. In this group of atypical patients, the precipitating and relieving factors were evaluated, retrospectively, after the source of pain had been identified, and it was found that these historical factors did not help to separate patients with cardiac disease from those with esophageal disease.

Case 2. Over the 3 years before consultation, Mrs. B., age 52, had been admitted to the hospital on five occasions when she was believed to have suffered a myocardial infarction. On each occasion her ECG and enzyme studies were normal. Her pain was epigastric and retrosternal, and radiated into her back and into her left arm as far as the elbow. She had this pain each day and intermittently it was severe. It was precipitated by exercise such as climbing stairs and using the vacuum cleaner at home. Her discomfort was more marked when she exercised following a meal. Antacids produced variable relief, and nitroglycerin was believed to relieve her pain, but it took 5 minutes to become effective. She did have moderate gastroesophageal dysphagia, indicating the presence of esophageal disease

Coronary angiography demonstrated a 25 per cent defect in one coronary artery, but this was not considered to be the cause of pain. On radiologic and manometric examination she had a hiatal hernia and acid perfusion studies reproduced her pain exactly.

Surgical correction of her hernia has given effective symptom relief, and 4 years later she remains well.

Other Symptoms of Hiatal Hernia and Reflux

Reflux to the Throat

Reflux of gastric content to the throat often has great diagnostic significance: 71.5 per cent of the 300 patients (Table 5.1) described

earlier reported this symptom, most frequently as a burning, sour or bitter taste. This form of reflux may occur at any time but is particularly common after eating and usually is associated with typical heartburn. It may appear with postural change or in bed at night owing to the increased effect in the horizontal position of gravity which allows fluid to run up to the esophagus. The patient often describes reflux with the "burping" that commonly follows eating.

Eructation

Eructation (burping), usually a mild symptom, can be induced in patients with gastroesophageal reflux by air swallowing. Air swallowing may be a reaction to nervous tension, may be secondary to excess salivation and the constant swallowing of saliva or may occur while eating. Once it is in the stomach, the accumulating air gives rise to a sensation of bloating, and because the gastroesophageal junction is incompetent the patients cannot prevent eructation. Occasionally the patient may be conscious of the bloating but may be unable to eruct. Such patients often resort to drinking carbonated beverages to induce more effective eructation.

As a symptom, eructation is usually mild, but in some it may be severe and constant, and a source of much discomfort or social embarrassment. The associated reflux may be accompanied by heartburn which adds to the patient's distress.

Hiccoughs

Occasionally hiccoughs (involuntary spasm of the diaphragm), which may have many possible causes, are associated with a hiatal hernia (31–33). These episodes are usually mild and do not constitute a significant component of the patient's complaints. Occasionally the hiccoughs are intractable, but no relationship has been demonstrated between intractable hiccoughs and gastroesophageal reflux. Attempts to correct hiccoughs by hiatal hernia repair are often unsuccessful.

The patient may report that the hiccoughing is associated with intermittent food sticking, but this type of hiccough represents air released from the esophagus, not diaphragmatic spasm.

In some patients a clear relationship can be

established between hiccoughs and a hiatal hernia.

Case 3. Mr. S. had had intermittent severe hiccoughs for 10 years. Episodes of hiccoughs lasted up to 10 days without relief. Reflux symptoms and intermittent dysphagia developed while hiccoughing. Radiologically a hiatal hernia was present. None of his past therapy had been of value, including swallowed local anesthetics and breathing CO_2 enriched air.

Initially he had some improvement from pharyngeal irritation with a nasogastric tube. When this failed, antacids and metaclopramide did give significant improvement, decreasing the frequency and severity of his symptoms. Because of the unreliability of surgical reflux correction in this disorder, surgery has not been considered.

Waterbrash

This excess of salivation associated with esophageal irritation was recognized in 30 per cent of our 300 patients. It was common in the presence of esophageal irritation from reflux, or that associated with food sticking. Aylwin (34) has proposed that the human produces excess alkaline saliva to neutralize gastric acidity. Indeed, the absence of saliva in the ill, dehydrated patient may explain in part the rapid progression of his esophageal disease.

Nausea and Vomiting

Of the 300 patients with hiatal hernias studied at Toronto General Hospital, 46.3 per cent had nausea and vomiting. Frequently these symptoms are a major source of distress and occasionally nausea and vomiting may dominate the clinical picture and may be responsible for considerable weight loss. In patients with gastroesophageal reflux who have had previous gastric surgery, particularly a Billroth II gastrectomy, and have associated gastritis, the nausea and vomiting become more frequent and more severe. Of 36 such patients studied after gastrectomy, 77 per cent had nausea and vomiting (35). In this particular situation the higher frequency of nausea and vomiting appears to be related to the concurrent association of gastroesophageal reflux and gastritis. The significance of these symptoms is difficult to assess, because they are also associated with other gastroesophageal disorders, such as peptic ulceration or gallbladder disease, which must be carefully excluded.

Hemorrhage and Anemia

Microcytic anemia has been reported in from 2 to 42 per cent (36–38) of patients with hiatal hernias. Commonly the anemia is mild but occasionally may be severe. Its exact cause has not been clearly elucidated (39–41). Esophagitis or generalized gastritis is not usually associated with anemia. An incarcerated hernia may bleed at the point where the stomach is compressed as it passes through the diaphragmatic crurae. Frank hematemesis or melena is rare. Windsor and Collis (38) have reported that surgical correction of the hernia relieves the anemia.

I have had experience with only 4 patients presenting with acute massive hemorrhage from the esophagus related to reflux. Three of these patients had a gastric-lined Barrett's esophagus with a penetrating ulcer and one had an ulcer at the gastroesophageal junction with recurrent hemorrhage. This last patient is worth considering as we were misled as to his primary diagnosis.

Case 4. Mr. N., age 44, had bled twice massively and was transferred to Women's College Hospital by air ambulance. He had minor past symptoms of reflux and radiologically had a hiatal hernia with a penetrating ulcer at the esophagogastric junction. Endoscopically a large vessel was visible in the ulcer crater. Using a transthoracic approach the fundus of stomach was mobilized and noted to have marked venous engorgement. His liver was palpably normal. He was treated by total fundoplication gastroplasty with oversew of the ulcer.

Because of a massive rebleed we performed angiography. His spleen was replaced by a grapefruit-sized mass with very high vascularity. This mass lesion was excised with the tail of spleen and proved to be a gastrinoma. His course since this second procedure has been uncomplicated. The clue to the diagnosis was the increased vascularity in the fundus of stomach.

Weight Loss

Weight loss is not characteristic of hiatal hernias and gastroesophageal reflux. Most patients supplement their diet with small and frequent meals or by drinking milk. Patients with the most marked weight loss usually have frequent vomiting or a severe associated dysphagia (42). Occasionally weight loss is severe and becomes a significant factor in determining therapy, particularly in children in whom nutritional deficiency may produce growth retardation.

In reviewing the symptoms of 359 patients with reflux requiring surgery, weight loss was significant (more than 10 pounds) in 56 patients (15.6 per cent).

Dysphagia—Mechanical

In patients with gastroesophageal reflux, mechanical dysphagia is due to a peptic stricture and characteristically occurs at the squamocolumnar junction. This junction lies in the gastroesophageal sphincter zone (Fig. 5.4) (43, 44), but in a gastric mucosa-lined (Barrett's) esophagus this point is more proximal and these patients develop a stricture immediately below the level of the tracheal carina (Fig. 5.5) (44). Of the 300 patients studied, 8.3 per cent had mechanical dysphagia (Table 5.4).

A stricture gives rise to dysphagia, the degree of which depends upon the size of the food bolus, the diameter of the lumen and the propulsive force of the esophageal musculature (Fig. 5.6). When disordered motor activity is severe as in schleroderma, the only propulsive force available is that of gravity; such dysphagia is much more marked than in a patient who has retained effective motor power in the esophagus.

Because mechanical dysphagia is related to the relative sizes of the bolus and the lumen, solid foods will be held up while liquids pass through without obstruction. Occasionally liquids will stick when motor spasm and a mechanical stricture combine.

The esophagus may regurgitate its contents when food sticks because this organ cannot tolerate retained food within its lumen. In disorders such as achalasia, food retention may be tolerated and give rise to the characteristic air-fluid level seen radiologically. In most other esophageal disorders, passive dilatation and food retention develop only in the late stages of disease. When food is regurgitated from the esophageal lumen, it retains its normal appearance and taste. The regurgitated bolus may contain considerable

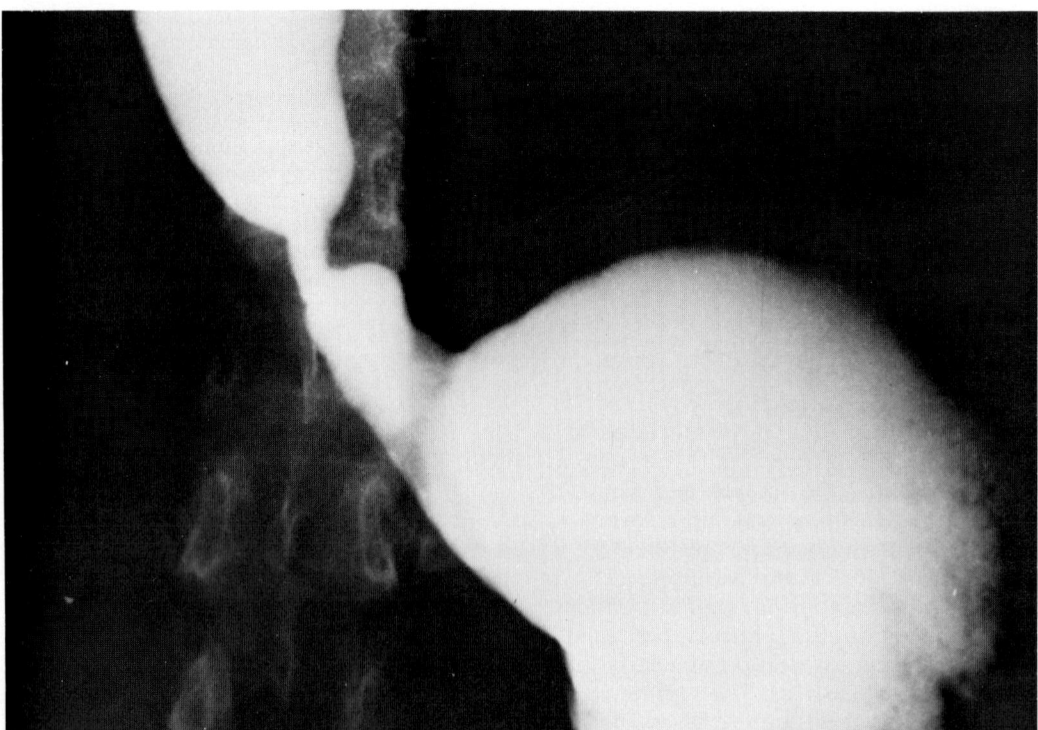

Figure 5.4. Stricture of Squamocolumnar Junction
This radiograph shows a small hiatal hernia. A stricture present at the squamocolumnar junction is approximately 1 cm in length and it narrows the esophageal lumen to less than one-third of its normal diameter.

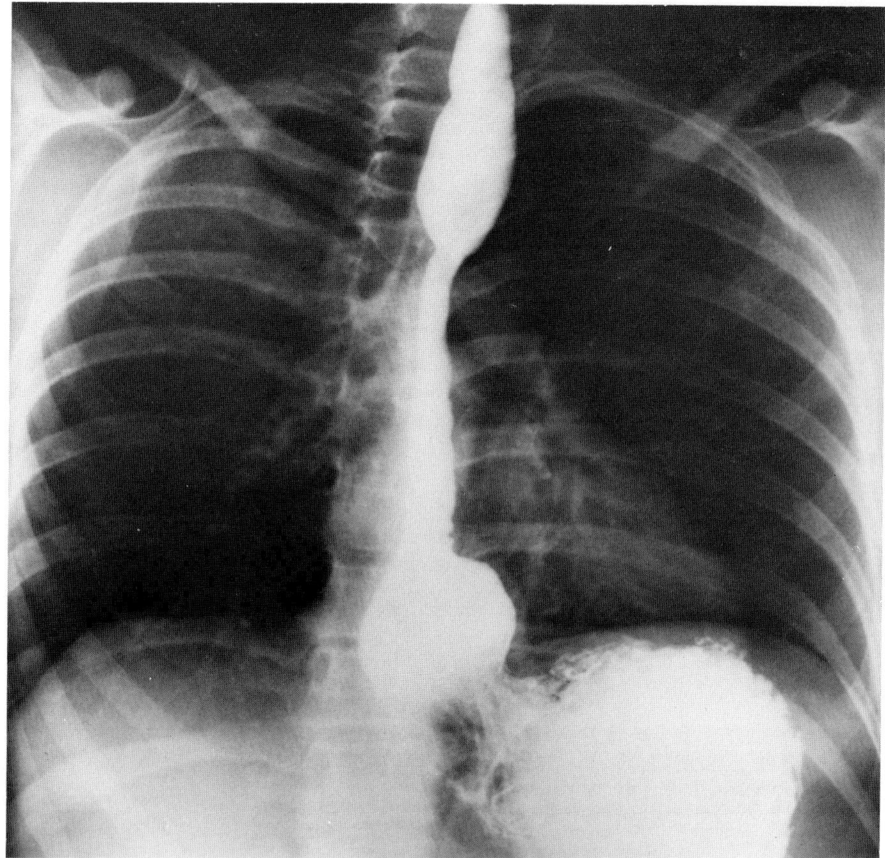

Figure 5.5. Barrett's Esophagus
In a Barrett's esophagus, the lower half of the esophagus is lined by columnar epithelium. Strictures, when they develop, are at the squamocolumnar junction, which is usually located at the tracheal level of the carina. In most instances there is a hiatal hernia.

frothy esophageal mucus and may occasionally be associated during the act of retching with gastroesophageal reflux and the taste of gastric content.

Dysphagia—Motor

Motor spasm may produce dysphagia (45, 46). This sensation, described as "food sticking," may be felt at any point in the esophagus, but all such sticking can be classed as either gastroesophageal or pharyngoesophageal dysphagia. Gastroesophageal dysphagia is centered behind the sternum, most commonly at its lower end, and pharyngoesophageal dysphagia at the level of the cricopharyngeus. In the 300 patients studied, gastroesophageal dysphagia occurred in 53.3 per cent and was confined chiefly to solids, although it can involve liquids (Table 5.4). The

degree of food sticking in motor dysphagia varies greatly, and in some patients it may be as severe as that associated with peptic stricture. Here regurgitation is less common than with a stricture, but when it does occur it has similar characteristics.

It is tempting to regard motor dysphagia as a phenomenon secondary to disordered motor activity (DMA). However, as noted earlier, no clear relationship can be established between the severity of motor dysphagia and the percentage of secondary DMA in the lower half of the esophagus.

In a group of 104 patients interviewed, this symptom was categorized as Type I dysphagia, where food sticking occurred less than once per week; Type II dysphagia where food sticking occurred up to once per day, and Type III dysphagia where food sticking

Table 5.4
Dysphagia in Hiatal Hernias (300 Patients)*

Dysphagia	Patients	
	no.	%
Total dysphagia	234	78
Mechanical dysphagia	25	8.3
Regurgitation	18	
Motor dysphagia	209	69.7
Gastroesophageal motor	160	53.3
Regurgitation	69	
Pharyngoesophageal motor	151	50.3
Coughing and choking	90	

* The incidence of dysphagia in patients with a clinically significant hiatal hernia is very high. In this series its severity varies from food sticking once per month to sticking with each swallowed bolus.

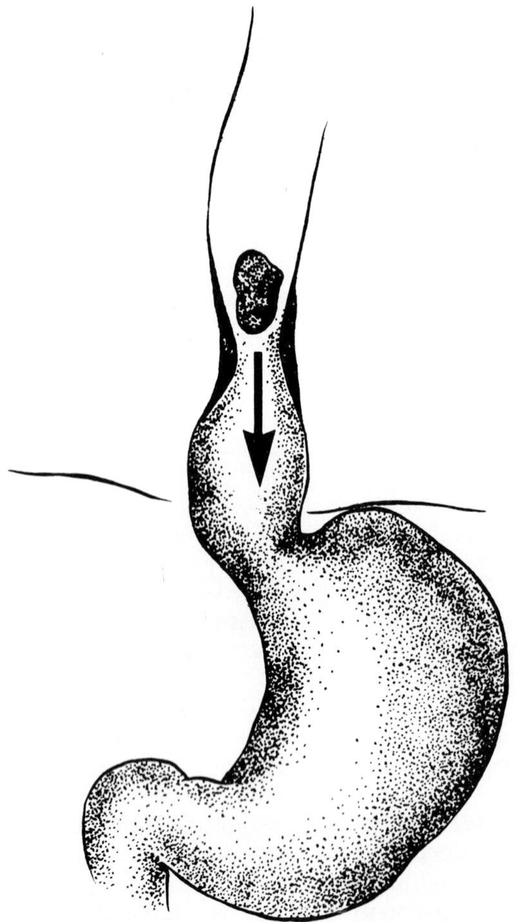

Figure 5.6
In the presence of a stricture the descent of the food bolus depends upon the length and diameter of the stricture lumen, the bolus size, gravity and the strength of esophageal motor power.

occurred more than once per day. Six patients with mechanical dysphagia from a peptic stricture were excluded from the study because the mechanical obstruction made it impossible to assess the motor component of their obstruction. No correlation could be shown when the type of dysphagia was compared with the percentage of DMA in the distal esophagus (Table 5.5). Dysphagia was as likely to occur in those with a low percentage of DMA as in those with a high percentage. While this study clearly shows that the percentage of disordered esophageal motor waves does not correlate with the presence of dysphagia, it does not indicate why the food becomes obstructed. As an alternate approach to the study of dysphagia, these patients were asked to swallow 1-cm marshmallow and 15-ml water boluses. At the moment when the patient experienced obstruction subjectively, the esophagus responded with a localized spasm and a diffuse rise in basal pressure (Fig. 5.7). This motor response may reflect the organ's sensitivity to the passage of the solid or liquid bolus, and the rise in pressure may be responsible for the obstruction. This study suggests that local esophageal spasm can produce obstruction, but it does not exclude the possibility that the

Table 5.5
Relationship of Dysphagia to Disordered Motor Activity (DMA) in Lower Esophagus*

Distal Esophageal DMA	No. Dysphagia		Dysphagia					
			Type I		Type II		Type III	
	no.	%	no.	%	no.	%	no.	%
0–40%	18	46	8	57	15	51	7	43
41–70%	13	33	4	28	6	20	7	43
71–100%	8	20	2	14	8	27	2	12
Total patients	39	99	14	99	29	98	16	98

* One hundred and four patients without previous esophageal surgery were assessed by history to determine the severity of their dysphagia. Six had a peptic stricture and were excluded from the study. In the remaining 98, the dysphagia, which was of a motor type, was categorized according to severity as: Type I, with food sticking less than once per week; Type II, with food sticking more than once per week and less than once per day; and Type III, with sticking daily. When the type of sticking was compared to the percentage of distal esophageal DMA as determined by manometric studies, no relationship could be demonstrated between the dysphagia and the severity of the secondary motor disorder.

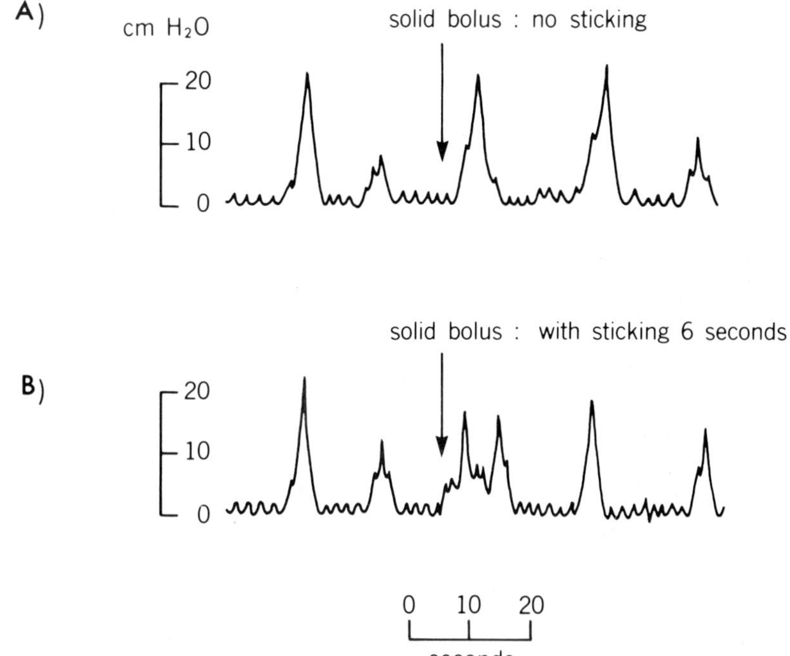

Figure 5.7. Bolus Sticking and Motor Activity
Secondary disordered motor activity of the esophagus. In A, a swallowed 1-cm marshmallow does not produce clinical sticking and there are no related motor changes. In B, the solid bolus does stick and there is a general increase in esophageal baseline pressure and disordered motor activity appears.

spasm is a response to obstruction rather than the cause.

Pharyngoesophageal dysphagia, which varied from "slight" and "occasional" to "very severe," was found in 50.3 per cent of the 300 patients studied. Clinically it is difficult to distinguish the actual impaction of food at the pharyngoesophageal junction from the referred sensation of food sticking at the gastroesophageal junction. We also know that distal esophageal obstruction can cause elevation of cricopharyngeal pressure and produce secondary discomfort. In addition, injection of liquid boluses to the esophagus will increase cricopharyngeal tone. The pressure elevation is more marked with decinormal hydrochloric acid than with saline. A few features of these two dysphagias help to make this distinction. First, when it sticks at the pharyngoesophageal junction, food may spill forward to the larynx, causing coughing or choking—a feature which clearly fixes such obstruction at the higher level. Secondly, if the patient is given a solid food bolus and asked to swallow, pharyngoesoph-

ageal obstruction will develop within 1 second, whereas gastroesophageal sticking is delayed for a full 6 to 8 seconds after the swallow (47, 48). These time intervals are directly related to the rate of food descent. If the patient reports sticking at 6 seconds and locates it at the pharyngoesophageal level, he is describing the referred sensation of obstruction or elevation of cricopharyngeal tone secondary to esophageal obstruction. This simple test is of great help in evaluating motor dysphagia.

Aspiration and Pharyngoesophageal Dysphagia

Aspiration is an important complication of pharyngoesophageal obstruction, and occasionally patients will report frequent spells of coughing and choking in which they expel both saliva and food (Fig. 5.8). In some patients pharyngoesophageal dysphagia is the dominant problem and, when severe, may produce considerable disability. These patients cannot eat in company because even

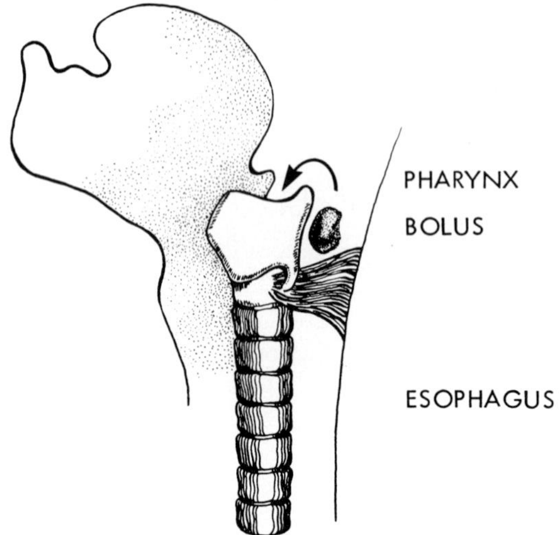

Figure 5.8. Pharyngoesophageal Dysphagia and Aspiration
Mechanism of food aspiration in patients with a hiatal hernia and pharyngoesophageal dysphagia is illustrated. When the food bolus hits the cricopharyngeus and cannot pass through the sphincter, it tends to spill forward into the larynx, thus inducing the coughing and choking of aspiration.

mild nervous tension provokes repeated aspiration and coughing.

The etiology of pharyngoesophageal dysphagia is obscure (49) and none of the many studies of the pharyngoesophageal junction have demonstrated a distinctive pattern related to food obstruction. The underlying cause is probably an imbalance between the pressures generated in the pharynx and the simultaneous relaxation of the cricopharynx. If the pressure peak generated by the pharyngeal motor wave does not equal or exceed the maximal relaxation of the cricopharynx, the bolus obstructs and the patient recognizes it as an inability to swallow. In most patients this phenomenon is intermittent, usually occurring early in the meal or with the first mouthful of liquids or solids; because of this intermittency, manometric studies of the pharyngoesophageal junction may not show any abnormality.

The following case illustrates the potential severity of pharyngoesophageal dysphagia.

Case 5. For at least 20 years, Mrs. H., age 56, had mild epigastric and retrosternal discomfort related to eating. These symptoms of pharyngo-esophageal dysphagia had not varied much during this time. They were present during all meals and were provoked by both liquids and solids. The symptoms had not progressed during this period, but the slightest distraction during her meal induced episodes of coughing and choking from aspiration. This threat was so severe that she could not eat in company and indeed, when she came to see me, reported that she could not eat with her own family.

Radiologically she had a small hiatal hernia with reflux. On manometric examination the motor changes were mild, and no abnormality could be demonstrated at the pharyngoesophageal junction. Subsequently a transthoracic hiatal hernia repair produced immediate partial relief of her symptoms and within 3 months her dysphagia resolved almost entirely. During the past 4 years she has remained well.

Aspiration

When encountered clinically, aspiration associated with gastroesophageal reflux is usually a chronic symptom that has been present for many years (50–55). This form of aspiration is quite different from that seen in patients with altered consciousness; the latter is more likely to be massive (56, 57), producing extensive lung soiling and an immediate threat to life. The aspiration encountered with reflux involves chronic lung soiling and secondary progressive lung injury. Such aspiration involves two important mechanisms.

1. The first is reflux and aspiration (58) that occurs predominantly at night. When the patient is asleep, the horizontal position encourages gravitational reflux, spillage of gastric content into the pharynx and further spillage into the larynx and trachea (51) (Fig. 5.9). With this acute stimulus, the patient wakens abruptly, coughing and choking, and with the taste of the aspirated bolus in his mouth. For most patients, this episode is so clear and so terrifying that they give an unmistakable history. Occasionally, aspiration may be silent, particularly in older patients.

2. The second mechanism operates in the presence of pharyngoesophageal dysphagia. When the bolus is held up at the cricopharyngeus because of the small capacity of the lower pharynx, the food spills forward, soiling the vocal cords and spilling into the tracheobronchial tree. The patient coughs and chokes and may regurgitate or vomit the food material (Fig. 5.8).

Each of these mechanisms produces sig-

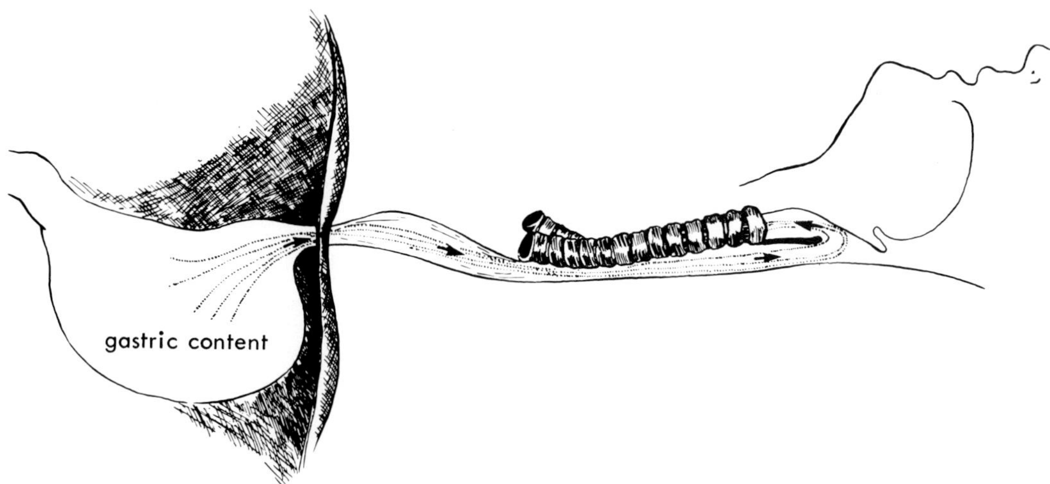

Figure 5.9. Night Reflux and Aspiration
When the patient is asleep and in the supine position, reflux may occur. If the refluxed bolus reaches the pharynx, forward spillage produces aspiration and the patient will waken coughing and choking.

nificant respiratory symptoms, and the precise effects of aspiration depend upon several variables: the quantity of the aspirate, the quality of the aspirate, the frequency of aspiration and the response of the tracheobronchial tree and lung to the aspirate. The quantity of the aspirate is difficult to judge from history, and attempts to measure its volume have been unsuccessful. Radioisotopes have been introduced recently. Given at night and scanned the following day, radioactive material may be detectable in the lungs. This technique, further refined, will add quantitative data to aspiration evaluation (59). The frequency of aspiration can be determined from the history of night aspiration, or of coughing and choking with swallowing. The quality of the aspirate, an important factor, has been analyzed to some degree.

Several workers have studied the effects of various aspirates in humans and in animals. Decinormal hydrochloric acid produces severe pneumonitis (60–62) and, in massive aspiration in humans, aspirate with a low pH is associated with a high mortality. Of the various components of pulmonary aspirate, hydrochloric acid has been most thoroughly studied; however, bile which is commonly found in the stomach is also highly irritating. For this reason we studied the effects of bile, hydrochloric acid and mixtures of bile and hydrochloric acid on the rabbit lung (63). The

aspirate was given in physiologic concentrations by direct intratracheal injections of volumes of 5 ml per kg. Rabbits were classified as those dying within 1 hour, within 24 hours, or surviving. Each animal was autopsied and its lungs were evaluated macroscopically and microscopically.

Hydrochloric acid of pH 1 killed all rabbits studied within 1 hour, but most of these animals died within a few minutes. The lungs were edematous and hemorrhagic at autopsy, but owing to the rapidity of the process showed little cellular infiltrate. This severe reaction is similar to that reported in other studies (60). Dilutions to pH 2 and greater produced no mortality and very little tissue change.

Bile in concentrations of 100, 50, 25, 12 and 6 per cent all produced death. The more concentrated bile killed all of the rabbits within 1 hour, whereas with the 6 per cent solution some rabbits lived up to 12 hours, and a few survived a concentration of 3 per cent bile. When 3 per cent bile was mixed with hydrochloric acid, pH 1.5, the mortality was increased slightly.

This study underlines the potential importance of bile in pulmonary aspirate and suggests that the combination of bile and hydrochloric acid may be even more lethal than the substances aspirated independently.

The effects of foodstuffs, such as mineral

oil, milk and particulate matter, vary with their chemical composition and their particulate size (64). Food may be aspirated both after reflux and with pharyngoesophageal dysphagia. The aspirate associated with reflux combines gastric and duodenal secretions with food, whereas in pharyngoesophageal dysphagia it consists of undigested food and saliva.

The sensitivity and degree of response of the end organ is obviously important; e.g. in the asthmatic, aspiration may prove to be a major additional stimulus to lung irritation and bronchospasm (65, 66). Recent studies suggest that a vagal reflex arch may trigger bronchospasm in the presense of gastroesophageal reflux. In most of these patients the aspiration has not *caused* the asthma, but it can pose a major load on an already reactive bronchial tree.

In the years 1969 to 1974, we studied 1000 consecutive patients (67) with hiatal hernias and gastroesophageal reflux, of whom 264 (26.4 per cent) gave a history of aspiration. In these 264 patients, the respiratory effects of aspiration were categorized as follows:

Cough and aspiration only,
Cough and voice change,
Recurrent acute respiratory infections,
Chronic respiratory infections, and
Asthma.

Aspiration was due to reflux and night aspiration in 110 patients, pharyngoesophageal dysphagia and aspiration in 54 patients, and both mechanisms operated in 100 patients (Table 5.6).

The severity of the respiratory symptoms could not be related to either the frequency or the type of aspiration as judged from history. Historical review allows the physician to estimate the frequency of aspiration, and an understanding of the mechanism lets him predict the type of aspirate. As noted earlier, with reflux the aspirate may contain food, gastric and duodenal secretion; with pharyngoesophageal dysphagia and aspiration, it contains saliva and undigested food content. This historic approach does not quantitate the amount of aspirated material.

Of the 264 patients noted above, 124 did not develop respiratory symptoms (Table 5.7) or respiratory disease, perhaps because the quality, quantity, the frequency of aspiration

Table 5.6 (67)
Aspiration and Hiatal Hernias (1000 Patients)*

Symptoms	Patients	
	no.	*%*
Aspiration	264	26.4
Reflux and aspiration	110	11
Pharyngoesophageal dysphagia and aspiration	54	5.4
Pharyngoesophageal dysphagia and reflux	100	10

* Aspiration was detected on the history in 26.4 per cent of 1000 consecutive patients with hiatal hernia. They complained of both pharyngoesophageal aspiration and reflux and aspiration. The frequency of aspiration varied from once per month to daily.

Table 5.7 (67)
Symptoms of Aspiration in Hiatal Hernias*

Patients with aspiration	264
No symptoms	124
Cough or voice change	89
Acute respiratory infections	15
Chronic bronchitis and bronchiectasis	2
Asthma	34

* Of 1000 consecutive patients with hiatal hernias, 264 had aspiration by history. Approximately one-half had respiratory symptoms that either were caused by or were aggravated by the aspiration.

or the response of the end organ did not exceed a critical level. Historically, we could not distinguish this group of patients from the 140 patients who developed symptoms. The distribution of symptoms in the latter group is outlined in Table 5.7: the majority developed cough or voice changes, but only a minority developed significant respiratory symptoms or disease.

Thirty-four of these 264 patients had asthma, but no clear relationship could be demonstrated between the development of asthma and the onset of aspiration symptoms. In most of these patients it was difficult to correlate the major asthmatic episodes with specific episodes of aspiration.

One hundred and twelve of these 264 patients with a history of aspiration were selected for operation because of their esophageal symptoms (Table 5.7). All have been followed up for periods varying from 1 to 4 years to determine the effects of surgical correction on the aspiration. The 89 patients with cough and voice change only were markedly improved. Patients with repetitive acute respiratory infections also improved, but they may develop additional respiratory symptoms in the future. The two patients with bronchiectasis were markedly improved, but a much larger group must be studied before any prediction can be made concerning the effects of surgical correction on bronchiectasis related to aspiration.

In patients in whom the development of respiratory symptoms can be clearly related to aspiration, surgical correction appears to give excellent results. Although these patients were selected for operation because of the poor response to standard conservative management of a hiatal hernia, a factor in selection in the future may be the presence of associated significant aspiration. Furthermore, the patient often regards this symptom as a serious threat, and in a significant number the associated lung disease is progressive unless the source of contamination is identified and removed.

Case 6. For 6 years, Mr. M., age 61 had had a persistent nonproductive cough. This cough, which occurred spontaneously or when he was speaking, was a great trial to him because as chairman of a company he had to conduct many meetings. When he consulted me, the cough was sufficiently severe that it interfered with his work and frequently he had to excuse himself and leave meetings because of it.

Treatment with steroids for several years had produced some initial improvement, but his cough remained a major problem. In the year preceding he had lost consciousness on several occasions during spells of coughing. During a review of his history, he reported occasional mild indigestion and described clearly night aspiration once or twice per week. He also had pharyngoesophageal dysphagia accompanied by episodes of coughing and choking 4 to 5 times per week. These symptoms of aspiration resolved completely following surgical correction of his hiatal hernia. He still has occasional mild episodes of coughing, but these no longer interfere with his work. This man's pharyngoesophageal dysphagia—the main cause of his symptoms—was obscured by the severity of the cough, but was readily identified on careful history taking.

The response of the asthmatics to hiatal hernia repair was disappointing. Each patient was selected for surgery because of reflux

symptoms and not in an effort to correct their asthma. Of the 28 operated upon symptoms of asthma did not improve in 11. Nine were slightly improved, 4 moderately improved and 4 markedly improved.

Case 7. Mrs. H., age 32, had a 9 months' history of recurrent bronchitis and episodes of bronchospasm. During the same period she had developed epigastric and retrosternal burning discomfort. She gave a clear history of night aspiration, and associated the episodes of aspiration with attacks of bronchospasm and with her respiratory infection. Pulmonary function tests showed a mild obstructive ventilatory defect.

Following hiatal hernia repair the symptoms of indigestion and aspiration have completely disappeared and she has no residual respiratory symptoms. The tests of pulmonary function have returned to normal. This is the only patient in the series of asthma patients who had total resolution of symptoms.

Case 8. Mrs. D., age 62, has had asthma for 2 years. Over the preceding 6 years she had developed "indigestion" and was able to give a clear history of reflux and aspiration. There was no demonstrable association between the episodic aspiration and her asthmatic attacks. A hiatal hernia was repaired because of the severity of her indigestion, and these symptoms have been effectively relieved. Her asthma and tests of pulmonary function were not affected by the hernial repair.

Only one patient has had return of pulmonary function to normal and 8 have had a slight improvement in function.

With increasing experience I am led to the conclusion that the majority of patients with asthma and aspiration do not show significant improvement in lung function following surgery. Many of these patients feel symptomatically improved. Part of this confusion is the difficulty in separating the chest tightness felt with bronchospasm from the tightness felt with reflux. Dyspnea is a common symptom in reflux and can occur completely unassociated with asthma symptoms. In the occasional patient where reflux is triggered by exertion, this becomes a very restricting symptom. In the asthmatic this heartburn-induced dyspnea, if present, will be relieved and may result in an apparent symptomatic improvement in their asthma.

Alternate explanations of the symptomatic improvement are possible, including bronchospasm triggered by vagal reflexes from the esophagus (68).

There is no doubt that the aspiration problem is most marked in children, and adolescent pulmonary disease is frequently described in the literature. This may be related in young children to their horizontal posture and may in part be related to the inability to obtain a clear history with resultant delays in diagnosis (69–73).

Aspiration is frequent in patients with gastroesophageal reflux. In our study of 1000 refluxing patients (67), 264 (27 per cent) had aspiration and, of these, roughly one-half developed respiratory symptoms. Approximately one-half of those developing respiratory symptoms developed significant and progressive lung damage which, if ignored, would go on to serious parenchymal injury. Unless these symptoms are carefully sought out and their cause recognized, they respond poorly to the standard management, that is, intermittent antibiotic therapy for the associated respiratory infections. The physician who deals with gastroesophageal reflux as a primary disease confronts this symptom directly; however, if he is dealing primarily with intermittent respiratory infection, neither he nor the patient may recognize the association between the respiratory complaints and the gastrointestinal symptoms.

Type II Hiatal Hernia

The symptoms in Type II (paraesophageal) hernia are usually much different from those described for Type I (7, 8). Reflux is unusual and the symptoms are related to distention of the intrathoracic gastric pouch. Distention produces left chest pain, often referred to the back, neck and arms. The distention is intermittent and often related to eating. Occasionally partial or total obstruction may develop at the diaphragmatic level and the patient then becomes acutely ill with symptoms of pain and dyspnea.

These hernias are frequently complicated by food stasis and mucosal ulceration; hence, hemorrhage and even perforation may follow. When the lumen is obstructed the hernia may strangulate and the necrotic stomach then perforates into the thoracic cavity (74, 75).

Type III Hiatal Hernia

In the Type III hiatal hernia, the patient's symptoms are usually those of the Type I hernia. This is a sliding hernia, but here the fundus of the stomach has rolled up into the chest together with the gastroesophageal junction.

The patient's history is of the greatest importance in the evaluation of esophageal disease because it usually permits a specific diagnosis. Even when the diagnosis cannot be made with certainty, the history provides the best guide to future investigation.

The symptoms outlined in this chapter vary greatly in intensity from patient to patient, and many of them, such as dysphagia, may be a minor component in the patient's history. Nevertheless, it is essential to recognize that this symptom complex is associated with esophageal dysfunction because such recognition leads directly to appropriate investigation and in time allows for decisive therapeutic intervention.

Having reviewed each symptom which commonly accompanies reflux, it is worth finally looking at how frequently each symptom becomes the presenting complaint. In 359 patients reviewed heartburn was the dominant symptom in 85.6 per cent, cricophayngeal dysphagia in 5 per cent, gastroesophageal dysphagia in 8 per cent, nausea in 0.8 per cent and aspiration with reflux in 0.3 per cent.

Heartburn is by far the most common primary complaint; however, although it may be typical, it is not as specific as recognizable reflux to the throat or dysphagia. Both reflux and dysphagia were present in 70.2 per cent, reflux alone in 14.5 per cent, dysphagia alone in 9.5 per cent, and neither of these symptoms in 5.8 per cent. By history alone, considering both recognizable reflux to the throat and dysphagia as specific esophageal symptoms, a diagnosis of esophageal disease could be made in 94.2 per cent of patients.

References

1. Botha, G. S. M.: *The Gastroesophageal Junction.* J & A Churchill Ltd., London, 1962.
2. Quincke, H.: Esophageal ulcers from digestive juices (Ulcus oesophagi ex digestione). Dtsch. Arch. Klin. Med., *24:* 72, 1879.

3. Tileston, W.: Peptic ulcer of the oesophagus. Am. J. Med. Sci., *132:* 240, 1906.
4. Hamperl, H.: Peptic esophagitis (Peptische ösophagitis). Verk. Dtsch. Ges. Pathol., *27:* 208, 1934.
5. Postlethwait, R. W.: *Surgery of the Esophagus.* Appleton-Century-Crofts. New York, 1979.
6. Harrington, S. W.: Esophageal hiatal diaphragmatic hernia. Surg. Gynecol. Obstet., *100:* 277, 1955.
7. Skinner, D. B., and Belsey, R. H. R.: Surgical management of esophageal reflux and hiatus hernia; long term results with 1,030 patients. J. Thorac. Cardiovasc. Surg., *53:* 33, 1967.
8. Hill, L. D., and Tobias, J. A.: Paraesophageal hernia. Arch. Surg. *96:* 735, 1968.
9. Ozdemir, I. A., Burke, W. A., and Ikins, P. M.: Paraesophageal hernia; a life-threatening disease. Ann. Thorac. Surg., *16:* 547, 1973.
10. Urschel, H. C., Jr., and Paulson, D. L.: Gastroesophageal reflux and hiatal hernia; complications and therapy. J. Thorac. Cardiovasc. Surg., *53:* 21, 1967.
11. Skinner, D. B.: Symptomatic esophageal reflux. Am. J. Dig. Dis., *11:* 771, 1966.
12. Field, P., and Stalker, K. J.: Incompetence of the cardiac sphincter without radiologic demonstration of hiatus hernia. Can. J. Surg., *11:* 412, 1968.
13. Hiebert, C. A., and Belsey, R.: Incompetency of the gastric cardia without radiologic evidence of a hiatal hernia. J. Thorac. Cardiovasc. Surg., *42:* 352, 1961.
14. Cohen, S., and Harris, L. D.: Does hiatus hernia affect competence of the gastroesophageal sphincter? N. Engl. J. Med., *284:* 1053, 1971.
15. Steiner, G. M.: Gastro-oesophageal reflux, hiatus hernia and the radiologist, with special reference to children. Br. J. Radiol., *39:* 135, 1977.
16. Brick, I. B., and Amory, H. I.: Incidence of hiatus hernia in patients without symptoms. Arch. Surg., *60:* 1045, 1950.
17. Wolf, B. S., Brahms, S. A., and Khilnani, M. T.: The incidence of hiatal hernia in routine barium meal examination. Mt. Sinai J. Med (NY) *26:* 598, 1959.
18. Atkinson, M.: The oesophagus and indigestion. Practitioner, *198:* 359, 1967.
19. Kramer, P.: The significance of dysphagia in diagnosis of esophageal disease. Med. Times, *97*(8): 148, 1969.
20. Davis, M. V.: Evolving concepts regarding hiatal hernia and gastroesophageal reflux. Ann. Thorac. Surg., *7:* 120, 1969.
21. Chernow, B., and Castell, D. O.: Diet and heartburn. J.A.M.A., *241:* 2307, 1979.
22. Palmer, E. D.: Serious heart disease simulated by hiatus hernia. U.S. Armed Forces Med. J., *8:* 477, 1957.
23. Bourne, G.: Cardiac pain from esophageal lesions. Lancet, *1:* 892, 1956.
24. Roberts, R., Henderson, R. D., and Wigle, E. D.: Esophageal disease as a cause of severe retrosternal chest pain. Chest, *67:* 523, 1975.
25. Master, A. M., Dack, S., Stone, J., and Grishman, A.: Differential diagnosis of hiatus hernia and coronary artery disease. Arch. Surg., *58:* 428, 1949.
26. Henderson, R. D., Wigle, E. D., Sample, K., and Marryatt, G.: Atypical chest pain of cardiac and esophageal origin. Chest, *73:* 24, 1978.
27. Mays, E. E., Dubois, J. J., and Hamilton, G. B.: Pulmonary fibrosis associated with tracheobronchial aspiration; a study of the frequency of hiatal hernia and gastroesophageal reflux in interstitial pulmonary fibrosis of obscure etiology. Chest, *69:* 512, 1976.
28. Brand, D. L., Martin, D., and Pope, C. E.: Esophageal manometrics in patients with angina-like chest pain. Am. J. Dig. Dis., *22:* 300, 1977.
29. Svensson, O., Stenport, G., Tibbling, L., and Wranne, B.: Oesophageal function and coronary angiogram in patients with disabling chest pain. Acta Med. Scand., *204:* 173, 1978.
30. Areskog, M., Tibbling, L., and Wranne, B.: Oesophageal dysfunction in non-infarction coronary care unit patients. Acta Med. Scand., *205:* 279, 1979.
31. Souadjian, J. V., and Cain, J. C.: Intractable hiccup; etiologic factors in 220 cases. Postgrad. Med., *43*(2): 72, 1968.
32. Salem, M. R., Baraka, A., Rottenborg, C. C., and Holaday, A.: Treatment of hiccups by pharyngeal stimulation in anaesthetized and conscious subjects. J.A.M.A., *202:* 126, 1967.
33. Bailey, H.: Persistent hiccup. Practitioner, *150:* 173, 1943.
34. Aylwin, J. A.: Physiological basis of reflux oesophagitis in sliding hiatal diaphragmatic hernia. Thorax, *8:* 38, 1953.
35. Henderson, R. D.: Gastroesophageal reflux following gastric operation. Ann. Thorac. Surg., *26:* 563, 1978.
36. Clerf, L. H., Shallow, T. A., Putney, F. J., and Fry, K. E.: Esophageal hiatal hernia. J.A.M.A., *143:* 169, 1950.
37. Grimes, O. F., and Stephens, H. B.: The surgical treatment of esophageal hiatus hernia. Am. J. Surg., *94:* 194, 1957.
38. Windsor, C. W. O., and Collis, J. L.: Anaemia and hiatus hernia; experience in 450 patients. Thorax, *22:* 73, 1967.
39. Mangla, J. C., Schenk, E. A., Desbaillets, L., Guarasci, G., Kubasik, N. P., and Turner, M. D.: Pepsin secretion, pepsinogen and gastrin in "Barrett's esophagus." Clinical and morphological characteristics. Gastroenterology, *70:* 669, 1976.
40. Safaie-Shirazi, S., and Hardy, B. M.: Treatment of reflux esophagitis resulting in massive esophageal bleeding. Arch. Surg., *111:* 365, 1976.
41. Engels, E., and Reismann, B.: Bleeding from hiatal hernia. Zentralbl. Chir., *101:* 1044, 1976.
42. Raptis, S., and Milne, D. M.: A review of the management of 100 cases of benign stricture of the esophagus. Thorax, *27:* 599, 1972.
43. Palmer, E. D.: The hiatus hernia-esophagitis-esophageal stricture complex. Am. J. Med., *44:* 566, 1968.
44. Allison, P. R., and Johnstone, A. S.: The oesophagus lined with gastric mucous membrane. Thorax, *8:* 87, 1953.
45. Ramirez, J., Guarner, V., and Pazimo, F.: Alterations in motility of the esophagus in peptic esophagitis. Am. J. Proctol., *19:* 67, 1968.
46. Polland, W. S., and Bloomfield, A. L.: Experimental referred pain from gastro-intestinal tract; esophagus. J. Clin. Invest., *10:* 435, 1931.
47. Henderson, R. D., Woolf, C., and Marryatt, G.: Pharyngoesophageal dysphagia and gastroesophageal reflux. Laryngoscope, *86:* 1531, 1976.

48. Henderson, R. D., and Marryatt, G.: Cricopharyngeal myotomy as a method of treating cricopharyngeal dysphagia secondary to gastroesophageal reflux. J. Thorac. Cardiovasc. Surg., *74:* 721, 1977.

49. Cherry, J., Siegel, C. I., Margulies, S. I., and Donner, M.: Pharyngeal localization of symptoms of gastroesophageal reflux. Ann. Otol. Rhinol. Laryngol., *79:* 912, 1970.

50. Davis, M. V., and Fiuzat, J.: Application of the Belsey hiatal hernia repair to infants and children with recurrent bronchitis, bronchiolitis and pneumonitis due to regurgitation and aspiration. Ann. Thorac. Surg., *3:* 99, 1967.

51. Chodosh, P. L.: Gastro-esophago-pharyngeal reflux. Laryngoscope, *87:* 1418, 1977.

52. Rachelefsky, G., Bryne, W., Strobel, C., et al.: Gastroesophageal reflux and recurrent pulmonary disease in children, abstracted. J. Allergy Clin. Immunol., *61:* 138, 1978.

53. Krantman, H. J., Rachelefsky, G. S., Lipson, M., and Fonkalsrud, E. W.: Recurrent pulmonary infiltrates, digital clubbing and failure to thrive in a 4-year-old boy. J. Allergy Clin. Immunol., *61:* 403, 1978.

54. Christie, D. L., O'Grady, L. R., and Mack, D. V.: Incompetent lower esophageal sphincter and gastroesophageal reflux in recurrent and acute pulmonary disease of infancy and childhood. J. Paediatr., *93:* 23, 1978.

55. Shermeta, D. W., Whitington, P. F., Seto, D. S., and Haller, J. A.: Lower esophageal sphincter dysfunction in esophageal atresia; nocturnal regurgitation and aspiration pneumonia. J. Pediatr. Surg., *12:* 871, 1977.

56. Dines, D. E., Baker, W. G., and Scantland, W. A.: Aspiration pneumonitis—Mendelson's syndrome. J.A.M.A., *176:* 229, 1961.

57. Marshall, B. M., and Gordon, R. A.: Vomiting, regurgitation and aspiration in anaesthesia; I. Can. Anaesth. Soc. J., *5:* 274, 1958.

58. Overholt, R. H., and Voorhees, R. J.: Esophageal reflux as a trigger in asthma. Dis. Chest, *49:* 464, 1966.

59. Reich, S. B., Earley, W. C., Ravin, T. H., et al.: Evaluation of gastropulmonary aspiration by a radioactive technique (Concise communication). J. Nucl. Med., *18:* 1079, 1977.

60. Cameron, J. L., Anderson, R. P., and Zuidema, G. D.: Aspiration pneumonia; a clinical and experimental review. J. Surg. Res., *7:* 44, 1967.

61. Greenfield, L. J., Singleton, R. P., McCaffree, D. R., and Coalson, J. J.: Pulmonary effects of experimental graded aspiration of hydrochloric acid. Ann. Surg., *170:* 74, 1969.

62. Cameron, J. L., Mitchell, W. H., and Zuidema, G. D.: Aspiration pneumonia; clinical outcome following documented aspiration. Arch. Surg., *106:* 49, 1973.

63. Henderson, R. D., Fung, K., Cullen, J. B., Milne, E. N., and Marryatt, G.: Bile aspiration; an experimental study in rabbits. Can. J. Surg., *18:* 64, 1975.

64. Gardner, A. M.: Aspiration of food and vomit. Q. J. Med., *27:* 227, 1958.

65. Ambiavagar, M., Chan, O. L., Pais, F. W., and D'Basm, B. E. G.: The acid aspiration syndrome. Singapore Med. J., *8:* 35, 1967.

66. Klotz, S. D., and Moeller, R. K.: Hiatal hernia and intractable bronchial asthma. Ann. Allergy, *29:* 325, 1971.

67. Henderson, R. D., and Woolfe, C. R.: Aspiration and gastroesophageal reflux. Can. J. Surg., *21:* 352, 1978.

68. Mansfield, L. E., and Stein, M. R.: Gastroesophageal reflux and asthma; a possible reflux mechanism. Ann. Allergy, *41:* 224, 1978.

69. Ashcraft, K. W., Goodwin, C., Amoury, R. A., and Holder, T. M.: Early recognition and aggressive treatment of gastroesophageal reflux following repair of esophageal atresia. J. Pediatr. Surg., *12:* 317, 1977.

70. Johnson, D. G., Herbst, J. J., Oliveros, M. A., and Stewart, D. R.: Evaluation of gastroesophageal reflux surgery in children. Pediatrics, *59:* 62, 1977.

71. Shapiro, G. G., and Christie, D. L.: Gastroesophageal reflux in steroid-dependent asthmatic youths. Pediatrics, *63:* 207, 1978.

72. Fonkalsrud, E. W., Ament, M. E., Byrne, W. J., and Rachelefsky, G. S.: Gastroesophageal fundoplication for the management of reflux in infants and children. J. Thorac. Cardiovasc. Surg., *76:* 655, 1978.

73. Leape, L. L., Holder, T. M., Franklin, J. D., Amoury, R. A., Ashcraft, R. A., and Ashcraft, K. W.: Respiratory arrest in infants secondary to gastroesophageal reflux. Pediatrics, *60:* 924, 1977.

74. Beardsley, J. M., and Thompson, W. R.: Acutely obstructed hiatal hernia. Ann. Surg., *159:* 49, 1964.

75. Bosher, L. H., Fishman, L., Webb, W. R., and Old, L.: Strangulated diaphragmatic hernia with gangrene and perforation of the stomach. Dis. Chest, *37:* 504, 1960.

CHAPTER 6

Hiatal Hernia and Gastroesophageal Reflux: Investigative Procedures and Assessment

Gastroesophageal reflux and the secondary effects of reflux account for most of the symptoms associated with a hiatal hernia. Usually patients with a hernia but without demonstrable reflux are either asymptomatic or have symptoms of minor severity. Conversely, reflux can exist and produce severe symptoms in a significant number of patients who do not have a radiologically demonstrable hernia.

The true incidence of reflux and the hiatal hernia complex has not been established, chiefly because the procedures used to make these diagnoses are themselves imprecise. In the past, radiology has been considered the most accurate of these investigations, and the reported incidence of hernia based on this procedure has varied from 1.3 to 45 per cent of the population (1). The extent of the problem is confused still further by studies which show severe reflux in the absence of a radiologically demonstrable hernia (2).

In clinical practice the purpose of investigation is to establish the source of symptoms and assess their severity and the effects of reflux on the esophagus. An accurate diagnosis and reliable assessment can be made in the majority of patients from a painstaking history and careful radiologic studies. More sophisticated evaluations by manometry, acid perfusion or endoscopy are reserved for patients with atypical symptoms and for those in whom severe symptoms call for intensive medical or surgical management.

The approach outlined in this chapter is the one I use at Women's College Hospital in the assessment of patients with a hiatal hernia or gastroesophageal reflux, and was developed over a number of years (3). The rationale of this approach can be illustrated in 124 patients who were fully investigated and found to require surgical correction of gastroesophageal reflux. Patients requiring surgery are used in this study because it is only in this group, with the addition of intraoperative examination, that esophageal wall changes from reflux and panmural esophagitis can be assessed. A complete history was obtained in each patient and, in addition, each had radiologic, manometric and endoscopic studies before undergoing a transthoracic hiatal hernia repair. At operation the esophageal wall was examined by palpation and a random muscle biopsy was taken to determine the presence of panmural esophagitis. Significant wall changes were considered to be present when the wall was clearly thickened and of a woody consistency. This change is easily recognized in advanced panmural esophagitis with stricture formation, but the surgeon must apply care and experience if this is to be recognized when less well developed. However, once they are recognized these changes are significant and highly specific.

History

The history which may be obtained in a patient with gastroesophageal reflux is outlined in Chapter 5. It is only necessary now to emphasize certain diagnostic features and demonstrate their value in assessing the severity of the pathologic changes associated with this defect. Certain symptoms are clearly esophageal and as such have considerable diagnostic value. Typical esophageal pain, like heartburn, cannot be considered pathognomonic because it is mimicked by disorders in related organs, but the patient's clear description of reflux and of the taste of gastric content in the pharynx and mouth is often specific enough to make the diagnosis of gastroesophageal reflux. Dysphagia, described at the pharyngoesophageal or gastroesophageal junctional level, clearly relates the complaint to the esophagus and, because of its frequency in gastroesophageal reflux, suggests this disorder. Minor symptoms including hiccoughs, burping, waterbrash, nausea and vomiting all strongly suggest esophageal disease, but can be simulated by other disorders.

Of these 124 patients, 94 (75.8 per cent) had dysphagia; 102 (82.2 per cent) clearly described reflux to the throat and 113 (91.1 per cent) had one or other of these cardinal symptoms. Although other esophageal disorders must still be excluded, these symptoms, if properly interpreted, locate the disorder in the esophagus, and raise a strong suspicion that the symptoms are related to gastroesophageal reflux.

The severity and chronicity of the patient's symptoms provide no guide to the assessment of structural changes in the esophagus. The symptoms of the 124 patients, described above, were assessed in terms of chronicity and frequency, and points were assigned to a maximum of 14 in any one patient (Table 6.1). Following complete investigation and during surgical correction, the degree of organic change was determined at operation by inspection and palpation of the esophageal wall for thickening, scar formation and shortening. This comparison showed no correlation between the severity of symptoms and the underlying structural changes (Fig. 6.1). Symptom severity was also compared with the presence of esophageal ulceration, and again the symptom severity did not accurately correlate with these advanced esophageal changes. Thus, it appears that symptoms are of great value in differential diagnosis but are of no value in assessing esophageal damage.

Radiographic Investigation of Hiatal Hernia and Gastroesophageal Reflux

In most patients radiography is the most common investigation and is often the only procedure needed. If the examination is done carefully using liquids and barium paste and adding a barium-soaked food bolus, an anatomic hiatal hernia or frank gastroesophageal reflux can be demonstrated in most patients (4–7). The esophagus is studied with the patient in both the horizontal and vertical po-

Table 6.1
Points System to Record Severity of Symptoms (Maximum 14)*

Heartburn	Mild 1; severe 2
Duration of symptoms	Less than 3 yr 1; more than 3 yr 2
Reflux to throat	1
Aspiration	1
Nausea and vomiting	Mild 1; severe 2
Hiccoughs; burping; waterbrash	1
Pharyngoesophageal dysphagia	Mild 1; severe 2
Gastroesophageal dysphagia	Mild 1; moderate 2; severe 3

* The points system was used to assess symptoms in 124 patients with esophageal disease. The severity of heartburn, nausea, vomiting and dysphagia was based on its frequency and duration. Reflux, aspiration, hiccoughing, burping and waterbrash were assigned 1 point if the patient reported them and no points if he did not. Nausea, vomiting, pharyngoesophageal and gastroesophageal dysphagia were given 1 point if mild and 2 points if the symptom was severe. The maximum in any patient was 14; the minimum was 1.

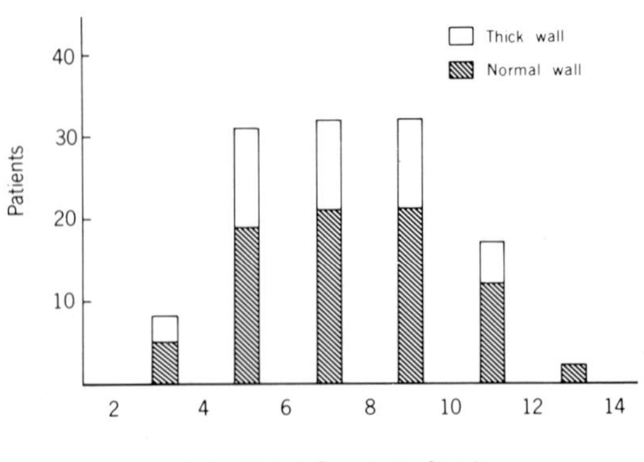

Figure 6.1. Clinical Symptoms vs. Esophageal Wall Thickness (124 Patients)
Severity of symptoms was compared with the presence or absence of esophageal wall thickening and shortening using a points system—minimum 1, maximum 14. There was no obvious correlation.

sition. The sphincter should be tested for reflux, both spontaneously and with the water siphon test (see below). It should be stressed that the "hernia" demonstrated on the radiograph is not necessarily the cause of the patient's symptoms; furthermore, this examination does not exclude gastroesophageal reflux as the cause of symptoms merely because it has not demonstrated a hernia.

Most barium examinations are recorded using "spot films" of highlights seen during the investigation. Some patients also require cineradiography to assess the pharyngoesophageal junction and esophageal motor function. During the study, spontaneous reflux may be recognized in the upright position but, at some stage in the investigation, the patient should be placed in a prone position with a sandbag beneath the upper abdomen and his head tilted downward. Reflux is easier to demonstrate in this position and, if necessary, water swallowed rapidly will produce relaxation in the gastoesophageal junction and reflux. This "water siphon" technique is a sensitive test and may induce reflux even in the normal subject; however, in patients with a symptomatic hiatal hernia, the reflux is more marked.

The principal radiologic diagnostic criterion for hiatal hernia is the demonstration of a gastric pouch above the level of the diaphragm. The pouch is recognized by its characteristic shape, its lack of motor function and the presence, within it, of recognizable mucosal folds (8, 9). Some patients with a hiatal hernia show a narrow fibrous band—Schatzki's ring—which delineates the squamocolumnar junction (Fig. 6.2) (10, 11). This ring of dense submucosal fibrous tissue lies at a variable position in close relationship to the gastroesophageal junction. Combined radiologic and manometric studies show that this ring may lie at the upper margin of the gastroesophageal junction (11) and may be demonstrated when the gastroesophageal junction is still maintained below the diaphragm (12). In short, the patient can have a Schatzki's ring without having a hiatal hernia; however, most patients who have such a ring have a hiatal hernia that can be clearly demonstrated.

When the lower esophagus is lined with gastric mucosa the squamocolumnar junction may lie at a much higher level. In this condition—the Barrett's esophagus—the squam-

ocolumnar junction lies immediately below the tracheal carina and a narrow stricture may be noted at this level (13, 14). This type of esophagus is almost invariably associated with a hiatal hernia, and its presence usually indicates long-standing esophageal disease. A radiologically thickened esophageal wall is also evidence of long-standing disease, but has to be differentiated from other causes of wall thickening, such as the muscular hypertrophy associated with diffuse esophageal spasm (DES) (15).

Criteria for the diagnosis of hiatal hernias are not absolute, and various radiologists accept different criteria. Hence, as noted earlier, the reported incidence of hiatal hernias in the asymptomatic population varies between 1.3 (16) and 45 per cent (1). This varied incidence reflects both changes in diagnostic criteria and differences in the care with which an anatomic hernia is sought. In addition to establishing an anatomic diagnosis, radiologic investigation may perform other important services; e.g., after a hernia is demonstrated, its size should be estimated and it should be classified as Type I, Type II or Type III. The radiologist should then search for strictures using a solid barium capsule or barium soaked food, which demonstrates mechanical obstruction. He should assess the reducibility of the hernia below the diaphragm by studying the subject in the vertical position. In addition, evaluation of esophageal motor function is of considerable importance in the differential diagnosis of disorders such as achalasia, primary disordered motor activity and scleroderma. At all times the radiologist must search carefully for malignancy and must view with particular suspicion any peptic stricture. Radiologic studies cannot exclude malignancy, and indeed can miss early malignancy (Fig. 6.3), but, in most instances, radiology will show changes that indicate the need for endoscopy and biopsy.

If the first examination has not demonstrated a hernia, a second radiologic study may show its presence. Finally, it should be remembered that in some patients the symptoms may be due to reflux occurring in the absence of a demonstrable hiatal hernia (17, 18).

Esophageal Scintigraphy

Technetium (^{99m}TC, DPTA) has recently been introduced as a method of studying

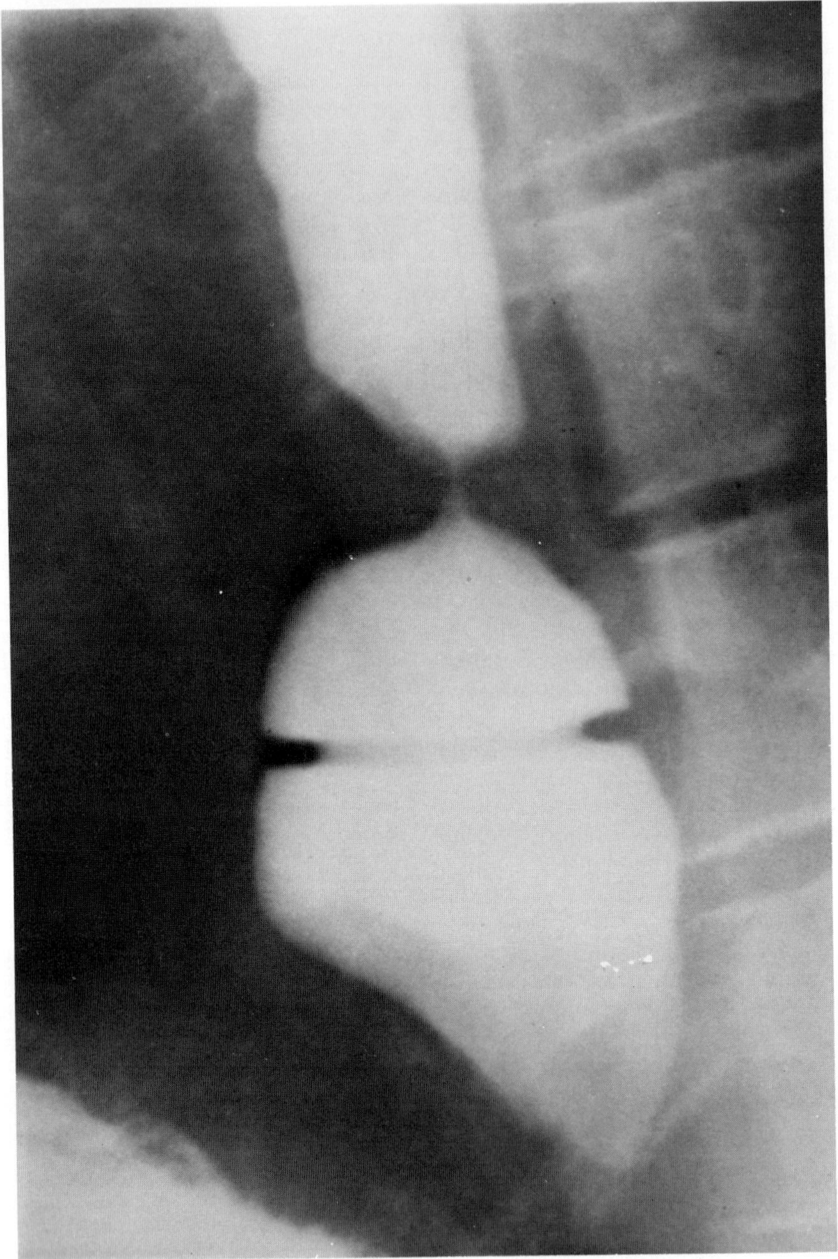

Figure 6.2.   Radiologic Hiatal Hernia and Schatzki's Ring
The radiologic study shows a small hiatal hernia. At the squamocolumnar junction there is a narrow bandlike stricture. Endoscopy confirmed that this stricture lay at the junction between the gastric mucosa distally and the esophageal mucosa proximally.

gastroesophageal reflux. The radioactive material is given as a swallowed bolus and can be detected by scanning techniques using a gamma camera. Reflux is demonstrated by the radioactivity in the refluxed bolus. Since the radiation level is measured it is possible to estimate the amount of swallowed material in the refluxed bolus and as such add a measure of quantitation to the study (19, 20). Although quantitation of reflux is desirable,

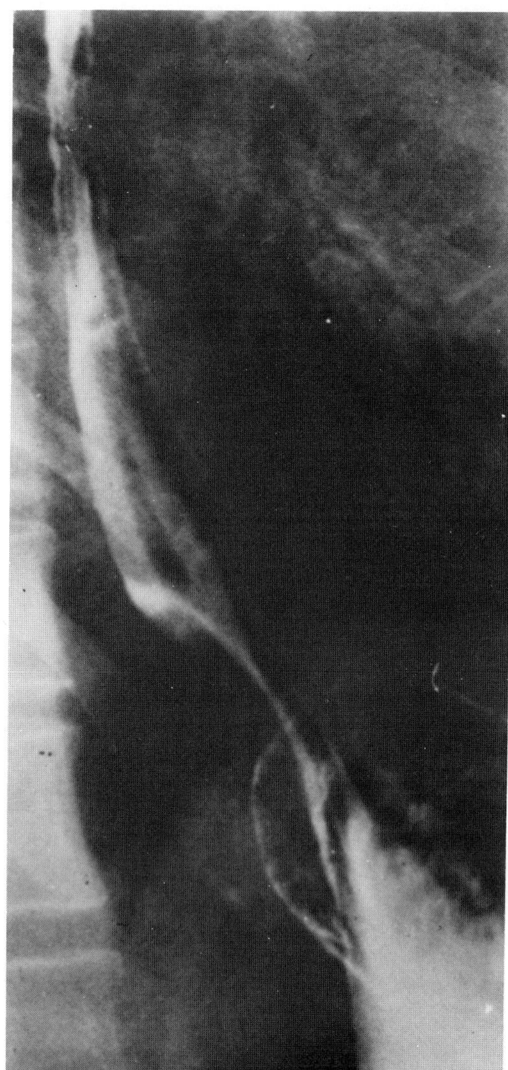

Figure 6.3. Barium Swallow—Hiatal Hernia and Carcinoma in Situ

Radiologic study of patient (Mrs. E.) shows the presence of a small hiatal hernia. The esophageal wall proximally was considered normal. On endoscopy the operator noted an area of surface irregularity 3 cm above the squamocolumnar junction; on biopsy and at subsequent resection this proved to be an in situ squamous carcinoma.

this method has not been studied enough to determine whether or not the findings are reproducible and if reproducible whether they can be used as a guide to patient care. Since the method does not delineate structure in as much detail as conventional radiography, it cannot be considered as a replacement for radiologic studies.

One adaptation of this technique is to study night aspiration. If the technetium is swallowed in the evening and the patient scanned the following day, the presence and amount of aspirated technetium can be detected by lung scan (21). Although this is a promising method of study, it is important to recognize that aspiration is an intermittent phenomenon and the absence of lung contamination does not exclude aspiration. Despite reports of documented aspiration using these methods, we have not been able to reproduce the findings in a limited number of patients studied.

Patient Study

Of the 124 patients with symptoms of esophageal disease mentioned earlier, 93 had radiologic studies that could be evaluated retrospectively. We evaluated them to determine whether they had a radiologic hiatal hernia and also whether there was any association between the radiologic findings and the presence of esophageal wall changes at the time of operation. All patients were studied by history, radiology, esophageal manometry and endoscopy, and at the time of operation we carefully examined and palpated the esophageal wall to determine whether the reflux had induced significant esophageal wall thickening from panmural esophagitis. Information obtained at operation was correlated with the radiologic findings assessed before surgery.

Sixteen (14 per cent) of the 93 patients we studied did not have a radiologically demonstrable hiatal hernia. Seven of the 16 had demonstrable reflux, and examination in the remainder was within normal limits. Of these 16 patients, 13 had a normal esophageal wall at operation and 3 had a thickened esophageal wall which indicated established panmural esophagitis. The thickening of the esophageal wall is secondary in inflammation and is often associated with shortening or with a peptic stricture from scar contracture.

We have also compared other radiologic features with the operative findings. In the group of 93 patients with hiatal hernia who had adequate radiologic studies, 58 were assessed as having a normal esophageal wall and at operation 35 had established panmural esophagitis (Table 6.2). Radiologic reducibility was determined before operation and

Table 6.2
Radiologic Findings vs. Wall Thickness (93 Patients)*

Hiatal Hernia	Normal Wall			Thick Wall		
	No.	Reducible	Reflux	No.	Reducible	Reflux
Not seen	13	13	6	3	3	1
Small	30	27	23	5	5	3
Medium	12	12	8	14	10	9
Large	3	3	2	13	1	7

* The radiologic features of the hiatal hernia were assessed by a radiologist. The radiologic appearance provided valuable assistance in predicting panmural esophagitis at operation only in those patients with a large and irreducible hiatal hernia.

compared to the operative findings. Of the 58 who had a normal esophageal wall, 55 had a radiologically reducible hiatal hernia. Of the 35 with panmural changes, only 19 had a radiologically reducible hernia. Thus, in this group at least, the incidence of panmural changes is clearly much higher in those patients with a radiologically irreducible hernia.

Hernia size and reducibility was also compared with panmural esophageal change. Sixteen of the 93 patients had hernias that extended higher than 20 cm above the diaphragm. Three of these had a normal wall at operation, and all three were radiologically reducible. Thirteen had panmural changes at operation, and 12 of these were irreducible. The finding of a large (greater than 20 cm) hernia and irreducibility gave a good indication of the presence of panmural esophagitis.

This study of 124 patients, although small, does show the value of radiology in both diagnosis and assessment. Eighty-six per cent of those studied had a radiologic hernia, and a further 7.5 per cent had demonstrable reflux. Reducibility and hernia size were also shown to be of some value in establishing the presence of panmural esophagitis before operation.

Endoscopy

Endoscopy allows the operator to visualize and stage the extent of mucosal damage from reflux. It should be emphasized that these changes are part of a dynamic process which can alter from one examination to the next. In addition to such staging, endoscopy and biopsy make it possible to exclude malignancy with a high degree of accuracy. Furthermore, the operator can extend the procedure, using flexible fiberoptic scopes, and evaluate the stomach and duodenum for inflammatory or malignant disease.

The pathologic changes in esophagitis have been studied extensively in both humans (22) and experimental animals (23, 24). The process begins in the mucosa and submucosa and spreads into the muscular layers to become a panmural esophagitis. Advanced esophageal change is accompanied by a diffuse inflammatory infiltrate, edema, fibrosis, increased vascularity and periesophagitis. As the fibrosis advances, the circumferential and longitudinal scars contract, producing circumferential strictures and shortening. These changes are confined chiefly to the lower esophagus and seldom progress above the level of the aortic arch.

Endoscopy visualizes the mucosal surface only and does not allow any assessment of deeper damage. However, it is possible to correlate mucosal changes with mural thickening and shortening, just as one can correlate mural changes and radiologic findings. For comparative purposes, esophagitis has been arranged in the following stages:

Normal
Stage I — chronic epithelial change or very mild inflammation
Stage II — acute inflammation of the esophageal mucosa without ulceration
Stage III(A) — ulceration in the lower 3 cm of esophagus
Stage III(B) — confluent ulceration of the esophagus extending above 3 cm
Stage IV — stricture formation.

Using this classification in the 124 patients studied before doing hiatal hernia repair, we compared the esophageal wall changes at operation with the changes seen at endoscopy. In Stages I, II and III(A) esophagitis, the mural changes were quite unpredictable. Twenty-eight of 106 patients with esophagitis categorized as Stages I to III(A) had thickening consistent with panmural esophagitis (Fig. 6.4). Eighteen patients with Stage III(B) or Stage IV esophagitis all had panmural changes. This study demonstrates the value of esophagoscopy in predicting wall thickness and shortening in patients with Stages III(B) and IV esophagitis. It also indicates clearly that the degree of structural change cannot be predicted from endoscopy alone because some patients with Stages I to III(A) had extensive panmural esophagitis.

Most endoscopic examinations are carried out using the fiberoptic flexible endoscopes. While these give excellent visualization they do not allow assessment of wall fixation, and the quality of biopsy may be inadequate. The rigid esophagoscope should be used in addition to the flexible endoscope when there is difficulty in evaluating a possible malignancy.

If dilatation is required, the rigid esophagoscope allows direct visualization and dilatation up to #26 Fr. Techniques of dilatation will be discussed in Chapter 7.

Endoscopy is essential if operation is being considered and indeed should be routine in such patients. This procedure permits some assessment of esophageal "pathology" and allows the operator to recognize a malignancy that may have been missed earlier.

In a more recent study of 359 consecutive preoperative endoscopies (25) 5 carcinomas were found, 2 not demonstrated radiologically. In addition, moderate gastritis was present in 16, duodenal ulcers in 14, gastric ulcers in 3, gastric polyps in 2, a gastric-lined esophagus in 4, ulcerative esophagitis in 36 and a peptic stricture in 26. In all, 106 patients had significant pathology (29.5 per cent).

This type of information is of critical importance, particularly when surgery is considered.

Esophageal Manometry

Manometric studies of the esophagus have considerable value in the diagnosis, differential diagnosis and assessment of esophageal disease (26, 27). The earliest of these methods used small balloons to detect pressure changes in the esophagus (28), but the pressure so detected was relative and not absolute. Open-ended catheters are now used to measure pressure and, with constant perfusion, these catheters record actual pressure (29). Alternately, miniature transducers incorporated in the esophageal manometric tubes also record actual pressure changes (30–33).

The manometric data reported in this text were obtained through PE 190 tubing with side holes and constant water infusion at 6.8 ml per tube per minute. Statham p23De strain gauges are used as sensing devices and the pressure changes are recorded on a Honeywell 1508 ultraviolet visicorder.

When a typical motor change is present, manometric study can be of considerable value in the detection of hiatal hernias. The following motor features are characteristic of this disorder.

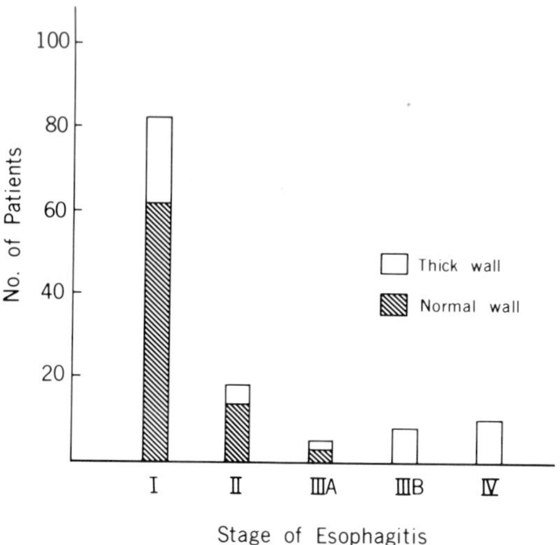

Figure 6.4. Endoscopic Staging and Wall Thickness
Esophagitis was staged at endoscopy. The presence of more than 3 cm of distal esophagitis (Stage III(B)) or a peptic stricture (Stage IV) correlated with the presence of a thick wall. Occasionally patients with Stage I to Stage III(A) esophagitis did have wall changes but these could not be predicted by endoscopy.

1. Double respiratory reversal (34, 35): These respiratory deflections, which change repeatedly from respiratory positive to negative, indicate vertical movement of the sphincter zone and variation in its ability to prevent reflux.

2. Apparent increases in the length of the gastroesophageal junction, shown manometrically, probably reflect elevations of gastric pressure in the hernia pouch, and this zone of gastric pressure may mimic the lower end of the gastroesophageal junction. A plateau of pressure and the appearance of two peaks of pressure also reflect an increase in intraluminal pressure at the diaphragm and an elevation of pressure in the short segment of stomach immediately below the sphincter (Fig. 6.5).

Actual movement of the hernia is manifested by pressure variability. The tone of the gastroesophageal junction is reduced in most patients with free reflux and with hernia (36, 37). Disordered motor activity in the body of the esophagus, an associated feature, varies in severity with the extent of esophageal damage from reflux.

Although manometry is of diagnostic value, the esophageal motor pattern may be normal or near normal in the presence of a hiatal hernia. Manometry is also valuable in differential diagnosis and in the assessment of the degree of esophageal wall injury from reflux.

Differential Diagnosis

Many esophageal motor disorders present with characteristic radiologic and endoscopic features; however, in achalasia, primary disordered motor activity, scleroderma and various abnormalities of the pharyngoesophageal junction, radiologic features may not provide a specific diagnosis. In these disorders manometry may settle the matter, and the chief decision in differential diagnosis is to distinguish these disorders from hiatal hernia. These patients commonly present with dysphagia and, in the absence of a typical radiologic pattern, manometry in conjunction with the history and radiologic features usually provides the specific diagnosis.

Case 1. The value of manometry is well illustrated by Mr. K., age 56. Twenty-five years before consultation he had developed severe dysphagia, and a diagnosis of achalasia was made from history and radiologic examination. He had a gastrostomy for feeding for a period of 6 months. Over the next 10 years his dysphagia continued and in 1960 and 1964 he had Heller myotomies.

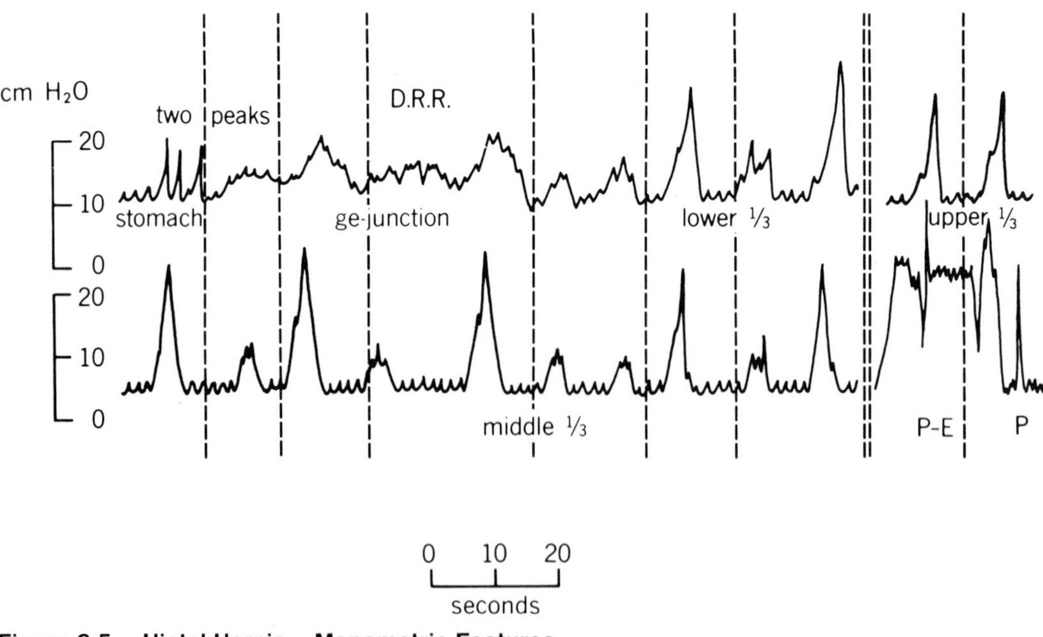

Figure 6.5.   Hiatal Hernia—Manometric Features
Manometric study in patient with a hiatal hernia. In the upper lead, gastroesophageal (ge) junction is 3 cm long and shows a pattern of two peaks of pressure, a reduced tone of 10 cm water, reduced deglutition response and double respiratory reversal (D.R.R.). The lower lead, which is 5 cm proximal in the body of the esophagus, shows considerable disordered motor activity of low amplitude, but with retained normal peristaltic motor waves. Each vertical line marks a 1-cm proximal move in the pressure tubes and the double vertical line indicates a major move to bring the pressure tubes into the proximal esophagus, cricopharyngeus (P-E) and pharynx (P). The pattern shown is typical of the hiatal hernia.

When first seen in 1970, he had severe dysphagia and symptomatic reflux. Radiology showed a narrowed gastroesophageal junction and endoscopy confirmed the presence of a stricture. At this stage the differential diagnosis was hiatal hernia with stricture, or achalasia with reflux and stricture following Heller myotomy. Manometric studies showed a low tone gastroesophageal junction secondary to myotomy. In the mid-body and upper esophagus, there were well-formed peristaltic motor waves which excluded the diagnosis of achalasia. Bouginage to #60 Fr returned his swallowing to normal. Two years later a hiatal hernia repair and gastroplasty were done because of continued reflux, and he has remained asymptomatic since that time.

In retrospect it seems self-evident that more complete evaluation at an earlier stage would have avoided this tragedy. When he was first seen, modern diagnostic tools were not available, but certainly the last few years of his distress were unnecessary. This patient exemplifies the need for careful evaluation of all esophageal patients before they are submitted to any type of operation.

Assessment of Esophageal Pathology

Assessment of esophageal wall changes is often crucial in the overall evaluation of the patient and his disorder. The two most characteristic features of hiatal hernia are the reduction in tone of the gastroesophageal junction and an increase in the degree of disordered motor activity in the lower half of the organ. The reduction in tone of the junction can be clearly correlated with the presence of reflux (38). Patients with reflux and established esophagitis also show an increase in the degree of disordered motor activity. In experimental animals these motor changes can be reproduced by perfusing the esophagus with mixtures of bile and decinormal hydrochloric acid. Under these circumstances the tone of the gastroesophageal junction falls and disordered motor activity increases to a degree which is proportional to the severity of the esophagitis so produced (39). When the irritating stimulus is removed and the esophagus allowed to recover, the motor changes also resolve. These changes are produced by esophagitis alone but, in the human, similar changes may be associated with hiatal hernia and gastroesophageal reflux.

Patient Study

All of the 124 patients with symptoms of esophageal disease mentioned earlier had manometric studies before operation. The tracings were analyzed with particular attention to the tone of the gastroesophageal junction and the percentage of disordered motor waves in the distal and the proximal half of the esophagus. Later, we compared the manometric data to the tissue changes seen at endoscopy and found at operation by direct inspection and palpation of the esophageal wall. No correlation was noted between the tone of the gastroesophageal junction and the presence or absence of esophageal wall thickening and shortening at operation. All of the patients in the study had clinical reflux, and in many the tone of the gastroesophageal junction was low.

The presence of disordered motor activity in the proximal half of the esophagus did not reflect esophageal pathology. This finding is not surprising because the endoscopic changes of esophagitis almost invariably are limited to the lower half of the organ. Low amplitude disordered motor activity in the distal half was closely related to esophageal pathology at operation as assessed by direct inspection and palpation. Of those patients with a normal esophageal wall, 90.6 per cent had less than 60 per cent disordered motor activity, and 77.6 per cent had less than 40 per cent disordered motor activity. Of patients with a thick esophageal wall, 94.6 per cent had more than 40 per cent disordered motor activity and 75.7 per cent had more than 60 per cent disordered motor activity (Fig. 6.6). In those patients with between 40 and 60 per cent disordered motor activity, preoperative predictions of wall thickness were inaccurate.

These predictions were accurate in 104 of the 124 patients who had not had previous hernia surgery. In the 20 patients with a recurrent hernia, assessment of wall thickness based on manometry was inaccurate.

Summary: Wall Changes and Investigative Findings

In the investigations described to the present, history, radiology, endoscopy and manometric evaluation have been used both for diagnosis and also to predict esophageal wall damage. History is critical in evaluating the severity of the patient's symptoms and the response of these symptoms to conservative management. The prime indication for surgical correction of gastroesophageal reflux is

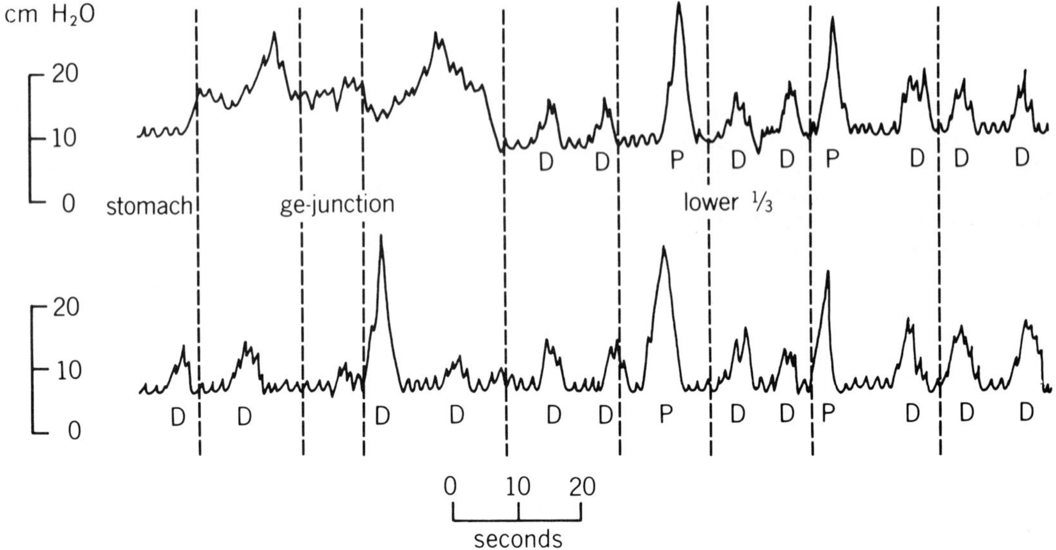

Figure 6.6.   Hiatal Hernia, DMA and Wall Thickness
Disordered motor activity (DMA) in the distal half of the esophagus allowed good prediction of esophageal wall thickening and shortening. Most of the patients with a thick wall had more than 60 per cent DMA and most with a normal wall had less than 40 per cent DMA. This patient had a hiatal hernia, 77 per cent DMA and a thick wall, D, disordered motor waves; P, peristalsis; ge, gastroesophageal.

pain and/or other symptoms which prove intractable after an adequate trial of conservative management. Radiology, manometry and endoscopy supply supplementary information, document esophageal changes and exclude other disorders. If the patient's symptoms remain severe despite conservative management, and operation is being considered, it becomes essential to be able to predict esophageal damage accurately. Radiologically a large hiatal hernia that is irreducible is almost always associated with secondary esophageal wall changes of thickening and shortening. By endoscopy, Stage III(B) ulcerative esophagitis or Stage IV esophagitis with stricture is also associated with wall thickening and shortening. Many patients with Stage I, II or III(A) esophagitis may have esophageal wall damage, but these changes are unpredictable. In such situations, supplementary manometric studies add an important dimension to the assessment of esophageal pathology. In any event, the combination of radiology, endoscopy and manometry allows the surgeon to predict accurately the changes in the esophagus and to select the most appropriate approach to surgical correction and the most appropriate method for repair of the hiatal hernia.

Acid Perfusion Studies

The patient with gastroesophageal reflux commonly presents with pain, and such pain may be difficult to distinguish from that which arises in related organs. Here perfusion of the esophagus with decinormal hydrochloric acid is valuable, because it reproduces esophageal pain (40) and localizes it to the esophagus. This test was devised to demonstrate the presence of esophagitis; however, experience has shown that perfusion will produce esophageal pain in the absence of endoscopic esophagitis and occasionally it will not produce pain when esophagitis is present. Pain reproduction during an acid "drip" is a valuable adjunct to diagnosis because it reproduces the cardinal symptom and localizes it to the esophagus. To carry out the test, the physician inserts a duodenal tube and positions it radiologically, or else conducts the test in conjunction with manometric studies. This latter approach allows him to correlate pain production with esophageal motor changes (41, 42) and hence strengthens the diagnosis. The addition of pH electrodes to the tube allows correlation of esophageal pH with the onset and relief of pain, and with esophageal motor changes.

My usual practice is to combine manometric and pH studies with acid perfusion of the esophagus (43). A standard manometric study is carried out before perfusion begins, then 200 ml of air in a bolus is injected into the stomach. In some patients the air bolus will produce typical pain, and in a few this can be correlated radiologically with distention of an esophageal hernia pouch. Perfusion is then carried out with 0.1 N hydrochloric acid at 6.8 ml per minute for a minimum of 25 minutes. If pain develops, water is perfused through the tube until the pH rises to 5 or until the pain is relieved. Repetitive perfusion with acid and water will permit the physician to correlate pain production with the acid perfusion because the pH is monitored throughout. When present, motor changes appear during periods of maximal pain production. This combined study is of particular value when both the patient and the examiner are fully aware of the symptoms present, and the patient then can spontaneously document the presence of pain. In patients with complicated pain problems this precise correlation is feasible only after a careful history has delineated the location and the factors which relieve it. In our study we had patients with multiple pains who could describe accurately the exact types of pain reproduced by the various stimuli.

Patients with gastric and duodenal disease sometimes give false positive responses to acid perfusion; hence, before accepting pain production to be esophageal, other gastrointestinal disorders must be excluded by radiologic or endoscopic investigation.

Although the physician must have a full understanding of the patient's pain before perfusion begins, the patient must remain unaware of the types of perfusate and the points at which pain would be anticipated. This correlation of pain with pH changes and motor changes gives an accurate assessment and avoids the pitfalls associated with the patient's anticipation.

Combined Cardiac and Esophageal Studies

These studies are particularly important in patients with atypical pain that could be either cardiac or esophageal. The term "atypical" in such patients is based on an unusual pain distribution or unusual precipitating or relieving factors. Commonly these patients have more than one type of pain, and each type must be clearly defined before proceeding to an acid perfusion study. In the period 1972 to 1974 we studied 105 patients with atypical chest pain. Many had been hospitalized previously and many had been treated inappropriately because of an inaccurate diagnosis. This study led us to conclude that esophageal and cardiac pain can be clearly distinguished, but only if both organs are investigated completely (44, 45).

Complete cardiologic and esophageal histories were elicited from each of these 105 patients, and the pain was carefully evaluated. Cardiac studies included coronary arteriography or multichannel exercise cardiography or both. The minimal esophageal studies included radiology, manometry and an acid perfusion study. After the various studies were completed, we assigned the patients to one of four groups: those with esophageal disease, those with cardiac disease, those with cardiac and esophageal disease, and those with neither disorder. Forty-three patients with esophageal disease had normal cardiac studies, but had gastroesophageal reflux radiologically and clear-cut pain production by acid perfusion. Twelve patients with cardiac disease had negative acid perfusion studies and positive exercise cardiograms or coronary angiograms. Twenty-two patients with both diseases had a positive acid perfusion study and positive cardiac studies. In the remaining 28 patients, who had no evidence of cardiac disease and a negative acid perfusion study, the pain arose from various sources some of which have yet to be identified.

As a result of experience accumulated during this study we now fully evaluate every patient who presents with atypical pain. If acid perfusion clearly reproduces his pain and he is being considered for hernia repair, we perform coronary arteriography to evaluate the degree of coronary artery disease. After this type of selection, 16 of these 105 patients with atypical pain underwent hiatal hernia repair. At present all have had satisfactory relief of their symptoms, suggesting that this method selects those with hernia and excludes those with associated cardiac disease. Patients with combined esophageal and cardiac disease occasionally have esophageal symptoms severe enough to require surgical correction of the hernia. In these, cardiologic assessment provides an accurate prediction of the risks involved in operation.

Previously (46, 47), many of the patients in this study had been considered to have cardiac disease and had been admitted to the hospital on several occasions and treated for myocardial infarction.

Case 2. During the 5 years before investigation, Mrs. B., age 56, had been admitted to hospital 8 times for chest pain. Nonspecific ECG changes had been demonstrated but no serum enzyme abnormalities. A coronary arteriogram showed a 25 per cent narrowing of the left anterior descending coronary artery but, because this was not considered severe enough to produce angina, her physician requested esophageal evaluation.

By history, her pain was epigastric and retrosternal and was precipitated both by eating and by exercise. It came on when climbing stairs and was relieved by 10 minutes of rest. Nitroglycerin was said to bring relief but required 10 minutes to produce an effect; this response was not typical of cardiac pain. She described reflux of bitter fluid to the throat occurring twice per week. Dysphagia was minor, but she did have food sticking at the gastroesophageal junctional level once or twice per week.

On radiologic examination she had a small hiatal hernia with reflux. Endoscopy was nonspecific. Manometric studies showed changes consistent with a hiatal hernia and there was a moderate degree of disordered motor activity. Acid perfusion produced her pain exactly and could be turned "off" and "on" by alternately acidifying and neutralizing the contents of her esophagus.

Her hiatal hernia was repaired surgically and she has remained free of symptoms in the 6 years since operation. Although this investigation is extensive, it is necessary in atypical cases to distinguish this type of pain from cardiac pain. Complete evaluation saves the patient from misdiagnosis and inappropriate therapy.

pH Reflux Test

Esophageal reflux can be classified as symptomatic, radiologic, endoscopic or manometric, or it can be assessed by using a pH probe and recording decreases in pH in the lower esophagus. pH during reflux can be studied by placing the electrode 5 cm above the gastroesophageal junction and inducing reflux by raised intra-abdominal pressure. Repetitive decreases in intraluminal pH are a good indication of reflux (48). The normal subject may exhibit reflux particularly after eating or during abrupt postural change; nevertheless, a clear fall in pH is a good index of gastroesophageal sphincter incompetence.

A more reliable method of assessing reflux is an overnight pH study (49) in which an electrode is left in the lower esophagus during the hours of sleep. In the normal subject reflux is transient, but in those with an incompetent sphincter it is repetitive and there is a delayed rise in esophageal pH. Both types of pH test are useful in evaluating reflux in difficult diagnostic situations, and are of particular value in the patient whose disorder cannot be confirmed radiologically yet whose historic or endoscopic findings strongly suggest reflux.

Twenty-four-Hour Reflux Testing

Twenty-four-hour pH reflux testing is an extension of these methods of study (50–52). Using 24-hour monitoring the response of the individual while awake and vertical can be studied and compared to reflux in the horizontal position and reflux following meals. In this test meals are designed which have a neutral pH and the patient can be asked to document various phenomena directly on the recording paper. The patient can then supply information which allows correlation of pH fall with heartburn, burping, lying or sitting.

Reflux can be shown to occur in the asymptomatic normal volunteer. The reflux demonstrated has to be quantitated to allow differentiation from the normal. One suggested method is to measure the number of reflux episodes in a vertical position, and in a horizontal position, also the percentage of time when the pH is below 4 and the longest duration of reflux. From these figures a reflux score is developed and used as an index of severity.

With both the overnight and the 24-hour test night reflux and aspiration can be correlated with coughing or with episodes of bronchospasm (53).

Acid Clearance Test

The acid clearance study measures the ability of the esophagus to clear an acid bolus (54). Secondary disordered motor activity is the characteristic response of the esophagus to reflux (55), and since these motor waves are non-propulsive they do not clear the esophagus effectively, particuarly in recumbency. The test delivers a bolus of 15 ml of decinormal hydrochloric acid at a specific level and then records the ability of the esophagus to clear the bolus. Manometric tubes and a pH electrode are placed 5 cm above the gastroesophageal junction, then the 15-ml bolus is instilled through a proximal manometric tube 10 cm above the electrode. With the patient swallowing at 30-second intervals, the tracing records the number of swallows required to raise the pH to 5.

This test has been applied to normal subjects and to patients with symptoms of reflux (56). Normal subjects clear the bolus in 10 swallows or less, whereas those with reflux require 15 to more than 40 swallows. Clearance time has been correlated with the presence of endoscopic esophagitis. Seventy per cent of patients with grossly visible esophagitis had abnormal clearance studies, whereas only 36 per cent of those who had no visible esophagitis had abnormal studies. The test is of considerable theoretical interest because it demonstrates how secondary disordered motor acitivity prolongs the clearance of the reflux bolus. It has some value in assessment of patients with gastroesophageal reflux because when clearance is grossly abnormal it suggests significant esophageal injury. The test is not specific enough to be of much clinical value at the present time.

Potential Difference

The electrical potential on the inner and outer aspect of the stomach wall differs markedly, depending on whether the stomach is at rest or is secreting. The potential difference across the esophageal wall is small and inconsistent; hence, studies of potential difference can demarcate the point of transition from gastric to esophageal mucosa. To determine potential difference, an intraluminal exploring electrode is filled with a concentrated solution of potassium chloride and agar (57, 58). The skin is used as a reference electrode. The sensitivity of this technique has been increased by various modifications. Hernandez and Beck (59) used Ringer's lactate solution in the exploring electrode and obtained a subdermal potential difference by scarifying the finger and immersing it in a saturated solution of potassium chloride.

The stomach is electrically negative, but at the squamocolumnar junction a change in potential difference appears and rises to a low positive electrical charge in the esophagus. Mucosal biopsy taken above and below the point of electrical change clearly shows that this change has taken place at the squamocolumnar junction (60). In patients with gastroesophageal reflux, the area over which the change in potential difference occurs is elongated and is shifted proximally. In those with esophageal ulceration, the potential difference falls, indicating that this test might be applied to the assessment of lesions of the esophageal mucosa (61). Also, the test may be useful as a screening procedure to detect abnormalities of the esophageal mucosa. Its applications to clinical practice have not yet been established.

Electromyography (EMG)

In esophageal disease electromyography is still an experimental procedure which has not yet been applied effectively to diagnosis. Using external esophageal electrodes, Hellemans and colleagues (62) have investigated normal esophageal motor function. Gastric and duodenal electrodes have been designed for medical use, but the application of EMG to clinical diagnosis awaits the development of a safe intraesophageal electrode (63).

The various studies described in this chapter can all be applied to the patient with gastroesophageal reflux. In general, the studies of proven clinical value are history, radiology, endoscopy, manometry and acid perfusion and pH studies.

In patients with mild symptoms a reliable diagnosis can often be made by history alone and the patient reassured. Radiology of the esophagus and stomach will be of confirmatory value and will exclude most disorders important in the differential diagnosis. In the minority of patients in whom they are necessary, extensive studies are indicated chiefly to exclude other major disease or to supply a more accurate assessment of disease severity before specific and more intensive management. If an operation seems to be necessary, the patient should have a complete evaluation because only accurate diagnosis will forestall inappropriate and often harmful therapy.

References

1. Wolf, B. S., Brahms, S. A., and Khilnani, M. T.: The incidence of hiatus hernia in routine barium meal

examinations. Mt. Sinai J. Med. N.Y., *26:* 598, 1959.

2. Field, P., and Stalker, M. J. B.: Incompetence of the cardiac sphincter without radiologic demonstration of hiatus hernia. Can. J. Surg., *11:* 412, 1968.

3. Henderson, R. D., and Pearson, F. G.: Preoperative assessment of esophageal pathology. J. Thorac. Cardiovasc. Surg., *72:* 512, 1976.

4. Kirklin, B. R., and Hodgson, J. R.: Roentgenologic characteristics of diaphragmatic hernia. A.J.R., *58:* 77, 1947.

5. Wolf, B. S.: Sliding hiatal hernia; the need for redefinition. A.J.R., *117:* 231, 1973.

6. Wolf, B. S.: Heartburn. The role of radiology. J.A.M.A., *235:* 1244, 1976.

7. Steiner, G. M.: Gastro-oesophageal reflux, hiatus hernia and the radiologist, with special reference to children. Br. J. Radiol., *50:* 164, 1977.

8. Berridge, F. R. Friedland, G. W., and Tagart, R. E. B.: Radiological landmarks at the oesophago-gastric junction. Thorax, *21:* 499, 1966.

9. Brombart, M.: *Clinical Radiology of the Oesophagus.* John Wright & Sons, Ltd., Bristol, 1961.

10. Schatzki, R., and Gary, J. E.: Dysphagia due to a diaphragm-like localized narrowing in the lower esophagus ("lower esophageal ring"). A.J.R., *70:* 911, 1953.

11. Wilkins, E. W., Jr., and Bartlett, M. K.: Surgical treatment of the lower esophageal ring. N. Engl. J. Med., *268:* 461, 1963.

12. Goyal, R. K., Bauer, J. L., and Spiro, H. M.: The nature and location of lower esophageal ring. N. Engl. J. Med., *284:* 1175, 1971.

13. Barrett, N. R.: The lower esophagus lined by columnar epithelium. Surgery, *41:* 881, 1957.

14. Allison, P. R., and Johnstone, A. S.: Oesophagus lined with gastric mucous membrane. Thorax, *8:* 87, 1953.

15. Henderson, R. D., Ho, C. S., and Davidson, J. W.: Primary disordered motor activity of the esophagus (diffuse spasm); diagnosis and treatment. Ann. Thorac. Surg., *18:* 327, 1974.

16. Brick, I. D., and Amory, H. I.: Incidence of hiatus hernia in patients without symptoms. Arch. Surg., *60:* 1045, 1950.

17. Crummy, A. B.: The water test in the evaluation of gastroesophageal reflux; its correlation with pyrosis. Radiology, *87:* 501, 1966.

18. Heibert, C. A., and Belsey, R.: Incompetency of the gastric cardia without radiologic evidence of a hiatal hernia. J. Thorac. Cardiovasc. Surg., *42:* 352, 1961.

19. Malmud, L. S., and Fisher, R. S.: Quantitation of gastroesophageal reflux before and after therapy using the gastroesophageal scintiscan. South Med. J., *71:* suppl. 1, 10-5, 1978.

20. Leisner, B., Witte, J., Kiefhaber, P., Eder, M., Pfeifer, J., Lang, G., and Mayr, B.: Functional scientigraphy in diagnosis of gastroesophageal reflux. Z. Gastroenterol., *16:* 235, 1978.

21. Reich, S. B., Earley, W. C., Ravin, T. H., et al.: Evaluation of gastro-pulmonary aspiration by a radioactive technique; concise communication. J. Nuc. Med., *18:* 1079, 1977.

22. Polish, E., and Sullivan, B. H., Jr.: Hiatal hernia and esophagitis. Am. J. Dig. Dis., *9:* 275, 1964.

23. Goldberg, H. I., Dodds, W. J., Gee, S., Montgomery, C., and Zboralske, F. F.: Role of acid and pepsin in acute experimental esophagitis. Gastroenterology, *56:* 223, 1969.

24. Henderson, R. D., Mugashe, F. L., Jeejeebhoy, K. N., Szczepanski, M. M., Cullen, J., Marryatt, G., and Boszko, A.: Synergism of acid and bile salts in the production of experimental esophagitis. Can. J. Surg., *16:* 12, 1973.

25. Henderson, R. D.: Results of esophageal investigation in 359 patients prior to surgical correction of reflux. Unpublished data.

26. Code, C. F., and Schlegel, T. F.: The pressure profile of the gastroesophageal sphincter in man; an improved method of detection. Mayo Clin. Proc., *33:* 406, 1958.

27. Edwards, D. A. W., and Rowlands, E. N.: Physiological observations in achalasia and their significance in methods of treatment. Gastroenterologia, *92:* 114, 1959.

28. Meltzer, S. J.: On the causes of the orderly progress of peristaltic movements in the esophagus. Am. J. Physiol., *2:* 266, 1899.

29. Pope, C. E.: A dynamic test of sphincter strength; its application to the lower esophageal sphincter. Gastroenterology, *52:* 779, 1967.

30. Millhon, W. A., Hoffman, D. E., Jarvis, P., Cross, J., Millhon, J. S., and Crites, N. A.: Preliminary report on Millhon-Crites intraesophageal motility probe. Am. J. Dig. Dis., *13:* 929, 1968.

31. Hay, D. J., Goodall, R. J. R., and Temple, J. G.: The reproducibility of the station pullthrough technique for measuring lower oesophageal sphincter pressure. Br. J. Surg., *66:* 93, 1979.

32. Earlam, R.: *Clinical Tests of Oesophageal Function.* Crosby Lockwood, Staples, London, 1975.

33. Dodds, W. J., Hogan, W. J., Arndorfer, R. C., and Dent, J.: Efficient manometric technic for accurate regional measurement of esophageal body motor activity. Am. J. Gastroenterol., *70:* 21, 1978.

34. Code, C. F., Kelley, M. L., Jr., Schegel, J. F., and Olsen, A. M.: Detection of hiatal hernia during esophageal motility tests. Gastroenterology, *43:* 521, 1962.

35. Hightower, N. C.: Esophageal motility in health and disease, Dis. Chest. *28:* 150, 1955.

36. Winans, C. S., and Harris, L. D.: Quantitation of lower esophageal sphincter competence. Gastroenterology, *52:* 773, 1967.

37. Haddad, J. K.: Relation of gastroesophageal reflux to yield sphincter pressures. Gastroenterology, *58:* 175, 1970.

38. Ramirez, J., Guarner, V., and Pazmino, F.: Alterations in motility of the esophagus in peptic esophagitis. Am. J. Proctol., *19:* 67, 1968.

39. Henderson, R. D., Mugashe, F., Jeejeebhoy, K. N., Cullen, J., Szczepanski, M., Boszko, A., and Marryatt, G.: The role of bile and acid in the production of esophagitis and the motor defect of esophagitis. Ann. Thorac. Surg., *14:* 465, 1972.

40. Bernstein, L. M., Fruin, R. C., and Pacini, R.: Differentiation of esophageal pain from angina pectoris; role of the esophageal acid perfusion test. Medicine (Baltimore), *41:* 143, 1962.

41. Siegel, C. I., and Hendrix, T. R.: Esophageal motor abnormalities induced by acid perfusion in patients with heartburn. J. Clin. Invest., *42:* 686, 1963.

42. Scharschmidt, B. F., and Watts, H. D.: The lower

esophageal ring and esophageal reflux. Am. J. Gastroenterol., *69:* 544, 1978.

43. Garabedian, M.: Uses of esophageal manometry and acid perfusion in the study of gastroesophageal reflux and hiatal hernia. Surg. Clin. North Am., *51:* 589, 1971.

44. Roberts, R., Henderson, R. D., and Wigle, E. D.: Esophageal disease as a cause of severe retrosternal chest pain. Chest, *67:* 523, 1975.

45. Henderson, R. D., Wigle, E. D., Sample, K., and Marryatt, G.: Atypical chest pain of cardiac and esophageal origin. Chest, *731:* 24, 1978.

46. Areskog, M., Tibbling, L., and Wranne, B.: Oesophageal dysfunction in non-infarction coronary care unit patients. Acta Med. Scand., *205:* 279, 1979.

47. Brand, D. L., Martin, D., and Pope, C. E.: Esophageal manometrics in patients with angina-like chest pain. Am. J. Dig. Dis., *22:* 300, 1977.

48. Tuttle, S. G., Bettarello, A., and Grossman, M. I.: Esophageal acid perfusion test and gastroesophageal reflux test in patients with esophagitis. Gastroenterology, *38:* 861, 1960.

49. Woodward, D. A. K.: Reflux pattern in hiatus hernia studied by prolonged indwellling electrodes. In *Surgery of the Esophagus: The Conventry Conference,* edited by R. A. Smith and R. E. Smith, p. 133. Butterworths, London, 1972.

50. DeMeester, T. R., and Johnson, L. F.: The evaluation of objective measurements of gastroesophageal reflux and their contribution to patient management. Surg. Clin. North Am., *56:* 39, 1976.

51. Johnson, L. F., and DeMeester, T. R.: Twenty-four-hour pH monitoring of the distal esophagus. A quantitative measure of gastroesophageal reflux. Am. J. Gastroenterol., *62:* 325, 1974.

52. Boesby, S., Madsen, T., and Sorensen, H. R.: Gastro-oesophageal acid reflux. Method for 12-hour continous recording of oesophageal pH with analysis of records. Scand. J. Gastroenterol., *10:* 379, 1975.

53. Hill, J. L., Pelligrini, C. A., Burrington, J. D., Reyes, H. M., and DeMeester, T. R.: Technique and experience with 24-hour esophageal pH monitoring in children. J. Pediatr. Surg., *12:* 877, 1977.

54. Booth, D. J., Kemmerer, W. T., and Skinner, D. B.: Acid clearing from the distal esophagus. Arch. Surg., *96:* 731, 1968.

55. Olsen, A. M., and Schlegel, J. F.: Motility disturbances caused by esophagitis. J. Thorac. Cardiovasc. Surg., *50:* 607, 1965.

56. Skinner, D. B., and Booth, D. J.: Assessment of distal esophageal function in patients with hiatal hernia and/or gastroesophageal reflux. Ann. Surg., *172:* 627, 1970.

57. Helm, W. J., Schlegel, J. F., Code, C. F., and Summerskill, W. H. J.: Identification of the gastroesophageal mucosal junction by transmucosal potential in healthy subjects and patients with hiatal hernia. Gastroenterology, *48:* 25, 1965.

58. Turner, K. S., Powell, D. W., Carney, C. N., Orlando, R. C., and Bozymski, E. M.: Transmural electrical potential difference in the mammalian esophagus in vivo. Gastroenterology, *75:* 286, 1978.

59. Hernandez, N. A., and Beck, I. T.: Gastroesophageal transmural potential difference measured by a new constant infusion method; the effect of skin scarification on this potential difference. Am. J. Dig. Dis., *14:* 206, 1969.

60. Meckeler, K. J. H., and Ingelfinger, F. J.: Correlation of electric surface potentials, intraluminal pressures, and nature of tissue in the gastroesophageal junction of man. Gastroenterology, *52:* 966, 1967.

61. Beck, I. T., and Hernandez, N. A.: Transmural potential difference in patients with hiatus hernia and oesophageal ulcer. Gut, *10:* 469, 1969.

62. Hellemans, J., Vantrappen, G., Valembois, P., Janssens, J., and Vandenbroucke, J.: Electrical activity of striated and smooth muscle of the esophagus. Am. J. Dig. Dis., *13:* 320, 1968.

63. Stoddard, C. J.: Current concepts of gastrointestinal motility and electrical activity. Br. J. Hosp. Med., *20:* 426, 1978.

CHAPTER 7

Medical Management of Hiatal Hernia: General Measures: Drug Therapy and Bougienage

Medical Management

The majority of symptoms in patients with gastroesophageal reflux are produced by the refluxed bolus (1, 2) (Table 7.1). Our treatment is aimed at avoiding reflux or reducing the irritant factors in the refluxed bolus. Reflux produces a variety of symptoms; however, the most common presenting symptom of reflux is heartburn. Occasionally dysphagia, nausea or vomiting may be the presenting and dominant symptom (Table 7.2). The major precipitating factors in the development of heartburn are the quality and quantity of food eaten and postural change. Occasionally exercise (especially posturally related) and hunger will precipitate heartburn (Table 7.3).

Treatment is based primarily on dietary adjustment, antacids to neutralize gastric acid and bed elevation to reduce night reflux. We now have medications that can be added in patients with refractory symptoms to further neutralize gastric acid or bile, to empty the stomach, to raise the tone of the high pressure zone (HPZ) or to speed up the healing of ulcerative esophagitis. These more complex medications should not be used unless the primary approach fails as they are expensive and may have side effects.

Diet

Both the quality and quantity of food eaten can be responsible for symptomatic heartburn. There is no absolute rule as to which food will produce symptoms and my approach has been to offer dietary advice, but to recognize that patient selection of appropriate foods should not be ignored. The patient has the symptom and quickly recognizes what foods give pain (3–6).

Certain foods are known to produce symptoms in the majority of patients with heartburn and any dietary regime should avoid these products. Other foods are usually tolerated well and can be used on a trial and error basis by the patient (Table 7.4). Why various foods give symptoms is not always clear, however, some of the symptoms can be explained by their action on gastric emptying, HPZ tone and acid secretion.

High gastric acidity lowers HPZ tone and alkalinity increases tone. Certain foods such as fatty meals, whole milk and carminatives have the direct affect of reducing tone. Fatty foods probably act by delaying gastric emptying and stimulating the cholecystokinin mechanism to reduce HPZ tone. Smoking, alcohol and carminatives act directly on the sphincter to lower tone.

Other food products produce esophageal pain and their action may be to cause local esophageal irritation. Such products include coffee and acidic fruit juices. These irritant foods are the "Bernstein Test" of eating.

Meal size is important and the majority of patients feel full early in the meal. Quite often, because of reduced meal size, they will rapidly become hungry and by trial and error start to eat small and frequent meals. Not uncommonly patients will so alter their diet that they begin to gain weight and this in itself may be a further aggravation. Weight loss is certainly recommended in the obese patient; however, the improvement in symptoms is very variable. I have on several occasions had patients whose first major symptoms developed while they were dieting.

The dietary recommendations should be to avoid all irritating foods, select a high-protein, low-fat diet from better tolerated food products (Table 7.4), reduce or stop alcohol (7) intake and smoking, eat small and frequent meals (usually six per day) and reduce weight if possible. Added to these recommendations food should not be eaten before going to bed and should be avoided before heavy exercise, particularly bending and lifting.

In the presence of severe dysphagia particulate size may be important; however, dysphagia often is motor in origin and simple reduction of food consistency may make no difference. The most profound dysphagias are often due to motor spasm.

Case 1. Mrs. S., age 66, had heartburn symptoms for 10 years and for 5 years had profound dysphagia. She had developed a severe peptic stricture which had been uncontrollable despite intermittent bougienage. When first seen she had been reduced to a diet of warm fluids for a period of 6 months. Despite this diet, she had maintained excellent nutrition. Radiologically and endoscopically her esophageal lumen was 1 to 2 mm in diameter and attempted dilatation was unsuccessful.

Table 7.1
Symptoms Present in Patients with Gastroesophageal Reflux*

Symptom	Occurrence
	%
Heartburn	96.6
Reflux to throat	71.5
Reflux and night aspiration	27.6
Dysphagia total	78.0
Peptic stricture	8.3
Motor dysphagia	69.7

* Heartburn, reflux to the throat and dysphagia are the three prime symptoms which allow a diagnosis of gastroesophageal reflux.

Table 7.2
Presenting Symptom in Patients with Reflux: Evaluation by History in 359 Patients with Severe Symptoms*

Symptom	Occurrence
	%
Heartburn	85.6
Gastroesophageal dysphagia	8.1
Cricopharyngeal dysphagia	4.9
Nausea	0.8
Bleeding	0.3
Aspiration	0.3

* Patients with reflux usually have several symptoms; however, one symptom dominates and is the presenting or chief complaint. In this table the commonest presenting symptom was heartburn.

Table 7.3
Precipitating Factors in 359 Patients with Reflux*

Factor	Occurrence
	%
Food	
Quality	97.8
Quantity	95.8
Posture	73.3
Exercise	14.8
Hunger	17.6

* Food and postural change are the commonest precipitating factors in patients with reflux. In a small number of patients symptoms are aggravated by exercise and hunger.

Table 7.4
Food and Heartburn*

	Irritant Foods	Well Tolerated Foods
Meat	Fatty or fried	Lean beef Chicken
Vegetables	Raw fruit and vegetables Acidic fruits	Potatoes, corn, apples, bananas
Liquids	Alcohol, carminatives (peppermint), acidic fruit juices, coffee, whole milk	Water, apple juice, decaffinated coffee, skimmed milk

* The foods labeled as irritants will produce heartburn in most patients with reflux symptoms. Those labeled as well tolerated are less likely to produce heartburn; however, there is much individual variability and in severely symptomatic patients even water may give distress.

We proceeded to surgical correction of reflux by total fundoplication gastroplasty using intraoperative retrograde dilatation. She now eats normally with no residual dysphagia.

This patient is important as she illustrates how with mechanical obstruction nutrition can be maintained. In some patients with motor dysphagia food intolerance is to both liquids and solids and weight loss may be severe. Occasionally nausea and vomiting predominate and again rapid weight loss may be present.

Bed Elevation

Reflux tends to occur at night (8). In the recumbent position, the effects of gravity are reduced and refluxed material will stay longer in the esophagus. Because the gravitational component of emptying is lost, the esophagus must rely chiefly on peristalsis. Elevation of the head of the bed on blocks 6 to 8 inches high will reduce reflux and greatly increase gravitational emptying. Parenthetically, it is important to stress that pillows alone are not a reliable means of elevation. Continuous pH monitoring demonstrates that with the bed elevated 13 inches, the frequency of pH falls below 5 and is significantly reduced. This simple maneuver may give quite marked relief of symptoms. The symptoms most likely to benefit from elevation are those of nocturnal heartburn, aspiration and pharyngoesophageal dysphagia. The frequent correction of pharyngoesophageal dysphagia after bed elevation alone suggests that night reflux and pooling at the pharyngoesophageal junction are important causes of this symptom.

Drug Therapy in Gastroesophageal Reflux

Antacids

Antacid therapy provides effective relief of pain in most patients with acid peptic disease and with reflux esophagitis (Table 7.5). However, there is no evidence that antacid therapy helps to heal a peptic ulcer or an esophageal ulcer (9). On theoretical grounds it might be argued that reduction in the acidity of the refluxed bolus should assist such healing. It has also been shown that antacids, by neutralizing the stomach contents, increase the pressure at the gastroesophageal junction (10, 11).

All antacids are not the same. Fordtran and associates (12) have compared various antacids both in vivo and in vitro, and this and similar studies have brought out certain points that should have a major bearing on the selection of medication for patients with reflux.

Calcium-containing antacids have a rebound effect, so that while initially neutralizing gastric acid they are followed by increased acid secretion and often an increase in the symptoms of reflux.

Many proprietary preparations combine anticholinergics with antacids. While anticholinergics tend to be effective only when administered at a level which produces a dry mouth and blurred vision, at lower doses they may produce a fall in gastroesophageal sphincteric tone and thus increase reflux.

The other antacids have been divided into those with major potency and those with minor potency as estimated by in vitro and in vivo studies (12). Under normal circumstances the physician should select an antacid of major potency. If diarrhea is a problem, magnesium salts should be avoided as these tend to make it worse. If the patient has cardiac disease an antacid low in sodium can be used. Antacids with an aluminum content (13) (aluminum hydroxide) prolong gastric emptying and should not be used in patients with pyloric outflow obstruction.

Liquid antacids are more readily mixed with gastric juices and are more effective than those taken in tablet form. Tablets can be used for their convenience, but they should be carefully chewed before swallowing.

When should an antacid be given? In general the peak of gastric acidification occurs 1 hour after eating, and this is the timing recommended in peptic ulcer disease (14). With gastroesophageal reflux, pain begins within 5 minutes of eating and antacid therapy most effectively reduces symptoms if it is taken at this time. The patient would be directed to take 30 ml of a potent antacid immediately after eating and before bed. When symptoms are severe, the antacids may be taken on an hourly schedule until the exacerbation subsides.

Metoclopramide

The actions of metoclopramide, a relatively new drug which was first synthesized in 1953 (15), have been extensively studied and estab-

Table 7.5
Drug Therapy of Gastroesophageal Reflux*

Drugs	Mode of Action	Value in Treatment	Complications
Antacids	Neutralize gastric acid; increase gastroesophageal tone	Effective	Rebound acid secretion with calcium; diarrhea with magnesium; fluid retention with sodium
Metoclopramide	Increases gastroesophageal tone; increases gastric emptying	Probable value	Drowsiness: extrapyramidal symptoms, seizures
Carbenoxolone	Prolongs life of gastric mucosal cell	Possible value	Sodium and fluid retention; potassium depletion.
Anticholinergics	Prolong gastric emptying; decrease gastroesophageal tone; decrease gastric acidity	No proof of value	Dry mouth; hazy vision
Cholinergics	Increase gastric emptying; increase gastroesophageal tone; increases gastric acidity	No proof of value	May aggravate peptic ulceration
Cholestyramine	Absorbs bile salts	Probably of value in bile reflux	Malabsorption
Cimetidine	H_2 blocking agent; reduces gastric acid	Effective	Central nervous system symptoms; fever; creatinine increase; decreased sperm count
Alginates	Mechanical barrier to reflux	Effective	Minor

* A wide variety of medications are available for the treatment of reflux; however, antacids are the most important and should be used in initial therapy.

lished (16, 17). Metoclopramide has been shown to enhance gastric emptying, increase the strength of the contraction of the gastric antrum, relax the duodenal cap and increase the synchronization between antral and duodenal motor activity (18). The drug also increases lower esophageal sphincter tone and the force of esophageal peristaltic contractions (19). It has no effect on gastric secretion, and acts as a powerful antiemetic. The actions of metoclopramide are antagonized by atropine (20).

Experimentally it has been demonstrated that metoclopramide acts directly on the ganglion cells of Auerbach's plexus (21), either by activating cholinergic ganglion cells or by suppressing inhibitory pathways.

Metoclopramide has been used in the management of gastroesophageal reflux on the presumption that faster gastric emptying and increased gastroesophageal sphincter tone should decrease reflux. It is given as a single 10-mg tablet 30 minutes before meals and may also be given at bedtime. Early clinical studies have been disappointing (22), but clearly more investigation is necessary. Although it is not possible to show a significant sustained HPZ tone increase with metoclopramide, there is a demonstrable symptom improvement in double blind controlled studies (23).

As reported to date, the side effects of metoclopramide are moderate, namely drowsiness, bowel disturbance, extrapyramidal symptoms, dizziness and faintness. The drug is contraindicated in early pregnancy (24).

My own experience with this drug has been mixed. In some patients the addition of metoclopramide, without any other alteration in management, has produced an immediate improvement in symptoms. It seems to be most effective when epigastric bloating is a dominant symptom. In other patients the drug is totally ineffective and a significant number of patients cannot tolerate it. There is no accurate method of predicting its effectiveness, and hence a trial of therapy seems necessary and worthwhile in each patient. Because of the development of extrapyramidal signs, I have avoided the use of this medication in older patients and particularly in patients with parkinsonism.

Carbenoxolone

Carbenoxolone was introduced for the management of gastric ulcer. The drug acts at its site of maximal absorption and reportedly increases the lifespan of gastric mucosal cells by 50 per cent. This drug has been applied to the treatment of esophagitis (25, 26), but the reports are not yet sufficient to establish its efficacy.

This drug has been used in the treatment of esophagitis with satisfactory results (27, 28). Recent reports of combining carbenoxolone with alginate compounds indicate effectiveness in healing esophageal ulceration. Although there are no extensive reports on this medication, its effectiveness with ulceration seems to be unique and superior to the reported effectiveness of antacids alone, cimetidine or metaclopramide. More evaluation is necessary, however, before this medication is introduced in routine medical management of reflux.

The biggest disadvantage of carbenoxolone (29) is its side effects. Taken as 50 mg four times per day, the drug may produce sodium retention, potassium depletion, fluid retention and hypertension. For these reasons carbenoxolone is contraindicated in patients with fluid retention, hypertension or cardiac disease.

Anticholinergic Drugs

These drugs, which have been used extensively in the management of duodenal ulcer, act by decreasing gastric acidity (30, 31). The classic agent in this group, atropine, has side effects, which include dryness in the mouth and blurring of vision. Synthetic drugs, such as methantheline (Banthine) and propantheline (Pro-Banthine), have fewer side effects.

Anticholinergics act by decreasing gastric acidity and also by decreasing gastric motor activity. Unfortunately, they also decrease the tone of the gastroesophageal junction (32, 33) and may actually enhance reflux. For this latter reason they cannot be recommended in the management of patients with symptomatic reflux.

Atropine specifically blocks the action of metoclopramide, and hence the two drugs cannot be used in combined therapy.

Cholinergic Drugs

Cholinergic drugs, such as bethanechol chloride, which have been used in the management of gastroesophageal reflux, act by stimulating vagal ganglia and produce increased gastric motor activity and increased gastroreflux junctional tone. In addition, bethanechol increases gastric acidity. Although improved gastric emptying and increased junctional tone may reduce reflux, this effect has to be balanced against increased gastric acidity (34).

Although occasionally bethanechol is used in the management of reflux, no long-term studies have ever proved its efficacy. Furthermore, since the motor actions of this drug are similar to those of metoclopramide, bethanechol has been supplanted to a considerable degree by the newer drug. In addition, metoclopramide has the major advantage that it does not increase gastric acid secretion. In my practice I have used bethanechol in patients who had symptomatic relief from metoclopramide, but who developed side effects from the medication necessitating discontinuance.

Cholestyramine

Therapy for gastroesophageal reflux may also include cholestyramine—a resin that reduces the bile salt content of the refluxed bolus by binding bile salts. Bile has been shown to contribute to gastric ulceration and when present in the stomach may worsen the effects of refluxed acid and pepsin on the esophagus (35, 36). Most patients with major bile reflux have had previous gastric surgery, but in some duodenogastric reflux may occur spontaneously. When the refluxed bolus contains bile the addition of cholestyramine may produce real benefit. Three grams of this powder are mixed with Jello or taken with orange juice, 3 times daily, usually 20 minutes after a meal. The powder has an unpleasant taste and has to be disguised in some highly flavored medium to make it palatable.

Cholestyramine is used with the same rationale as antacids, or to neutralize the irritant component of the refluxed bolus. Although highly effective in some patients, the individual patient usually must recognize a significant symptomatic improvement before he is willing to continue such an unpalatable medication.

Usually the medication is ineffective as bile is only one constituent of the refluxed bolus. I have found cholestyramine most effective in patients with total gastrectomy and pure bile reflux. In this situation, occasionally complete symptomatic relief can be achieved.

Cimetidine

This is the newest and one of the most significant additions to the management of gastroesophageal reflux in the past 10 years. Cimetidine acts by producing an H_2-receptor blockade and is capable of producing a marked reduction in gastric acidity (37, 38). In duodenal ulcer disease there is an improved rate of healing as compared to placebo therapy or antacids. In gastric ulcer disease the results are not as clear; however, it is probably still effective. Patients with gastroesophageal reflux have been studied fairly extensively; however, its efficacy in these patients is not completely established.

Double blind studies show a significant symptomatic improvement; however, there is evidence that despite improved symptoms in the average patient, esophageal ulceration is not healed (39–43).

The medication is taken as 300 mg three times per day at meals and also at night (1200 mg total dose). This dose level can be continued for 3 months and then should be reduced to a single tablet at bed time.

Side effects have been reported including increased symptoms upon drug withdrawal. There are occasional central nervous system effects of confusion, slurred speech, delerium and hallucinations; however these are most common with high dosage and in patients with neural impairment. There are also reports of fever and of creatinine elevation (44).

Generally the drug is well tolerated and most of the troublesome problems are found in elderly patients. The biggest concern with this medication is a recent report of suppression of spermatogenesis in young males. If this report is further confirmed, the usefulness of the medication will be significantly impaired (45).

Breast pain and breast enlargement has been reported in patients on high dose cimetidine for Zollinger-Ellison syndrome (46). There is a suggestion that renal allograft rejection may be more frequent in patients on cimetidine (47); however, this has not been completely established (48).

Alginate

Alginate* with aluminum hydroxide, magnesium trisilicate and sodium bicarbonate is available in tablet form for the control of gastroesophageal reflux. Four tablets, chewed and swallowed with water, act as a high-viscosity, low-density foam layer on the surface of the stomach content and interfere with the reflux process.

This unique substance was first described in Sandmark in 1963 (49) and has gradually gained acceptance as an effective medication for reflux control. When the product is chewed and contacts with water, its carboxyl group reacts with sodium bicarbonate to release carbon dioxide. The released carbon dioxide forms a foam which layers on the surface of gastric secretion and food content.

Clinical studies have demonstrated its effectiveness in reflux control and laboratory studies with pH probes and radiologic controls have demonstrated that reflux can be reduced (50–55).

In my own clinical experience, some patients will get relief from alginates when more standard antacid therapy has failed.

Combined Medical Management

Medical management of gastroesophageal reflux combines dietary control and bed elevation with the liberal use of antacids. In the majority of patients this is the limit of therapy and should be given a significant trial before the addition of metaclopramide or cimetidine is considered. These newer medications should be reserved for failure of initial therapy as their introduction adds the risk of side effects and in addition results in considerable expense to the patient (Table 7.6).

There is no reliable estimate of the percentage of the general population who have

* Gaviscon, Marion Laboratories, Inc., Kansas City, MO.

Table 7.6
Treatment Schedule

1. Diet:
   - a. Weight reduction
   - b. High-protein and low-fat diet
   - c. Small frequent meals
   - d. Avoidance of late evening meals
2. Drug therapy:
   - a. Antacids
   - b. Metoclopramide
   - c. Cholestyramine (in presence of bile reflux)
   - d. Avoidance of anticholinergics
3. Bed elevation: Elevate head of bed 6 to 8 inches (pillows are inadequate)

gastroesophageal reflux. Probably in most patients the symptoms are so mild that medical advice is never sought. These patients modify their diet by eliminating foods they recognize as producing irritation and add proprietary antacids. A small group, 10 to 20 per cent, need more extensive investigation and management and only a minority of these require an operation to correct reflux because of the failure of conservative management.

Esophageal Dilatation

Esophageal dilatation is a very important addition to the medical management of peptic strictures of the esophagus (56, 57). The techniques of dilatation are not universal knowledge, and there is much concern about the potential of perforation and the ensuing major problems. Properly conducted, esophageal dilatation can be simple and safe. In the majority of patients after the initial dilatation, this procedure can be continued on an outpatient basis.

Experience and judgment are critical to safe dilatation; however, once acquired they allow appropriate use of the various techniques with very little risk.

Dilatation can be performed using direct vision, indirect dilatation with mercury weighted bougies or a guide system to direct the bougie through the stricture. Dilatation is possible at the time of surgery through a gastrotomy. Each of these methods will be reviewed (Table 7.7).

Direct Vision Esophageal Dilatation

This usually requires a general anesthetic and the passage of a rigid esophagoscope. It is possible to use the rigid esophagoscope under local anesthesia, but the technique is uncomfortable for the patient. Using this method the stricture can be visualized, biopsied and brushed if necessary to exclude malignancy and gum elastic bougies passed up to #26 Fr. The diameter of the dilatation can be increased to #32 Fr by separately passing two gum elastic tipped bougies on a wire shaft through the stricture and then dilating by simultaneously withdrawing the bougies (Fig. 7.1).

The lumen size achieved by such dilatation is small; however, often this is enough to break the margins of a tight stricture and

Table 7.7
Methods of Dilatation*

Direct vision dilatation	Gum elastic
Indirect dilatation	Gum elastic
	Hurst mercury
	Malloney mercury
Guided dilatation	Plummer sound
	Tucker bougies
Intraoperative dilatation	Hegar dilators

* The majority of patients are dilated by indirect techniques or using direct vision dilatation at endoscopy. The other described techniques are rarely necessary.

allow continuance of dilatations with mercury weighted bougies. Under the same anesthetic once the lumen is dilated to #26 to #32 Fr, the esophagoscope may be withdrawn and indirect bougienage continued often up to #60 Fr.

Great care must be taken in dilatation under general anesthesia as the patient's pain response is absent and excessive force can disrupt the esophageal wall. With peptic strictures of the esophagus, the surrounding esophageal wall is thickened and fibrosed so that with care, dilatation is safe. In nonpeptic strictures such as seen following repair of a tracheoesophageal fistula, the scar is thin and the surrounding esophageal wall is not as fibrosed. These strictures are easy to dilate and equally easy to perforate so that dilatation must be done with extreme caution.

Indirect Dilatation

In most strictures dilatation can be carried out under local anesthesia with the patient sitting. I rarely use sedation and give only 30 cc of 2 per cent lidocaine (Xylocaine) viscous to gargle. Hurst bougies previously were the most popular; however, their dilating tip is rounded and much less effective than the taper tipped Malloney bougie. Both of these bougies are very pliable and depend for their dilating force on mercury filling.

Initial dilatation is with a bougie only slightly wider than the radiologic stricture. One can rapidly move up through the bougie size to reach full dilatation of #60 Fr. The great majority of strictures I have dilated can be brought to a #60 Fr in one or two sessions of dilatation. In most patients the passage of

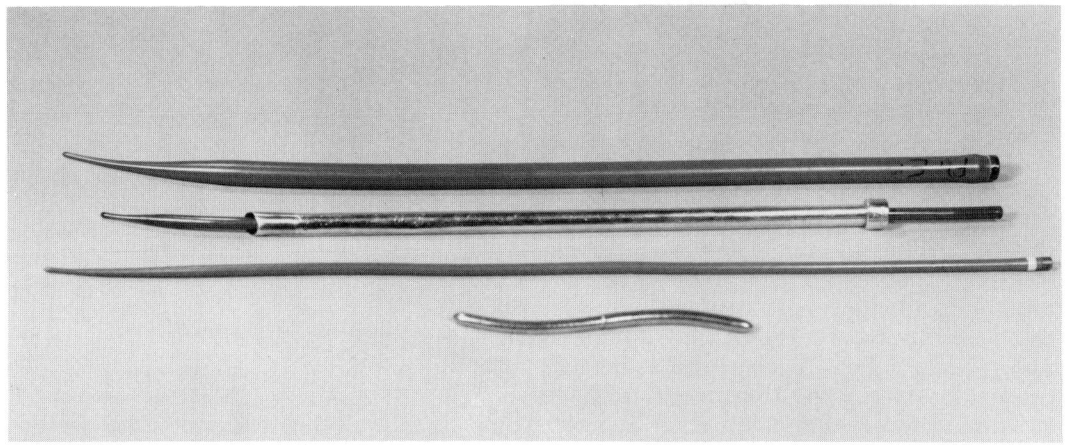

Figure 7.1
Standard Pilling rigid esophagoscope illustrates the size of bougies available for dilatation. A #30 Fr bougie fills the lumen of the esophagoscope. Below there is a #30 Malloney bougie and a Hegar dilator of comparable size. The large bougie above the esophagoscope is a #60 Fr Malloney bougie; when it is used for dilatation it must be passed blind.

two to three bougies is adequate at any one time.

With mercury bougies of small diameter the dilating effect is poor and I rarely use bougies of less than #36 to #40 Fr size. A large, taper tipped bougie will dilate with its tip and obviate the necessity of the very small size. Initial dilatation is usually performed in hospital; however, repeat dilatations can be done in the outpatient department or in the office. In more than 1000 such dilatations under local anesthesia with careful avoidance of the use of force, I have never had a perforation.

Case 2. Mr. R., age 76, had moderate reflux symptoms and developed a peptic stricture with severe dysphagia to solids. Because of cardiac disease he has not been considered for surgical correction of reflux.

Initially he was endoscoped under a local anesthesia with direct biopsy and brushings to exclude malignancy. He had extensive esophageal ulceration and a stricture estimated at #40 Fr lumen size. He was dilated with #42 to #46, #50 and #52 bougies at the time of endoscopy. This was well tolerated, and he was discharged for home 4 hours after the procedure.

Subsequently over the past 2 years he has required dilatation at 3-month intervals. He is now dilated to #60 Fr on each occasion. This is done under local anesthesia (2% viscous Xylocaine) in the outpatient department and his only prepara-tion is taking a liquid breakfast 5 hours before the procedure. This is well tolerated and causes only mild inconvenience to the patient.

Guided Dilatation

Various methods have been developed (58) for guided dilatation of esophageal strictures. The simplest method is to have the patient swallow a silk thread. Fifteen feet of thread on a spool can be passed at approximately 3 inches per hour. Once the thread is securely in the small bowel this can then be used to guide olive tipped bougies through the stricture (Fig. 7.2). The metal bougie tips range from #12 to #60 Fr.

Tucker bougies can be used in a similar fashion. Using retrograde dilatation a thread is passed and brought out through a gastrostomy. The attached bougie can be pulled orally and through the gastrostomy for dilatation (Fig. 7.3).

I have had very little experience with either of these techniques, having in almost all cases successfully achieved dilatation with the described direct and indirect methods.

Intraoperative Dilatation

If adequate dilatation cannot be achieved by the techniques described above, it is possible to dilate the stricture with the esophagus exposed in the operating room. In patients in whom surgery is indicated for management of reflux (if the simple techniques described are not successful), at the time of thoracotomy the fundus of stomach and lower esophagus can be mobilized, a small gastrotomy incision made and retrograde dilatation carried out using Hegar dilators. Almost all strictures can be dilated in this manner and if the esophagus is split appropriate surgical procedures can be carried out at the same time. Once this initial dilatation has been completed and reflux control achieved, then follow-up dilatation, if necessary will keep the esophagus fully patent while the tissue heals and the stricture resolves.

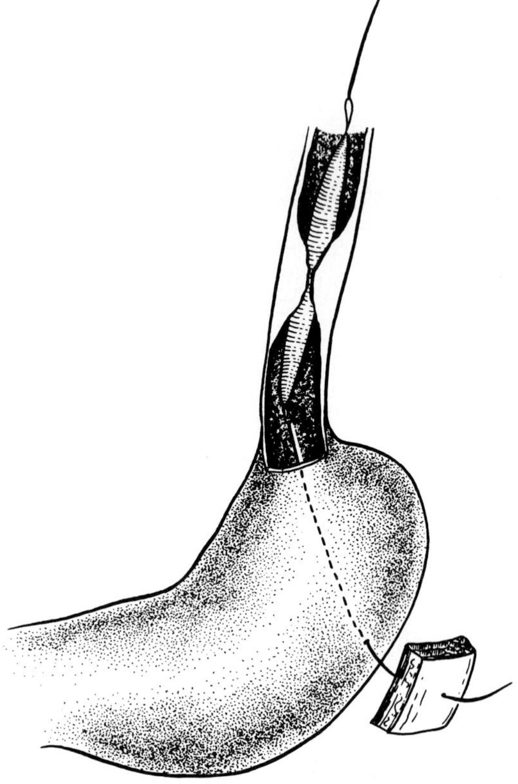

Figure 7.3
Tucker bougies are rarely used. A guide thread can be passed via a gastrostomy and used to pull the dilator through the stricture.

Medical Management of Strictures

Peptic stricture (excluding Schatzki rings) is an end stage of esophageal disease. If the patient is fit for surgery, this should be the method of management. In a few patients, where reflux symptoms are not severe or where concomitant disease contraindicates surgery, then long-term bougienage is effective and safe (59, 60).

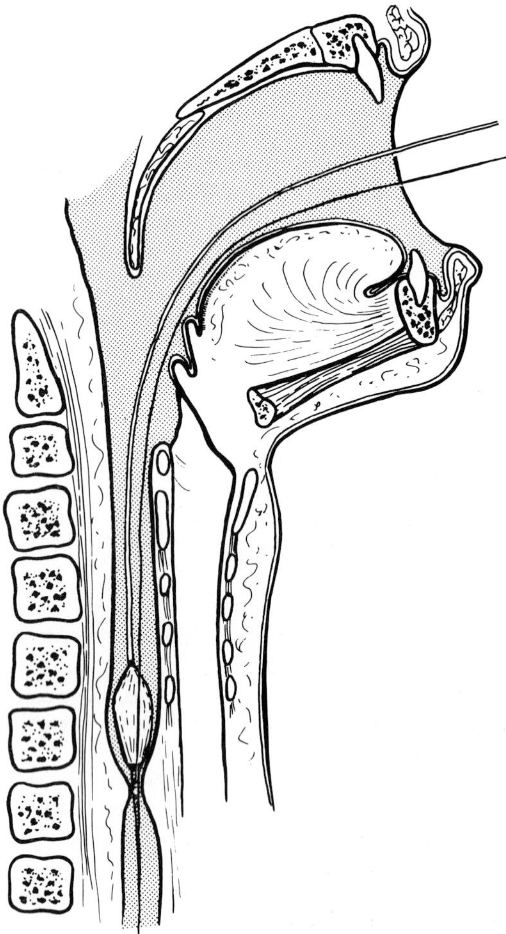

Figure 7.2
Olive-tipped bougies can be used for dilatation of different strictures, although the indications for use are very few. A guide string is passed and used to carry the tip of the dilator through the stricture.

References

1. Skinner, D. B., Belsey, R. H. R., Hendrix, T. R., and Zuidema, G. D. (Editors): *Gastroesophageal Reflux and Hiatal Hernia.* Little, Brown & Co., Boston, 1972.
2. Grossman, M. I.: Gastrointestinal hormones. Physiol. Rev., *30:* 33, 1950.
3. Chernow, B., and Castell, D. O.: Diet and heartburn. J.A.M.A., *241:* 2307, 1979.
4. Nebel, O. T., and Castell, D. O.: Lower esophageal sphincter pressure changes after food ingestion. Gastroenterology, *63:* 778, 1972.
5. Jennewein, H. M., Waldeck, F., Siewert, R., et al.: The interaction of glucagon and pentagastrin on

lower oesophageal sphincter in man and dog. Gut, *14:* 861, 1973.

6. Dennish, G. W., and Castell, D. O.: Inhibitory effect of smoking on the lower esophageal sphincter. N. Engl. J. Med. *284:* 1136, 1971.

7. Mayer, E. M., Grabowski, C. J., and Fisher, R. S.: Effects of graded doses of alcohol upon esophageal motor function. Gastroenterology, *75:* 1133, 1978.

8. Stanciu, C., and Bennett, J. R.: Effects of posture on gastro-oesophageal reflux. Digestion, *15:* 104, 1977.

9. Blumenthal, I. S.: Digestive disease as a national problem; III. Social cost of peptic ulcer. Gastroenterology, *54:* 86, 1968.

10. Castell, D. O., and Harris, L. D.: Hormonal control of gastroesophageal-sphincter strength. N. Engl. J. Med., *282:* 886, 1970.

11. Higgs, R. H., Smyth, R. D., and Castell, D. O.: Gastric alkalinization; effect on lower-esophageal-sphincter pressure and serum gastrin. N. Engl. J. Med., *291:* 486, 1974.

12. Fordtran, J. S., Morawski, S. G., and Richardson, C. T.: *In vivo* and *in vitro* evaluation of liquid antacids. N. Engl. J. Med., *288:* 923, 1973.

13. Hurwitz, A., Robinson, R. G., Vats, T. W., Whittier, F. C., and Herrin, W. F.: Effects of antacids on gastric emptying. Gastroenterology, *71:* 268, 1976.

14. Badley, B. W. D.: Some aspects of medical management of gastrointestinal disease; Part II. Can. Med. Assoc., J., *112:* 331, 1975.

15. Justin-Besancon, L., Laville, C., and Thominet, M.: Le métoclopramide et ses homologues; introduction à leur étude biologique. C. R. Acad. Sci. (Paris), *258:* 4384, 1964.

16. Johnson, A. G.: Controlled trial of metoclopramide in the treatment of flatulent dyspepsia. Br. Med. J., *2:* 25, 1971.

17. Robinson, O. P. W.: Metoclopramide—a new pharmacological approach? Postgrad. Med. J., *49:* (Suppl. 4); 9, 1973.

18. Johnson, A. G.: The action of metoclopramide on human gastroduodenal motility. Gut, *12:* 421, 1971.

19. Matsuo, H.: Study of the action of mechanism of Primperan. In *Third Japanese Symposium on Therapy and New Drugs*, p. 56, 1966.

20. Jacoby, H. I., and Brodie, D. A.: Gastrointestinal actions of metoclopramide; an experimental study. Gastroenterology, *52:* 676, 1967.

21. Dilawari, J. B., and Misiewicz, J. J.: Action of oral metoclopramide on the gastroesophageal junction in man. Gut, *14:* 380, 1973.

22. Venables, C. W., Bell, D., and Eccleston, D.: A double-blind study of metoclopramide in symptomatic peptic esophagitis. Postgrad. Med. J., *49:* (Suppl. 4), 73, 1973

23. McCallum, R. W., Ippoliti, A. F., Cooney, C., and Sturdevant, R. A. L.: A controlled trial of metoclopramide in symptomatic gastroesophageal reflux. N. Engl. J. Med., *296:* 354, 1977.

24. Robinson, O. P. W.: Metoclopramide—side effects and safety. Postgrad. Med. J., *49:* (Suppl. 4), 77, 1973.

25. Lipkin, M.: *Carbenoxolone Sodium*, edited by J. H. Baron and F. H. Sullivan, Butterworths, London, 1970.

26. Sircus, W.: Progress report; carbenoxolone sodium. Gut, *13:* 816, 1972.

27. Reed, P. I., and Davies, W. A.: Controlled trial of a carbenoxolone/alginate antacid combination in re-flux oesophagitis. Curr. Med. Res. Opin., *5:* 637, 1978.

28. Reed, P. I., and Davies, W. A.: Controlled trial of a new dosage form of carbenoxolone (Pyrogastrone) in the treatment of reflux esophagitis. Am. J. Dig. Dis. *23:* 161, 1978.

29. Archambault, A., Farley, A., Gosselin, D., Martin, F., and Birkett, J. P.: Evaluation of duogastrome (carbenoxolone sodium) for the treatment of duodenal ulcer. A multicentre study. Can. Med. Assoc. J., *117:* 1155, 1977.

30. Barman, M. L., and Larson, R. K.: The effect of glycopyrrolate on nocturnal gastric secretion in peptic ulcer patients. Am. J. Med. Sci., *246:* 325, 1963.

31. Sun, D. C. H.: Long-term anticholinergic therapy for prevention of recurrences in duodenal ulcer. Am. J. Dig. Dis. (N.S.), *9:* 706, 1964.

32. Lind, J. F., Crispin, J. S., and McIver, D. K.: The effect of atropine on the gastroesophageal sphincter. Can. J. Physiol. Pharmacol., *46:* 233, 1968.

33. Kelley, M. L., and Friedland, H. L.: Gastroesophageal sphincter pressures before and after oral anticholinergic drug and placebo administration. Am. J. Dig. Dis., *12:* 823, 1967.

34. Roling, G. T., Farrell, R. L., and Castell, D. O.: Cholinergic response of the lower esophageal sphincter. Am. J. Physiol., *222:* 967, 1972.

35. Moffat, R. C., and Berkas, E. M.: Bile esophagitis. Arch. Surg., *91:* 963, 1965.

36. Cross, F. S., and Wangensteen, O. H.: Role of bile and pancreatic juice in production of esophageal erosions and anemia. Proc. Soc. Exp. Biol. Med., *77:* 862, 1951.

37. Malagelada, J. R., and Cortot, A.: H_2-receptor antagonists in perspective. Mayo Clin. Proc., *53:* 184, 1978.

38. Schlippert, W.: Cimetidine; H_2-receptor blockade in gastrointestinal disease. Arch. Intern Med., *138:* 1257, 1978.

39. Powell-Jackson, P., Barkley, H., and Northfield, T. C.: Effect of cimetidine in symptomatic gastro-oesophageal reflux. Lancet, *2:* 1068, 1978.

40. Finkelstein, W., and Isselbacher, K. J.: Drug therapy; cimetidine. N. Engl. J. Med., *299:* 992, 1978.

41. Feldman, M., and Richardson, C. T.: Histamine H_2-receptor antagonists. Adv. Intern. Med., *23:* 1, 1978.

42. Behar, J., Brand, D. L., Brown, F. C., Castell, D. O., Cohen, S., Crossley, R. J., Pope, C. E., and Winans, C. S.: Cimetidine in the treatment of symptomatic gastroesophageal reflux. A double blind controlled trial. Gastroenterology, *74:* 441, 1978.

43. Kravitz, J. J., Snade, W. J., and Cohen, S.: Effect of histamine and histamine antagonists on human lower esophageal sphincter function. Gastroenterology, *74:* 435, 1978.

44. Cimetidine (Tagamet); update on adverse effects. Med. Lett., *20 (18):* 77, 1978.

45. Van Theil, D. H., Gavaler, J. S., Smith, W. I., and Paul, G.: Hypothalamic-pituitary-gonadal dysfunction in men using cimetidine. N. Engl. J. Med. *300:* 1012, 1979.

46. Hall, W. H.: Breast changes in males on cimetidine (Letter to the Editor). N. Engl. J. Med., *295:* 841, 1976.

47. Zammit, M., and Toledo-Pereyra, L. H.: Cimetidine for kidney transplantation; experimental observations. Surgery, *86:* 611, 1979.

48. Charpentier, B., and Fries, D.: Cimetidine and

renal—allograft rejection (Letter to the Editor). Lancet, *1:* 1265, 1978.

49. Sandmark, S.: Hiatal incompetence studies on mechanics and principles of examination for hiatus hernia and gastro-oesophageal reflux. Acta Radiol. Suppl. 219, 1, 1963.

50. McHardy, G., et al.: Reflux esophagitis in the elderly, with special reference to antacid therapy. J. Am. Geriatr. Soc., *20:* 293, 1972.

51. McHardy, G.: A multicentric, randomized clinical trial of Gaviscon in reflux esophagitis. South Med. J., *71:* Suppl. 1, 16, 1978.

52. Barnardo, D. E., Lancaster-Smith, M., Strickland, I. D., and Wright, J. T.: A double-blind controlled trial of "Gaviscon" in patients with symptomatic gastro-oesophageal reflux. Curr. Med. Res. Opin., *3:* 388, 1975.

53. Amdrug, E., and Jakobsen, B. M.: Reflux esophagitis treated with Gaviscon. Acta Chir. Scand. Suppl. 396, 16, 1969.

54. Stanciu, C., and Bennett, J. R.: Alginate/antacid in the reduction of gastro-oesophageal reflux. Lancet, *1:* 109, 1974.

55. Beckloff, G. L., Chapman, J. H., and Shiverdecker, P.: Objective evaluation of an antacid with unusual properties. J. Clin. Pharmacol. *12:* 11, 1972.

56. Bolstad, D. S.: The management of strictures of the esophagus. Ann. Otol. Rhinol. Laryngol., *75:* 1019, 1966.

57. Payne W. S., and Olsen, A. M. *The Esophagus.* Lea & Febiger, Philadelphia, 1974.

58. Plummer, H. S.: The value of a silk thread as a guide in esophageal technique. Surg. Gynecol. Obstet., *10:* 519, 1910.

59. Lanza, F. L., and Graham, D. Y.: Bougienage is effective therapy for most benign esophageal strictures. J.A.M.A., *240:* 844, 1978.

60. Lanza, F. L.: Conservative management of esophageal stricture using dilatation and antireflux therapy. South Med. J., *71:* Suppl. 1, 8, 1978.

CHAPTER 8

Hiatal Hernia and Gastroesophageal Reflux: Indications for Surgery and Choice of Approach

There are two major indications for the surgical management of a hiatal hernia and reflux. The most common is failure of adequate medical management, but, in addition, certain complications, when recognized, may make operation necessary.

As noted earlier, medical management includes dietary control, bed elevation, antacids and possibly the addition of metoclopramide. This program should be continued under careful supervision for several months before any consideration is given to operation, because during this time symptoms may be abolished or reduced to a tolerable level. However, if severe symptoms persist, the correct operation offers an excellent chance of effective and permanent control (Fig. 8.1).

Large Type I or Type II hernias should be treated surgically as these tend to be complicated by strangulation, ulceration, hemorrhage and perforation (1, 2). Because of these problems, surgery carries a much smaller risk than conservative management if the patient's general condition permits operation. Hemorrhage and perforation may also occur with ulceration in a Barrett's esophagus and even more rarely massive bleeding can occur from an ulcer at the gastroesophageal junction (3–5). Other complications, such as recurrent anemia, peptic stricture and aspiration, while they do not constitute absolute indications for surgery, may be severe enough to produce major disability if not corrected medically. Because of these potential complications, surgery is indicated at an earlier stage.

Microcytic anemia may persist even after good control of other symptoms has been achieved. Such anemia may develop without evidence of ulceration, and presumably the blood is lost from inflamed gastric mucosa in the hernia sac. In this situation surgical repair of the hernia has been reported to give effective relief (6–8).

Although a peptic stricture is usually dilatable, it develops only in the presence of advanced disease and hence is likely to recur after dilatation (9). Occasionally, when the patient is first seen, his stricture may be so severe that adequate dilatation is not possible, and without surgical correction the patient would have to carry on with a sharply reduced caloric intake. Under these circumstances, an operation offers effective relief of dysphagia.

Aspiration from reflux (10–12) or from pharyngoesophageal dysphagia may respond well to conservative management, but if it should persist and continue to produce significant pulmonary symptoms, operative repair may be necessary to prevent lung soiling and to arrest the progress of the pulmonary disease.

Every surgeon sees many examples of advanced esophageal disease that require early surgery. The two patients described below illustrate this group well.

Case 1. Mr. Z., age 55, had minor indigestion, which had occurred intermittently over a 10-year period. He had a major "bleed" from a previously undiagnosed duodenal ulcer and was submitted to gastrectomy. At that operation the surgeon performed a vagotomy, hiatal hernia repair and Billroth II resection. Before leaving the hospital this patient developed dysphagia and over the following month this symptom progressed to the point where he could take only liquids. For 6 months he was treated for a peptic stricture by intermittent

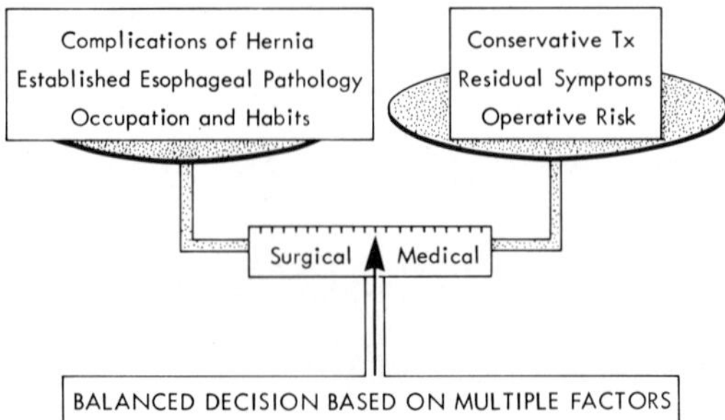

Figure 8.1.   Balanced Decision: Surgical vs. Medical Treatment (Tx)
The chief indication for operation is failure of medical management. The other factors that have to be considered vary so much from patient to patient that there can be no "routine" approach to hiatal hernia repair.

dilatation, but this procedure did not relieve his symptoms. When I first saw him he had a narrow stricture 10 cm long and had a recurrence of his hiatal hernia. Dilatation under general anesthesia to a #30 Fr gave slight symptomatic relief, but this was not sufficient to ensure a reasonable dietary intake. Further surgery was recommended, and at thoracotomy the stricture was dilated up to #50 Fr, using Hegar dilators through a gastrotomy. His reflux was controlled by a gastroplasty and he is now asymptomatic and eating normally.

Case 2. Five years before consultation, Mrs. M., age 58, had had a right upper lobectomy for localized bronchiectasis. She did well for 2 years and then developed recurrent respiratory infections with cough and massive sputum production. When I first saw her she had been under intensive medical management; she had been in the hospital for a month, but continued to produce copious yellow sputum and to run a fever. At this stage it was recognized that she had severe reflux and night aspiration, which persisted despite elevation of the head of her bed. She now had extensive bronchiectasis in her right lung, but the left lung was free of disease.

Because medical management had failed, the hiatal hernia was repaired surgically. Over the following month in the hospital her sputum production dramatically decreased and she was discharged on long-term antibiotics and physiotherapy. In the 2 years since she has remained well; she has had an occasional respiratory infection with slight continued sputum production, but has been free of esophageal symptoms.

These cases illustrate extreme examples of persistent major symptoms and demonstrate the effectiveness of surgical treatment in such patients.

Barrett's Esophagus

The Barrett's esophagus (13, 14) merits separate mention. This gastric mucosal-lined esophagus was described by Allison and Johnstone (15) and by Barrett in 1953 (14); it is being increasingly recognized as an important end stage of esophageal disease. Although its exact etiology is not fully understood, there is evidence that gastric mucosal replacement occurs after extensive esophageal ulceration. Congenital islands of gastric mucosa can occur in the esophagus; however, most patients with an extensive gastric lining have a long history of reflux symptomatology. Recently, gastric mucosal lining has been shown to occur following esophagogastric anastomosis, and it has also been shown to progress in patients with active reflux and ulceration (16, 17).

The importance of the Barrett's esophagus lies in its potential for complications. Penetrating ulcers behave more like gastric ulcers with bleeding and perforation. The new squamocolumnar junction is commonly associated with stricture.

Adenocarcinoma of the esophagus is significantly increased in frequency and recently has been reported as occurring in 8.6 (17) to 26.3 per cent (18); however, this frequency may be exaggerated by case selection, in that patients with adenocarcinoma will present for treatment of their malignancy. There is no long-term follow-up of patients with known gastric lining to determine the incidence of carcinoma development.

When patients with a Barrett's esophagus are seen, the mucosal changes must be considered premalignant and long-term follow-up of such patients is essential to minimize the risks of a developing carcinoma.

Choice of Surgical Approach

Once surgical repair has been chosen to correct gastroesophageal reflux, the operation must be planned and the procedure tailored to the needs of the individual patient. For hernia repair there are three possible exposures—transabdominal, transthoracic or thoracoabdominal; each has certain advantages. Before making a choice the surgeon must consider two factors. First, does the patient have both intrathoracic and intra-abdominal disease that requires simultaneous surgical corrections (19)? If disease is present in both cavities, this may decide the choice of approach. The second consideration is whether a complete repair is feasible through the approach chosen.

There are many examples of coexisting lesions which can be corrected simultaneously, e.g., through an abdominal approach a hernia repair can be performed and the gallbladder removed (20), and through a thoracic approach pulmonary or esophageal resections may be done. More frequently multiple abdominal pathology is present; however, in one patient, a woman, age 60, a small apical scar, biopsied at the time of hernia repair, was found to be alveolar cell carcinoma. She underwent lobectomy followed by hernia repair. In this instance I chose the thoracic approach because of the lung lesion, but the necessary esophageal repair was carried out simultaneously.

An important factor in the choice of approach is the individual surgeon's ability to carry out the specific operative correction. There are two major reasons for choosing a thoracic approach. First, it has real advantages in the presence of a recurrent hernia because the dissection necessary to mobilize the esophagus cannot be done easily from the abdomen. Secondly, the presence of an irreducible hiatal hernia is a major contraindication to abdominal repair. An irreducible hernia usually requires either a thoracic or thoracoabdominal exposure. These conclusions, although accepted by most surgeons, remain controversial.

Hill and colleagues (21) believe that all hernias can be reduced and held in a reduced position by his repair (Fig. 8.2). Others, who advocate the Belsey or Nissen (22–26) repair or a gastroplasty, insist that peptic scarring can make a hernia irreducible. Belsey, who bases his views on a 10-year follow-up, believes that in the presence of panmural esophagitis and esophageal shortening, the incidence of recurrence after his repair will be as high as 45 per cent (27). Current surgical opinion and my own experience during long-term follow-up support Belsey's view, namely, that reduction and abdominal repair should not be attempted in patients with esophageal shortening. If this view is accepted, the choice of approach to repair depends, at least in part, on the clinical assess-

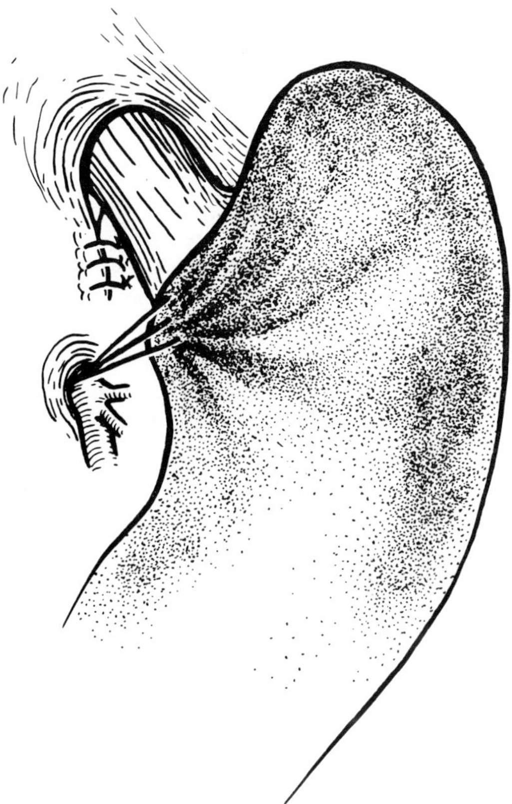

Figure 8.2
The Hill transabdominal hiatal hernia repair closes the diaphragmatic curve, then partially wraps the lower esophagus with sutures from the seromuscular layer of the proximal stomach. These seromuscular sutures are tethered to the median arcuate ligament, immediately above the celiac axis.

ment of esophageal pathology before repair. Chapter 6 reviewed the evidence that panmural esophagitis with esophageal shortening was common in patients who had the following findings on assessment:

1. Large and radiologically irreducible hernia.
2. Stage III(B) and Stage IV esophagitis.
3. Manometry showing more than 60 per cent distal disordered motor activity.

These criteria help the surgeon select those patients most likely to have esophageal wall changes characteristic of panmural peptic esophagitis; one's choice of surgical approach will be strongly influenced by this possibility.

Transabdominal Hiatal Hernia Repair

This, the most common approach to hernia reduction and repair, is of particular value in those patients who require surgical correction of coexisting abdominal disease. It is the repair of choice for most abdominal surgeons, and for them the advantage of familiarity makes it the most appropriate approach.

The transabdominal operations offered for the patient with esophageal shortening due to panmural fibrosis and scarring include the Hill repair (previously noted) and the Nissen fundoplication (Fig. 8.3) (28). The Nissen repair wraps the stomach around the lower esophagus, but allows the plicated lower esophagus to slide into the chest. With this approach the gastroesophageal junction remains in the chest but the gastric fundoplication acts as a flap valve and effectively prevents reflux.

Transthoracic Hiatal Hernia Repair

The prime indications for a thoracic approach are a) when concomitant thoracic pathology is suspected or b) when adequate

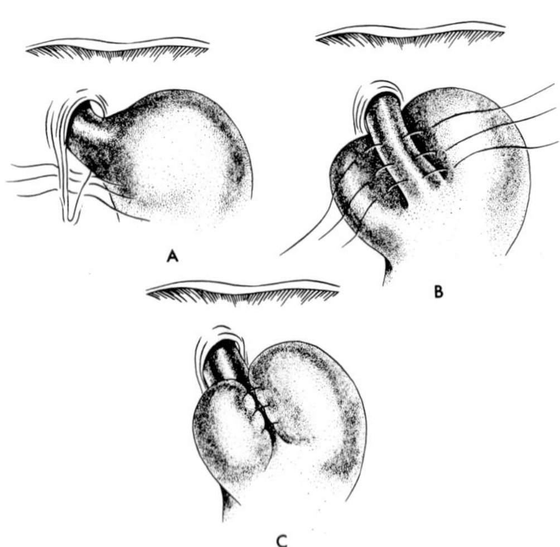

Figure 8.3.   Nissen Fundoplication
The Nissen hiatal hernia repair involves mobilization of the gastric fundus and a complete wrap of the fundus of stomach around the distal 5 cm of esophagus. This procedure can be used to hold the esophagus below the diaphragm, or can be modified to allow the plicated esophagus to lie in the thoracic cavity. Repair can be done through either a transthoracic or transabdominal approach.

mobilization and reduction do not seem possible via the abdominal approach.

The Belsey repair (Fig. 8.4) or Nissen fundoplication can be performed through the chest (9). In addition, when the hernia is found to be irreducible, the surgeon can modify the operative procedure and carry out a gastroplasty (Fig. 8.5) or an alternative esophageal plastic procedure (24, 25). If correction calls for an esophageal resection and bowel replacement, the diaphragm or costal margin can be split to give the thoracic and abdominal exposure necessary for bowel mobilization (Fig. 8.6).

The thoracic approach allows adequate inspection and palpation of the esophagus, and better mobilization of the intrathoracic esophagus. A direct approach is advocated in most surgical diseases, and the application of this principle to the esophagus has several obvious advantages.

Occasionally, direct inspection and palpation may be essential for accurate diagnosis. The two patients described below illustrate this point.

Case 3. Mrs. M., age 61, presented with a long history of gastroesophageal reflux and a history of mechanical dysphagia—namely, sticking of solid food and regurgitation for 6 months. Radiologic examination demonstrated a peptic stricture immediately above the gastroesophageal junction. On endoscopy direct visualization and biopsy showed only chronic inflammatory changes, with no evidence of malignancy. The lesion was approached through the thorax with the intention of performing a gastroplasty. At operation closer inspection and palpation of the esophagus revealed a hard plaque at the site of the stricture, namely, an invasive squamous cell carcinoma. The costal margin was divided and an esophagogastrectomy performed without delay.

The important point here is that an esophageal cancer was missed despite careful preoperative evaluation, and the correct diagnosis was made only because of the complete exposure achieved by the thoracic approach. If an abdominal approach is used to manage complicated esophageal problems, this type of diagnostic difficulty will not be recognized.

Case 4. Mr. R., age 51, had a short history of gastroesophageal reflux. Six months earlier he had developed intractable motor dysphagia with sticking of both liquids and solids and frequent regurgitation. On radiographic examination he had a 6-cm hiatal hernia with moderate gastroesophageal reflux, but no other abnormality. On endoscopy there was reflux but no evidence of esophageal ulceration. Manometry showed a gastroesophageal junction of normal tone with well-preserved relaxation in response to deglutition. He had a severe disorder of motor activity in the lower two-thirds of his esophagus, in which the motor waves were of moderate amplitude. At this stage the clinical diagnosis was "gastroesophageal reflux and a hiatal hernia."

At thoracotomy we noted his esophagus was thickened and spastic. These changes, which could be recognized only on direct inspection and palpation, changed the diagnosis to diffuse esophageal spasm (DES), and extended esophageal myotomy was performed at once.

Once again the true diagnosis was not suspected before operation and would not have been made if the repair had been attempted through a transabdominal approach. Although most patients with DES have characteristic manometric features, this particular patient was sufficiently atypical to mislead us before exploration. In many centers manometric studies are not yet available, and without this aid the risk of misdiagnosis of primary motor disorders is even greater.

This second case also illustrates the value of a thoracic approach, and the increased diagnostic accuracy made possible through direct inspection and palpation of the esophagus.

Arguments advanced against the thoracic approach include impairment of respiratory

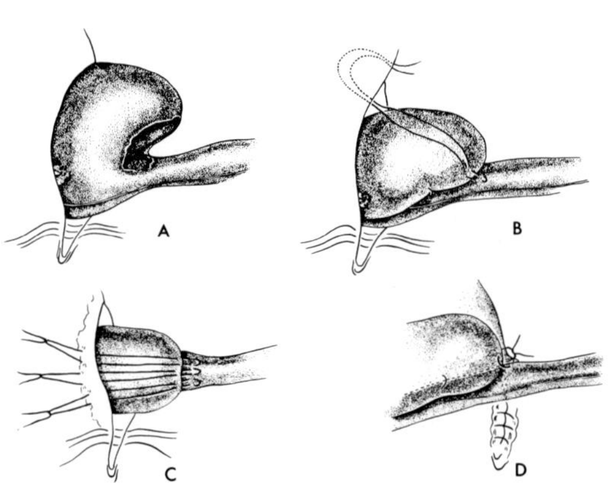

Figure 8.4.   Belsey Repair
The Belsey hiatal hernia repair is performed via a transthoracic approach. The fundus of stomach is mobilized (A) and the esophagogastric fat pad removed. A fundoplication is prepared and sutures are passed through the diaphragm (B and C). The hernia is reduced and fixed in position by its diaphragmatic sutures and by closure of the crura (D).

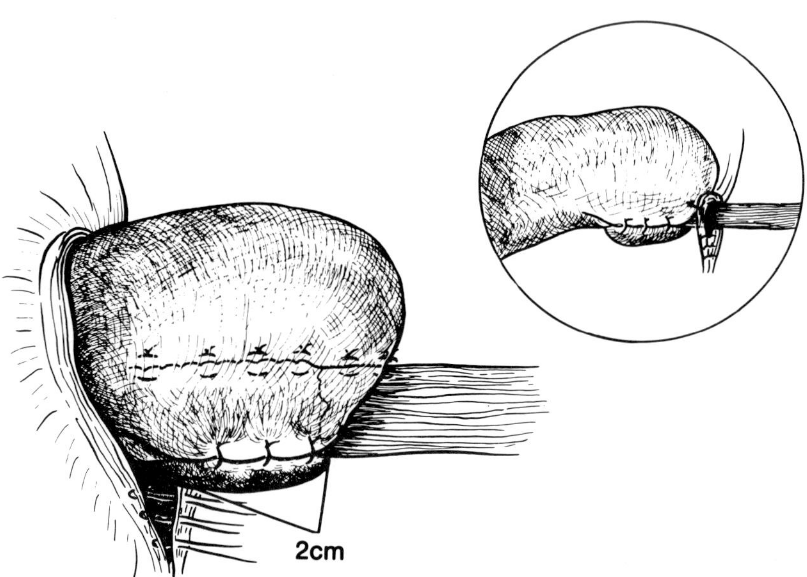

Figure 8.5.   Transthoracic Total Fundoplication Gastroplasty
The total fundoplication gastroplasty (TFG) incorporates the gastroplasty tube, completely wrapped by fundus of stomach. Details of this operative procedure are described in Chapter 11.

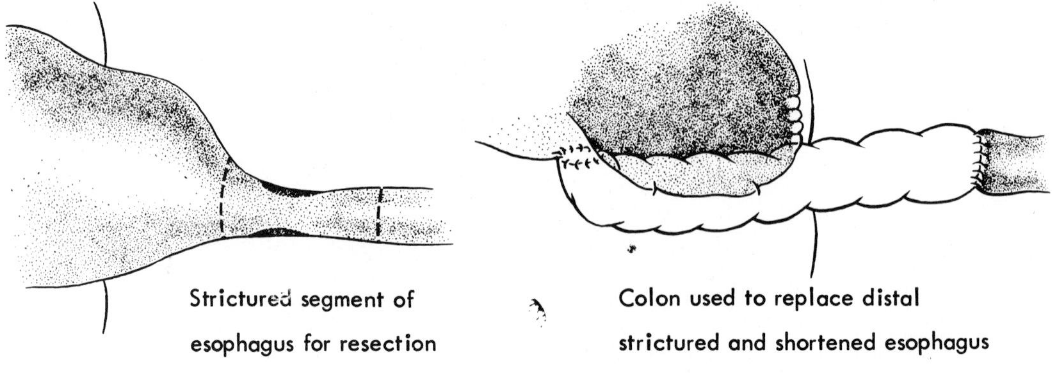

Figure 8.6.   Bowel Replacement of Lower Esophagus
Replacement of esophagus with bowel is of particular value when the esophagus is shortened and constricted by scarring. The distal esophagus is resected and the esophagogastric junction oversewn. A segment of splenic flexure of colon, vascularized by the ascending branch of the left colic artery, is used to replace the resected esophagus.

function and postoperative incisional pain. Respiratory function is restricted to an equal degree by a high abdominal approach, so that this objection should not affect the choice (29). Postoperative wound pain is more frequent following thoracotomy, but it can be reduced considerably by avoiding undue spreading of the wound margins, and by protecting the neuromuscular bundles during incision and retraction.

Thoracoabdominal Approach

The thoracoabdominal approach is advantageous in the patient with recurrent hiatal hernia because it allows direct dissection of the esophagus above and below the diaphragm, thus avoiding unnecessary traction and blunt manipulation (30). This approach is also valuable where a transthoracic repair is considered necessary but where, in addition, the patient requires gastric or cholecystic surgery. There are fewer indications for the approach, but when it is used it does not add significantly to the operative morbidity or mortality.

There is no single optimal surgical approach. The individual surgeon should choose an approach based on his assessment of the esophageal pathology and his own personal experience and expertise. A clearer delineation of the various indications will be reached only after careful long-term follow-up of patients and the assessment of the late results of the various operative procedures.

References

1. Hill, L. D., and Tobias, J. A.: Paraesophageal hernia. Arch. Surg., *96:* 735, 1968.
2. Ozdemir, I. A., Burke, W. A., and Ikins, P. M.: Paraesophageal hernia; a life-threatening disease. Ann. Thorac. Surg., *16:* 547, 1973.
3. Radigan, L. R., Glover, J. L., Shipley, F. E., and Shoemaker, R. E.: Barrett esophagus. Arch. Surg., *112:* 486, 1977.
4. Safaie-Shirazi, S., and Hardy, B. M.: Treatment of reflux esophagitis resulting in massive esophageal bleeding. Arch. Surg., *111:* 365, 1976.
5. Engels, E., and Reismann, B.: Bleeding from hiatal hernia. Zentralbl. Chir., *101:* 1044, 1976.
6. Clerf, L. H., Shallow, T. A., Putney, F. J., and Fry, K. E.: Esophageal hiatal hernia. J.A.M.A., *143:* 169, 1950.
7. Grimes, O. F., and Stephens, H. B.: The surgical treatment of esophageal hiatus hernia. Am. J. Surg., *94:* 194, 1957.
8. Windsor, C. W. O., and Collis, J. L.: Anaemia and hiatus hernia; experience in 450 patients. Thorax, *22:* 73, 1967.
9. Skinner, D. B., and Belsey, R. H.: Surgical management of esophageal reflux and hiatus hernia; long term results with 1030 patients. J. Thorac. Cardiovasc. Surg., *53:* 33, 1967.
10. Klotz, S. D., and Moeller, R. K.: Hiatal hernia and intractable bronchial asthma. Ann. Allergy, *29:* 325, 1971.
11. Henderson, R. D., Fung, K., Cullen, J. B., Milne, E. N. C., and Marryatt, G.: Bile aspiration; an experimental study in rabbits. Can. J. Surg., *18:* 64, 1975.

12. Gardner, A. M.: Aspiration of food and vomit. Q. J. Med., *27:* 227, 1958.
13. Barrett, N. R.: The oesophagus lined by columnar epithelium. Gastroenterologia, *86:* 183, 1956.
14. Barrett, N. R.: The lower esophagus lined by columnar epithelium. Surgery, *41:* 881, 1957.
15. Allison, P. R., and Johnstone, A. S.: The oesophagus lined with gastric mucous membrane. Thorax, *8:* 87, 1953.
16. Hamilton, S. R., and Yardley, J. H.: Regeneration of cardiac type mucosa and acquisition of Barret mucosa after esophagogastrostomy. Gastroenterology, *72:* 669, 1977.
17. Naef, A. P., Savary, M., and Ozzello, L.: Columnar-lined lower esophagus; an acquired lesion with malignant predisposition. Report on 140 cases of Barret's esophagus with 12 adenocarcinomas. J. Thorac. Cardiovasc. Surg., *70:* 826, 1975.
18. Radigan, L. R., Glober, J. L., Shipley, F. E., and Shoemaker, R. E.: Barrett esophagus. Arch. Surg., *112:* 486, 1977.
19. Mustard, R. A.: The surgical treatment of esophageal hiatus hernia. Am. J. Surg., *119:* 674, 1970.
20. Mustard, R. A.: A survey of techniques and results of hiatus hernia repair—collective review. Surg. Gynecol. Obstet., *130:* 131, 1970.
21. Hill, L. D., Tobias, J., and Morgan, E. H.: Newer concepts of the pathophysiology of hiatal hernia and esophagitis. Am. J. Surg., *111:* 70, 1966.
22. Polk, H. C.: Indications for, technique of, and results of fundoplication for complicated reflux esophagitis. Am. Surg., *44:* 620, 1978.
23. Woodward, E. R.: Surgical considerations in reflux peptic esophagitis. Front. Gastrointest. Res., *3:* 126, 1978.
24. Henderson, R. D.: The gastroplasty tube as a method of reflux control. Can. J. Surg., *21:* 264, 1978.
25. Henderson, R. D.: Reflux control following gastroplasty. Ann. Thorac. Surg., *24:* 206, 1977.
26. Vansant, J. H.: Surgical management of hiatal hernia with esophageal reflux. Am. Surg., *44:* 179, 1978.
27. Skinner, D. B., Belsey, H. R., Hendrix, J. R., and Zuidema, G. D. (Editors): *Gastroesophageal Reflux and Hiatal Hernia.* Little, Brown & Co., Boston, 1972.
28. Clarke, J. M., Rayl, J. E., and Woodward, E. R.: Experience with the Thal and Nissen operations in the treatment of reflux esophagitis with stricture; a preliminary report. Am. Surg., *35:* 89, 1969.
29. Beecher, H. K.: Effect of laparotomy on lung volume; demonstration of new type of pulmonary collapse. J. Clin. Invest., *12:* 651, 1933.
30. Collis, J. L.: A review of surgical results in hiatus hernia. Thorax, *16:* 114, 1961.

CHAPTER 9

Transabdominal Hernia Repair

Reducible Hiatal Hernia— Transabdominal Approach

The terms "reducibility" and "irreducibility" are applied to describe the position of the hernia within the thoracic cavity and the ability of the surgeon to reduce the herniated stomach below the diaphragm. In most patients a hiatal hernia can be demonstrated radiologically only by increasing the abdominal pressure. When this pressure is removed and the patient stands upright, the hernia pouch, if it is reducible, descends below the diaphragm. In some patients, however, the hernia pouch is fixed within the thoracic cavity and does not reduce even with the patient standing—a situation referred to as "radiologic irreducibility."

Radiologic irreducibility is not the same as surgical irreducibility. When he operates, the surgeon mobilizes the gastroesophageal junction and at this stage the hernia pouch can be placed below the diaphragm. Such mobilization and reduction is the cornerstone of most surgical approaches to correction of gastroesophageal reflux. A few patients remain in whom, despite mobilization, the hernia cannot be reduced. In these patients, panmural esophagitis and scar formation in the esophageal wall have fixed the hernia within the thoracic cavity and produced esophageal shortening. Of course, reducibility and nonreducibility are relative terms. In some patients complete mobilization of the esophagus may allow reduction under tension. The decision whether a hernia is surgically reducible or irreducible therefore becomes a point of debate, and at present we do not have sufficient clinical data to allow a definitive statement. For example, Hill and colleagues (1) have stated that all hernias are reducible through an abdominal approach and that all can be repaired using his methods. Belsey maintains the opposite view, believing that repair under tension predisposes to hernia recurrence (2). When he reduced the hernia and did his repair under tension, the incidence of recurrence was 45 per cent despite his great experience.

This chapter will describe the transabdominal approach to the reducible hernia, which is applicable to patients with a radiologically demonstrable hiatal hernia and those with only demonstrable reflux symptoms.

Surgical methods for the control of gastroesophageal reflux can be divided into repairs where the esophageal wall is normal, and repairs where the esophageal wall is shortened secondary to panmural esophagitis. The three major groups of transabdominal procedures are the Hill repair, the Nissen repair, and a variety of other fundoplications. Other surgical approaches may have some merit, but they have never been studied with effective follow-up, so that their long-term value remains to be established. Experimental hernia repairs have been described which use intercostal muscle or fascia lata (4) to support the gastroesophageal junction and, theoretically, they should prevent reflux, but these methods have not been widely accepted. Operations based on tissue-supporting procedures using Teflon mesh and silastic rings (5, 6) have not had an effective follow-up, and on theoretical grounds must be approached with reserve because of risk that infection and scar formation may produce esophageal obstruction. Intercostal muscle bundles have also been used to wrap lower esophagus. This method was devised to create a motor active wrap around lower esophagus. While no follow-up has been published, Demos (7) states that the results continue to be satisfactory. The Nissen and Boerema gastropexy, which tethers the stomach to the anterior abdominal wall, has been used frequently, although it has not been fully evaluated. The Hill and Nissen repairs, the gastropexy and various abdominal fundoplications will be described and evaluated in this chapter to give some perspective on their relative merits. The Allison (8, 9) repair, which can be done transabdominally, is primarily described as a thoracic approach and will be outlined in Chapter 10.

Theoretical Considerations

In patients with a reducible hiatal hernia, all operative procedures aim at producing an intra-abdominal segment of the esophagus, and most repairs combine with this some form of diaphragmatic crural repair. Many repairs add fundoplication, which wraps the fundus of stomach around the esophagus and has a dual effect; it creates an acute angle of entry of esophagus to stomach and also produces a mass of esophagus and stomach which cannot pass through the repaired hiatus.

The several repairs combine these techniques in various ways and emphasize different components of the repair in the prevention of reflux (10). Since the major source of symptoms is reflux, the major criterion for success is control of reflux, and with the control of gastroesophageal reflux, other esophageal symptoms subside. The important questions in evaluating the claims made for the various techniques are these:

1. Why does one repair successfully control reflux, while other repairs fail?
2. Does some single component of the repair effectively prevent reflux, or does the success of a repair depend purely on its ability to prevent recurrence of a hiatal hernia and to maintain an intra-abdominal segment of esophagus?
3. Is a fundoplication necessary to prevent reflux, or is its major function the addition of a mass of stomach which stabilizes the esophagus below the diaphragm?

Mechanical Properties of Hernia Repair

Prevention of recurrence requires that the esophagus be fixed permanently in its reduced position. Hill's repair tethers the esophagus to the arcuate ligament, using the phrenoesophageal ligament and adjacent fatty tissue on the lesser curvature (Fig. 9.1). The strength of these tissues may explain the success of this repair.

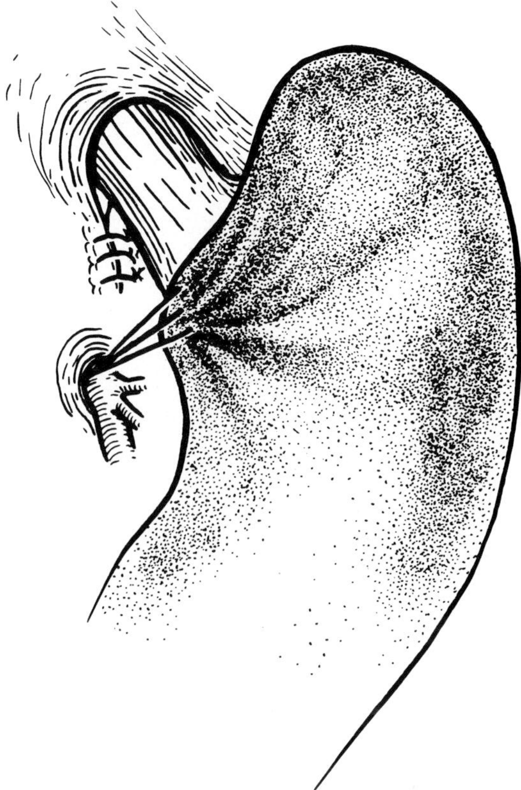

Figure 9.1
The Hill repair incorporates diaphragmatic closure with a fundoplication, tightening fundus around lower esophagus and anchoring it to the median arcuate ligament.

In the Nissen repair (Fig. 9.2) a fundoplication wraps the lower esophagus completely in gastric fundus. The sutures holding the stomach in place are anchored in gastric wall which, because of its serosal surface, holds them more effectively than would the esophagus.

Most repairs appose the diaphragmatic crura which narrow the esophageal diaphragmatic canal and prevent the esophagogastric fundoplication from slipping back into the thoracic cavity. Many procedures also anchor the fundus of stomach to the undersurface of the diaphragm. However, inherent weakness in the tissues involved reduces the security of repairs; indeed, more than any other factor, the differences between the success of various hiatal hernia repairs may reflect the relative tissue strengths of the materials used.

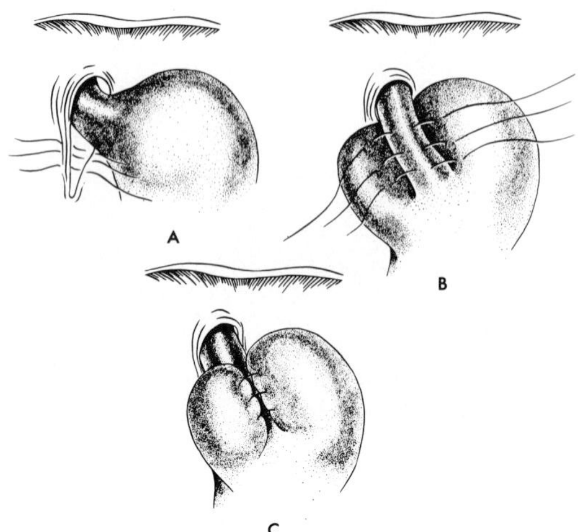

Figure 9.2. Nissen Repair
The Nissen (34) hiatal hernia repair mobilizes the esophagus and the proximal greater curvature of stomach. The diaphragmatic crura are approximated and the fundus of the stomach is then passed around the esophagus to totally envelop the distal 5 cm of esophagus.

Physiologic Effects of Hernia Repair

In reviewing the physiologic effects of hernia repair two closely related topics must be considered. Many surgeons add vagotomy (11, 12) and pyloroplasty to the hernia repair and in recent years highly selective vagotomy (HSV) (13) has also been advocated. The second consideration is division of the hepatic branch of the vagus.

Vagotomy is not indicated either in truncal form or as HSV unless there is peptic ulcer disease necessitating this addition. If the hernia repair is adequate and reflux controlled, there can be no gain from this addition. Added vagotomy exposes the patient to the risks of dumping and postvagotomy diarrhea and reduces the responsiveness of the high pressure zone (HPZ) to gastric distention. In addition, if the hepatic branch of the vagus is divided as part of a vagotomy or to gain exposure to the crura, the incidence of cholelithiasis rises (14).

Following reflux control procedures, significant changes in the HPZ have been demonstrated (15–17). These occur with the Nissen, the Hill and the Belsey Mark IV repair and are now also being documented with the Belsey gastroplasty and total fundoplication gastroplasty (TFG: Nissen gastroplasty). In discussing physiologic control of reflux (Chapter 4) I outlined the results obtained in 359 patients with TFG and 240 with follow-up manometry done 3 to 12 months after surgery. The HPZ tone rose from a preoperative level of 12.04 cm H_2O to a postoperative level of 18.35 cm H_2O—a rise of 52.41 per cent.

Similar results have been reported by other investigators and attempts made to correlate HPZ tone increase with effective reflux control. In our preoperative studies 72 (20.4 per cent) patients had a normal tone HPZ and 29 (8.2 per cent) had a high tone HPZ and yet all patients had intractable reflux unresponsive to conservative management. Although postoperatively HPZ tone was significantly increased, some remained below normal (15 to 20 cm H_2O with a water-perfused manometric catheter system). Postoperatively 71 had an HPZ tone below 15 (29.6 per cent), 99 were normal (41.2 per cent) and 70 were above normal (29.2 per cent) (Fig. 9.3) (Table 9.1). None of these patients had symptomatic reflux, none refluxed by pH study during manometry and in 335 follow-up radiologic studies none had radiologic reflux.

Results reported with the Belsey, Hill and Nissen repairs tend to be similar with all showing an increase in HPZ tone. Most likely these tone increases are the result of effective reflux control and esophageal healing.

Disordered motor activity (DMA) in the lower half of the esophagus is related, at least in part, to the damaging effects of reflux. In the group of 359 with TFG we measured preoperatively lower esophageal DMA and compared this postoperatively in the 240 patients studied. DMA was 44.7 per cent preoperatively and fell to 31.6 per cent following surgery (a decrease of 29.3 per cent). These figures are further evidence of esophageal healing following reflux control.

There is some evidence that hiatal hernia repair may "overcorrect" gastroesophageal competence; e.g., following fundoplication up to 12 per cent (18, 19) of patients cannot "burp" and complain of the "gas bloat" syndrome. This complaint usually resolves spontaneously in a few weeks, but in a few patients remains a significant problem. The inability to burp is good evidence of gas retention by an excessively competent antireflux mechanism. It has also been shown in cadaver studies that fundoplication prevents reflux

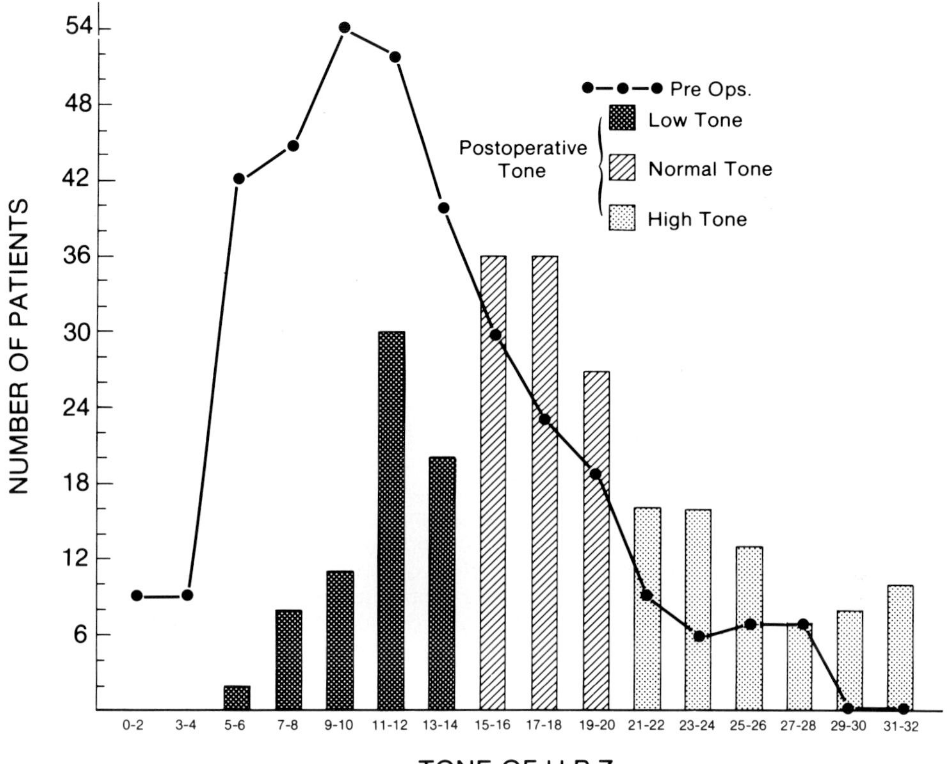

Figure 9.3. HPZ Tone in 240 Patients Before and After Total Fundoplication Gastroplasty
The pre- and postoperative HPZ pressures are displayed showing a substantial pressure increase following reflux control.

Table 9.1

HPZ Tone—Results of TFG*

HPZ Tone	Below Normal	Normal	Above Normal
	%	%	%
Preoperative	71.4	20.4	8.2
Postoperative	29.6	41.2	29.2

Average preoperative tone 12.04 cm H_2O; average postoperative tone 18.35 cm H_2O

* Preoperative and postoperative manometric studies show a major increase in HPZ tone following reflux control. Even in patient with major reflux before surgery, 28.6 per cent had a normal or high tone HPZ.

when the stomach is distended (20). These clinical and experimental findings suggest that fundoplication does play an active part in reflux control, but do not prove that this added reflux control is necessary.

The Hill, Belsey and Nissen repairs all appear to give effective control of reflux. However, we have no convincing evidence that satisfactory control must be achieved by simple creation of an intraabdominal segment of esophagus, as in the Allison repair (21). Fundoplication gives added support to the antireflux mechanism, but its main effect may be to create a more stable repair and one that is less likely to break down and produce a recurrence of reflux. As originally described, the Hill repair produces an intraabdominal segment of esophagus which, without fundoplication, effectively controls reflux. Hill's unsupported intra-abdominal segment of esophagus strongly suggests that an intra-abdominal segment alone is enough to prevent reflux.

Esophageal manometric studies in experimental animals show that a tubed segment of stomach of #50 Fr diameter has an intrinsic tone of 10 cm H_2O. A 2.5- to 6-cm segment of such a gastric tube maintained below the diaphragm will effectively control reflux in the absence of a gastroesophageal sphincter. In this situation reflux control is produced by the segment of stomach even without fundo-

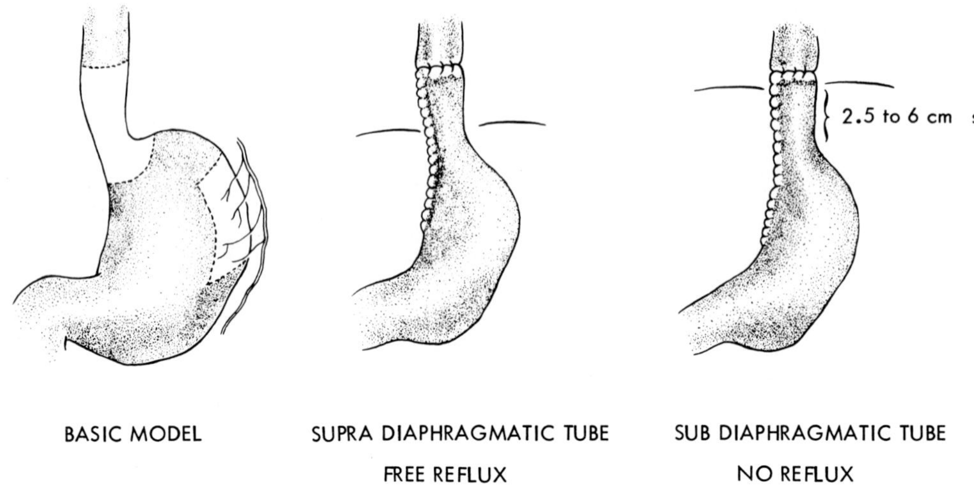

Figure 9.4. Experimental Study: Tubed Gastric Segment of Reflux Control
In this experimental study (22) the distal 5 cm of esophagus and proximal 2 cm of stomach are excised. A tube is created along the greater curvature of stomach vascularized by the short gastric vessels, and this tube is used to replace the distal esophagus. When the tubed gastric segment is totally intrathoracic, free reflux occurs, despite the presence of a constant pressure barrier of 10 to 15 cm of water in the tube. If 2.5 to 6 cm of the tube is maintained below the diaphragm, reflux is prevented.

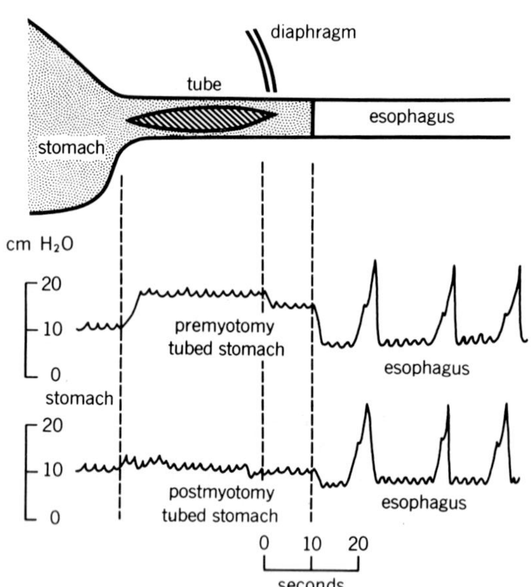

Figure 9.5. Tubed Gastric Segment and Myotomy
In this experimental study (22) a 6-cm segment of tube maintained below the diaphragm prevents reflux. This tube has a constant pressure of 10 to 15 cm of water. Myotomy, which reduces the tubal pressure to 0 cm of water, permits free reflux.

plication. However, if this segment is placed above the diaphragm, free reflux occurs (22). Reflux also occurs if this segment is myotomized and its tone reduced, even though the segment is maintained below the diaphragm (Figs. 9.4 and 9.5).

In summary, hiatal hernia repair effectively controls gastroesophageal reflux, although the exact mechanisms underlying such control have not been established. It remains to be determined whether the effectiveness of a repair depends on mechanical fixation, improvement in esophageal motor function, the addition of a fundoplication, or whether each of these factors contributes something essential (23).

Transabdominal Repair

In each transabdominal repair, the approach to and mobilization of the gastroesophageal junction are much the same. The surgeon makes a standard upper abdominal midline or left paramedian incision, conducts a general exploration of the abdomen and carefully inspects the hiatal hernia. It is customary to assess the crural margins and record the size of the esophageal hiatus. One can insert two fingers into the normal hiatus, and this space tends to increase with hernia size. In a small hiatal hernia there are no specific landmarks to mark the presence of a hernia, and the decision to operate is based on the preoperative recognition of gastroesophageal reflux.

The gastroesophageal junction is mobilized by dividing the phrenoesophageal ligament. After local dissection, a finger can be passed round the distal esophagus to draw it into the abdominal cavity. The esophagus can be mobilized further by dividing the proximal short gastric vessels on the greater curvature and the small branches of the left gastric artery to the liver on the lesser curvature. This branch of the left gastric artery runs with the hepatic branch of the vagus. Although it occasionally has to be divided, it should, if possible, be preserved as the risk of developing cholelithiasis is significantly increased (14).

Following mobilization the esophagus can be palpated and the crural margins inspected again. The surgeon can visualize and palpate the esophagus only to a limited degree and must rely on preoperative assessment to determine the degree of pathologic change. He can assess esophageal reducibility at this stage and also the degree of thickening and vascularity of the accessible intrathoracic esophagus.

Hill Repair

The Hill repair consists of two steps (Fig. 9.1). The arcuate ligament is carefully identified at the points where the diaphragmatic crura divide. He identifies the celiac axis to avoid damaging it during suturing. Sutures will be placed from the phrenoesophageal ligament to the arcuate ligament but, before that step, reducibility is carefully assessed. If necessary, and to improve reducibility, the surgeon may perform a truncal vagotomy and an associated pyloroplasty. In the presence of panmural esophagitis, some added esophageal length can be obtained by dividing the vagal nerve.

The diaphragmatic crura are approximated with interrupted sutures. The main sutures to the phrenoesophageal ligament are now placed by rotating the gastroesophageal junction to expose both the anterior and posterior aspects of the lesser curvature and phrenoe-sophageal ligament. The sutures, which are inserted first in the anterior phrenoesophageal ligament, transfix the serosa and muscular layers of the stomach, then pass through the posterior phrenoesophageal ligament. These sutures are now anchored to the arcuate ligament. One or two more stitches are placed, then tied in such a way as to hold a 3-cm segment of esophagus below the diaphragm.

Two sutures are placed to anchor the gastric fundus to the lateral esophageal wall, increasing the gastroesophageal junctional angle. Hill asserts that the angle is unimportant, but these final sutures keep the stomach from herniating through the now-approximated diaphragmatic crura.

Intraoperative Manometry

Hill has pioneered a technique of intraoperative manometry (24–27) which he feels is of critical importance in correcting reflux. This method has been used in 200 patients with gastroesophageal reflux. The lower esophageal sphincter pressure is measured before surgery. His repair is then carried out and the fundoplication sutures, which approximate anterior and posterior seromuscular layers on the esophagogastric junction are sutured but not tied. The sutures are then tied under manometric control and the tension increased until a manometric reading of 50 to 57 cm H_2O is obtained. Postoperatively pressures of 15 to 25 cm H_2O result from this degree of tension. In follow-up evaluation including reflux testing no patient with a postoperative HPZ tone above 15 cm H_2O has been shown to have reflux.

Other reports of this technique are now available; however, long-term assessment of its value is still lacking. The critical postoperative pressure of 15 cm H_2O certainly does not apply to Nissen fundoplication, as in my experience 29.5 per cent of 240 patients studied following TFG had mean pressures below 15 cm H_2O and none of those had reflux. The Nissen wrap does create a flap valve mechanism transmitting gastric pressure to esophagus, and this may protect against reflux in the presence of a low tone sphincter which could in part account for the difference. Certainly with a Nissen type of wrap this method of intraoperative recording seems to have little value.

Orringer et al. (28) have used the same method in studying their patients with Nissen gastroplasty and find that the data obtained have no statistical relevance. Cooper (29) has used the method with the Belsey gastroplasty and reports that the data obtained are not statistically valid.

Recognizing that the esophagus is extensively handled and mobilized, the patient is anesthetized and narcotized and has a varying level of induced paralysis necessary for abdominal surgery, I find it very hard to believe that muscle tone can be recorded reproducably. Reproducability with manometry is very difficult in the conscious patient and varies from system to system. When one adds the variables of anesthesia I would feel that the data obtained at most measures the degree of lumen constriction produced by tightening the final fundoplication sutures. This pressure then abruptly and without explanation changes postoperatively.

Results of the Hill Repair

As mentioned previously, Hill claims that, using his method of repair and the transabdominal approach, all hiatal hernias are reducible. This operation has been in use since 1959. After an 8-year follow-up of 149 patients, Hill reported no recurrences and 96.7 per cent good or excellent results (30). In 36 patients with peptic stricture, who usually have panmural esophagitis and shortening, he categorized the results in 30 (83.3 per cent) (31) as good or excellent. Within 6 months of surgical correction these patients no longer required bouginage, indicating that the stricture had resolved after correction of reflux. In some of these patients Hill added vagotomy and pyloroplasty, which further frees the lower esophagus and allows easier reduction of the hernia.

Although the results reported for this operation are excellent, further follow-up is clearly necessary to establish its long-term value. We require further experience particularly in those patients with peptic stricture. The overall incidence of successful repair (83.3 per cent) for the Hill operation is not as high as that reported for gastroplasty.

In 1976 Hill (25) reported that 511 patients had been treated surgically with 5 anatomic recurrences. Reflux was present in 6 per cent of the last 100 patients. The improvement in

his results he relates to the use of intraoperative manometry.

Other authors have variable results with the Hill repair recording anatomic recurrences of up to 23 per cent (32, 33) with symptomatic recurrence of 18 per cent and esophagitis of 9 per cent. This particular report is a long-term follow-up (maximum 8 years) and includes 65 patients. The unsatisfactory results were reported in patients with complicated disease such as Barrett's esophagus, alkaline reflux from previous gastric surgery or recurrence from previous hiatal hernia repair. The high incidence of recurrence can easily be accounted for by the use of a transabdominal repair without esophageal lengthening in this type of disease. This same experience has been reported by Hill in that good or excellent results were obtained in only 83.3 per cent using his repair in patients with esophagitis and shortening.

The success of the Hill repair seems to depend more on the strong mechanical fixation of the esophagogastric junction to the arcuate ligament. Although Hill stresses the importance of intraoperative manometry, the pressures he is recording are very similar to those obtained with successful repairs using any of the standard transabdominal approaches and most likely would occur whether or not manometry was used intraoperatively.

Nissen Fundoplication

The Nissen fundoplication (Fig. 9.2) uses the same approach and mobilization as the Hill repair except that it may divide more of the short gastric vessels to obtain adequate mobilization of the gastric fundus. The diaphragmatic crura are approximated with interrupted sutures. Gastric fundus is then rolled around the esophagus, bringing the fundus behind and then forward at the lesser curvature. Three or more sutures are now placed from the seromuscular layer of stomach, through the muscular esophagus and to the rolled portion of stomach on the lesser curve. When these sutures are tied, the esophagus is completely surrounded by a tube of stomach, is anchored below the diaphragm by the stomach mass and cannot pass through the sutured crura (34).

This method of repair, which has been widely practiced, apparently gives satisfactory clinical results. After repair some patients complain of dysphagia; hence the surgeon must take care not to narrow the distal esophagus by the gastric wrap. At the time of fundoplication, a #50 Fr Malloney bougie can be passed through the esophagus to avoid narrowing the esophageal lumen. The surgeon must also take care to fully mobilize the gastric fundus because, without this, the wrap may be done under tension, again producing dysphagia. The dysphagia problem undoubtedly can be produced by a tight wrap; however, the length of the wrap may be of equal importance. Technical details of the method of wrap will be described in the section on total fundoplication gastroplasty.

As noted earlier, by its excessive competence, this operation may produce the "gas bloat" syndrome in up to 12 per cent of patients, but this complaint usually resolves gradually over a few months. Mild dysphagia has been reported in 16 per cent of patients but is a persistent problem in only 2 per cent (18). A 7 per cent recurrence rate has been reported—a result which is comparable to that approached by similar operative approaches.

Recurrence of Standard Nissen

The Nissen procedure is one of the most popular now in use, and it has been documented as being the most effective in reflux control. As has been shown with the results of TFG, the HPZ pressure rises significantly; however, with the method of fundoplication, a new element of reflux control is introduced. Because of the total wrap any increase in gastric pressure will completely surround the lower esophagus, and this transmitted pressure accounts for the efficacy of the procedure. As will be noted later, the fundoplication may slip into the chest and still maintain competence because of its flap valve mechanism.

There are certain specific problems with the Nissen procedure (35, 36) which have not been resolved. The inability to burp or vomit is reported in some series. This difficulty is variable and even when present may be a minor complaint. Gas bloat—which is a term used for early satiety and fullness—can occur with any procedure but is most common after the Nissen. Recently, a higher incidence of

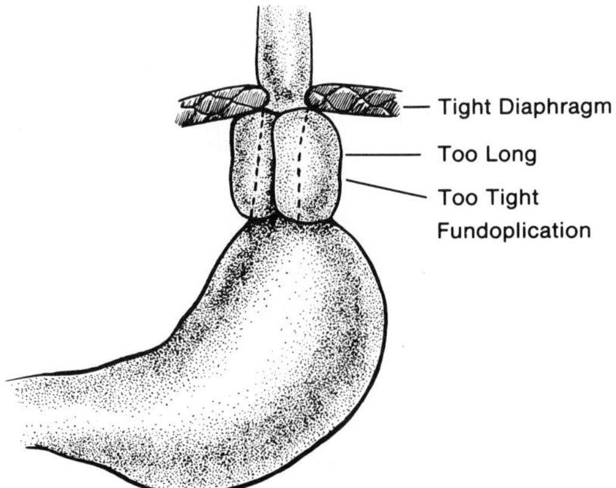

Figure 9.6. Standard Nissen—Tight Repair
A tight Nissen repair is difficult to diagnose clinically. Tightness may be due to diaphragmatic narrowing or a tight fundoplication. Too long a fundoplication is probably the most common cause of dysphagia following Nissen wrap.

gastric ulceration (37, 38) has been reported; however, the reporting is not yet sufficient to indicate that this is a major problem.

In my experience the biggest difficulty with the Nissen procedure is to recognize when anatomic recurrence has taken place. There are three specific problems which can be differentiated:
   a) Tight repair (39, 40)
   b) En mass recurrence with wrap intact or with wrap breakdown
   c) Intussusception recurrence (Fig. 9.7)

The tight repair may be caused by too tight a fundoplication, too tight a diaphragmatic closure or may also be due to too long a wrap. Too long a wrap produces a degree of competence which prevents both food descent and reflux.

Case 1. Mr. M., age 41, had a transabdominal Nissen fundoplication 1½ years before he was seen for evaluation. Dysphagia preoperatively had been mild and intermittent; however, postoperatively it became constant and occurred with both liquids and solids. Regurgitation occurred intermittently, and he required endoscopy for food impaction on three occasions.

He had been bougienaged to #60 Fr on six occasions with slight improvement for 2 to 3 days followed by recurrence of symptoms. During this time he lost 30 pounds in weight.

Past radiologic studies were considered normal. At the time of bougienage no resistance was felt to the passage of the bougie. He was referred because

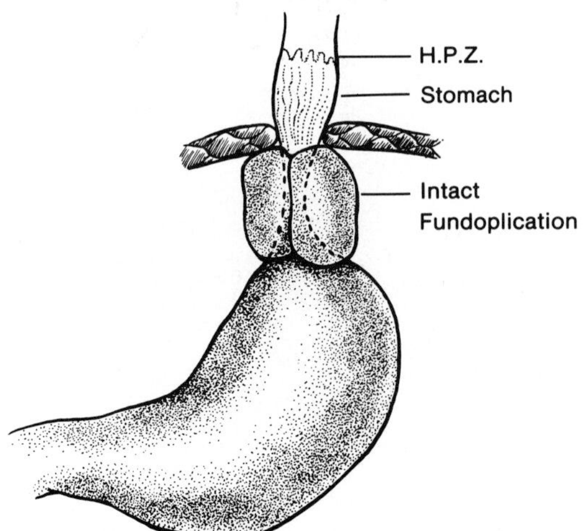

Figure 9.7. Standard Nissen—Intussusception Recurrence
Intussusception recurrence is rare and difficult to diagnose. Fundus of stomach becomes detached from lower esophagus and the esophagogastric junction then migrates through the fundoplication. Since the stomach is bulky it becomes progressively compressed by the fundoplication, producing dysphagia.

of difficulty in diagnosis and his marked weight loss.

Manometric studies showed no evidence of hernia recurrence and the HPZ tone was high normal (25 cm H_2O). Endoscopy was normal apart from some residual mucus in the esophagus and mild inflammatory changes at the gastroesophageal junction. Radiology with liquids was normal showing no evidence of recurrence or reflux. When he was given a barium sandwich it obstructed at the gastroesophageal junction and was regurgitated (Fig. 9.8).

The history and findings are classical for a tight repair either at the level of the diaphragm or in the Nissen fundoplication. His fundoplication was not tight and was of normal length at the time of thoracoabdominal rerepair. The diaphragmatic crura were too tight, and part of this was due to suture reaction with local small, sterile abscesses.

This patient illustrates all the problems of a tight repair. Tightness is not usually recognizable endoscopically or radiologically unless solids are swallowed. Since the constricting force is muscle, it stretches open with the passage of a #60 bougie, but the muscle fibers are not disrupted and will close down shortly after the bougie is removed. Improvement following bougienage lasts 2 to 3 days only.

En mass recurrence of a standard Nissen is not uncommon. Some of these patients remain asymptomatic if the fundoplication is intact as with this method of wrap reflux is well controlled. Even with reflux control and an intact en mass recurrence I have had patients who developed dysphagia, postprandial fullness and nausea. When recurrence develops and the fundoplication breaks down, patients usually develop symptomatic reflux similar to their preoperative condition.

Intussusception recurrence is the most difficult to diagnose; however, the following patient illustrates the problem well.

Case 2. Mrs. P., age 53. This patient had a transabdominal Nissen fundoplication for reflux. She had minor postoperative difficulties but then progressed well for 6 months. At that time she developed progressive dysphagia, initially to solids and later to both liquids and solids. I examined her at the time when her dysphagia was intermittent and not too severe. Manometrically her HPZ tone was high normal at 22 cm H_2O. Radiologically she was normal including studies with a barium sandwich. Endoscopy was normal and she was bougienaged to #60 Fr with temporary relief. Over the next 3 months her symptoms became progressively more severe, and she was reduced to a liquid diet. Radiologically it was now possible to show solid food obstruction; however, liquid barium studies were normal. Endoscopically gastric mucosa was visible above the point of competence.

A thoracoabdominal TFG was performed, and she had a typical intussusception Nissen recurrence. The fundoplication was intact; however, stomach was pushing through the fundoplication and into the chest. Since the stomach is bulky it becomes progressively compressed and the patient develops a "motor obstruction" only temporarily helped by bougienage.

These three types of Nissen recurrence must be recognized as they can give rise to major symptoms unresponsive to conservative management. Many patients are left without effective treatment because of failure in diagnosis. The main points of differentiation are outlined in Table 9.2.

Variations on the Nissen

Variations have been described in the Nissen (41, 42) fundoplication technique where instead of the full fundoplication the zone of fundol approximation is reduced to 1 cm or less. This procedure has theoretical advantages in that reflux control may be accom-

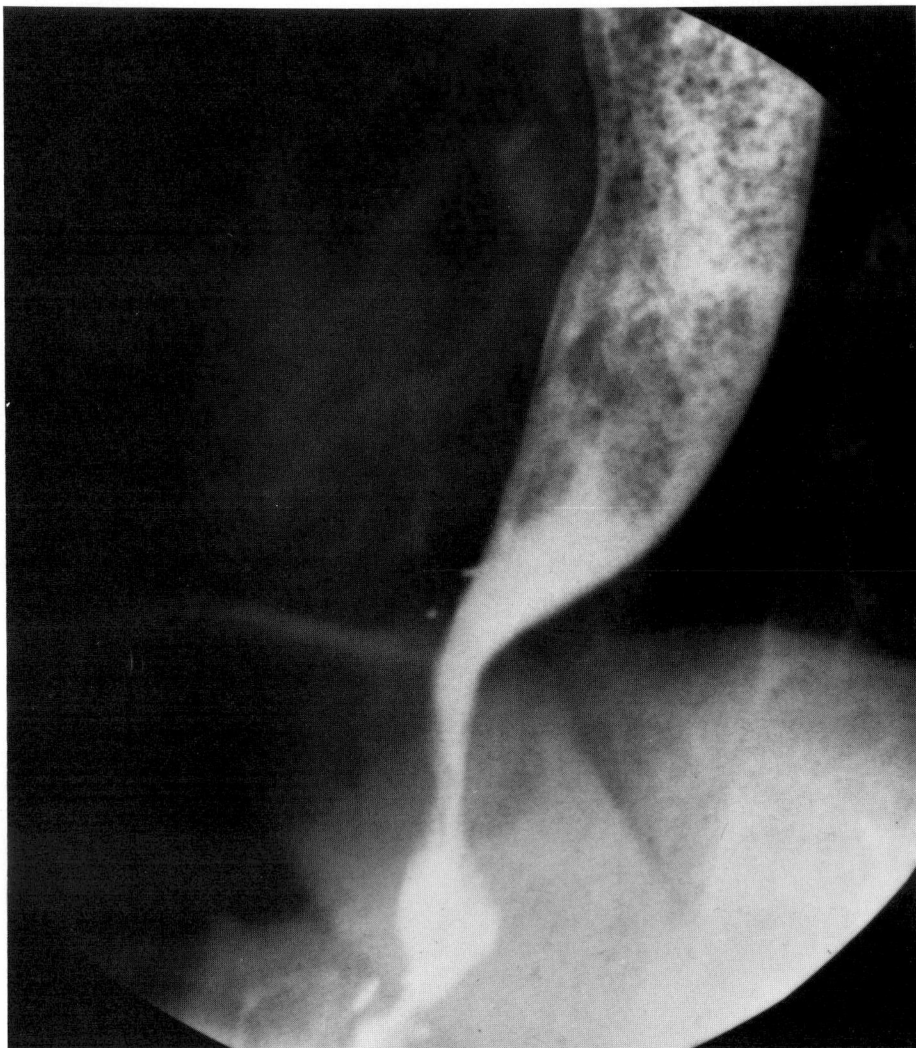

Figure 9.8
Obstruction from a tight repair or intussusception recurrence may be difficult to diagnose. The liquid barium swallow may be normal; however, when a barium sandwich is added, obstruction can be demonstrated.

plished without as much risk of dysphagia, difficulty in burping and inability to vomit. There are no long-term studies with this procedure and one would anticipate the usual recurrence rate of 10 to 20 per cent in experienced hands.

Other Fundoplication Procedures

Several operations achieve control of reflux by combining diaphragmatic repair and fundoplication (Fig. 9.9). The chief difference between these various procedures is the design of the fundoplication; the procedure used most commonly follows closely the technique of Belsey's fundoplication, wrapping the stomach around the anterior half or two-thirds of the esophagus.

Mobilizing the esophagus for this repair follows the methods previously described (43). The gastric fat pad should be carefully removed. Posterior crural sutures are placed and tied following completion of the fundoplication. The fundoplication, which is begun along the left lateral wall of esophagus, employs three layers of three sutures that approximate the seromuscular coat of stomach to the muscular coat of the esophagus. A final

Table 9.2
Nissen Recurrence—Investigative Findings*

Nissen Recurrence	Onset Symptoms	Dominant Symptom	Manometry HPZ	Liquid Radiology	Solid Radiology	Endoscopy	Bougienage
Intact fundo-plication	Delayed	Nil	Normal	Recurrence	Recurrence	Recurrence	
Breakdown fundopli-cation	Delayed	Reflux	Low tone	Recurrence	Recurrence	Recurrence	
Tight repair	Immediate	Dysphagia	High tone	Normal	Obstruction	Normal	Transient relief
Intususscep-tion recur-rence	Delayed	Dysphagia	High tone	Normal	Obstruction	Normal	Transient relief

* Using history, radiology, manometry and endoscopy it is possible to differentiate between a tight repair, intussusception or anatomic recurrence.

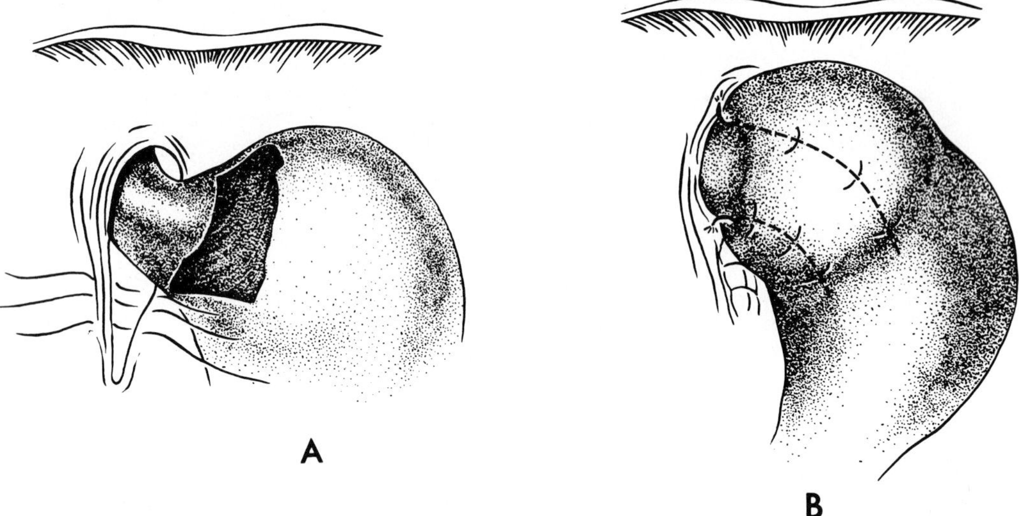

Figure 9.9. Standard Fundoplication
Reducible hiatal hernia is treated by standard transabdominal fundoplication (44), a common form of hernia repair. Following mobilization and removal of the esophagogastric fat pad, the operator approximates the diaphragmatic crura and does a two-thirds anterior fundoplication. The stomach is then sutured to the undersurface of the diaphragm.

layer of sutures from stomach to diaphragm gives added strength to the repair.

This abdominal approach, which has the features of a Nissen fundoplication but avoids the total wrap of stomach around esophagus, is reported to give satisfactory results. Mustard (44) described 97 such patients whom he had followed up for 3 to 10 years. Of this group, 58 (60 per cent) had other abdominal pathology, e.g., duodenal ulcer or gallstones, which was corrected as part of the operation. Sixty-eight patients had good or excellent results and 19 had fair or poor results. (Ten were lost to follow-up). The patients with fair or poor results had such complaints as post-vagotomy diarrhea, persistence of symptoms and, in four (5 per cent), anatomic recurrence.

This result (5 per cent recurrence) compares favorably with results reported for the Nissen and the Hill repairs; however, this operative approach needs more extensive study before a final judgment can be rendered.

Gastropexy

As an approach to hernia repair, gastropexy is unique because it incorporates none

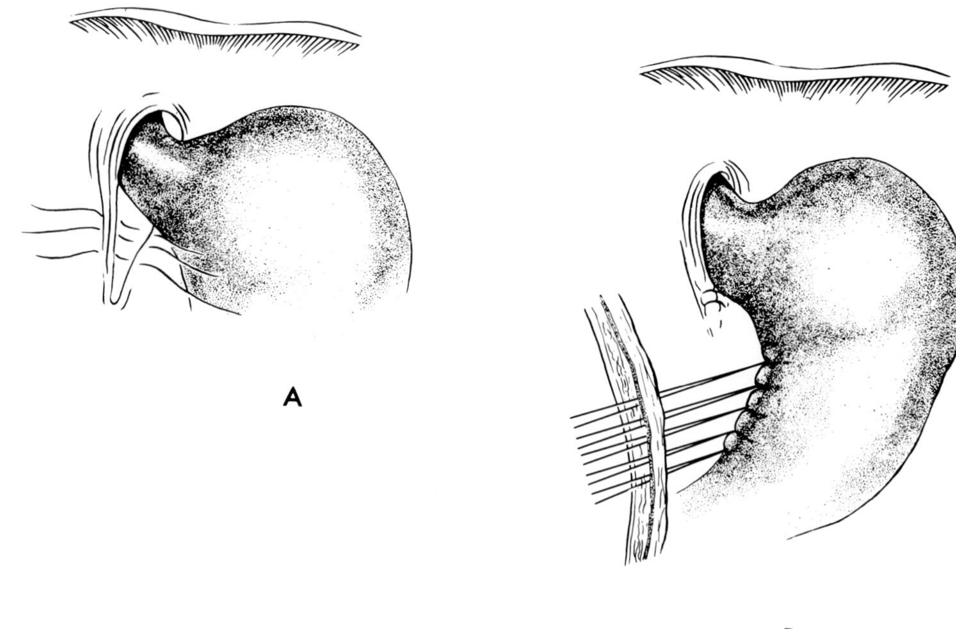

Figure 9.10. Gastropexy
Gastropexy, as described by Boerema (49), incorporates mobilization and repair of the diaphragmatic crura, with suturing of the lesser curvature of stomach to the anterior abdominal wall.

of the principles of other abdominal repairs (Fig. 9.10). This operation can be done by simple fixation of the lesser curvature of stomach to the anterior abdominal wall or with the addition of a diaphragmatic crural repair (45, 46).

When the crura are not being repaired, the stomach is drawn down into the abdominal cavity, thus reducing the hiatal hernia by traction. Silk sutures are placed from the lesser curvature of stomach to the anterior abdominal wall above the left lobe of liver. During this suturing constant tension is used to maintain hernia reduction. In 65 patients followed up for 2 months to 4 years, Ziperman and Lau (47) reported a recurrence of symptoms in 6.6 per cent. This recurrence rate is high in view of the short follow-up and the lack of documented follow-up investigation (48).

Boerema (49) has described a more exacting operative repair in which he dissects and mobilizes the hiatal area and adds a crural repair. He studied 500 cases between 1952 and 1969. In a paper describing 100 of these patients, he reported that 5 per cent had a recurrent hernia. His mortality rate was 1 per cent, but no deaths were directly related to operative complications.

These various operations—namely, the Nissen, Hill, abdominal fundoplication and gastropexy—are among those commonly used for transabdominal hernia repair. At first glance it would seem simple to compare morbidity, mortality and recurrence rates of each and then to choose one operative approach. Unfortunately the method of reporting data varies greatly from one study to another and the duration and thoroughness of follow-up also vary. For this reason it is difficult to answer satisfactorily the question What is the best abdominal hernia repair? The answer must depend upon continued follow-up of patients treated by the various procedures and development of criteria to chart symptomatic and anatomic recurrence. In such a review, repairs with each technique which fail must be analyzed and described with the same clarity and detail as the earlier successes.

References

1. Hill, L. D., Tobias, J., and Morgan, E. H.: Newer concepts of the pathophysiology of hiatal hernia and esophagitis. Am. J. Surg., *111:* 70, 1966.

2. Skinner, D. B., Belsey, H. R., Hendrix, J. R., and Zuidema, G. D. (Editors): *Gastroesophageal Reflux and Hiatal Hernia.* Little, Brown & Co., Boston, 1972.

3. Demos, N. J., Timmes, J. J., and DiBianco, J.: Experimental study of a new operation for the treatment of reflux esophagitis. J. Thorac. Cardiovasc. Surg., *54:* 832, 1967.

4. Brain, R. H. F., and Maynard, J.: Fascia lata graft repair of esophageal hiatal hernia. Am. J. Surg., *115:* 488, 1968.

5. Merendino, K. A., and Dillard, D. H.: Permanent fixation by Teflon mesh of the size of the esophageal diaphragmatic aperture in hiatus hernioplasty; a concept in repair. Am. J. Surg., *110:* 416, 1965.

6. Angelchik, J. P., and Cohen, R.: A new surgical procedure for the treatment of gastroesophageal reflux and hiatal hernia. Surg. Gynecol. Obstet., *148:* 246, 1979.

7. Demos, N.: Personal communication.

8. Allison, P. R.: Hiatus hernia; a 20 year retrospective survey. Ann. Surg., *178:* 273, 1973.

9. Gardner, R. J., Bonnabeau, R. C., and Warden, H. E.: Surgical repair of gastroesophageal reflux with sliding hiatal hernia. Am. J. Surg., *133:* 554, 1977.

10. Henderson, R. D.: Gastroesophageal junction in hiatus hernia. Can. J. Surg., *15:* 63, 1972.

11. Jones, N. A., and Anders, C. J.: A new approach to the surgical treatment of reflux oesophagitis. Ann. R. Coll. Surg. Engl., *61:* 48, 1979.

12. Angorn, I. B., Dimopoulos, G., Hegarty, M. M., and Moshal, M. G.: The effect of vagotomy on the lower oesophageal sphincter; a manometric study. Br. J. Surg., *64:* 466, 1977.

13. Jordan, P. H., Jr.: Parietal cell vagotomy facilitates fundoplication in the treatment of reflux esophagitis. Surg. Gynecol. Obstet., *147:* 593, 1978.

14. Csendes, A., Larach, J., and Godoy, M.: Incidence of gallstones development after selective hepatic vagotomy. Acta Chir. Scand., *144:* 289, 1978.

15. Lind, J. F., Burns, C. M., and MacDougall, J. T.: "Physiological" repair for hiatus hernia—manometric study. Arch. Surg., *91:* 233, 1965.

16. Moran, J. M., Pihl, C. O., Norton, R. A., and Rheinlander, H. F.: The hiatal hernia-reflux complex; current approaches to correction and evaluation of results. Am. J. Surg., *121:* 403, 1971.

17. Henderson, R. D., Mugashe, F., Jeejeebhoy, K. N., Cullen, J., Boszko, A., Szczepanski, M., and Marryatt, G.: The motor-defect of esophagitis. Can. J. Surg., *17:* 112, 1974.

18. Woodward, E. R., Rayl, J. E., and Clarke, J. M.: Esophageal hiatus hernia. Curr. Probl. Surg., *1:* 62, 1970.

19. Clarke, J. M., Rayl, J. E., and Woodward, E. R.: Experience with the Thal and Nissen operations in the treatment of reflux esophagitis with stricture; a preliminary report. Am. Surg., *35:* 89, 1969.

20. Watkins, D. H., Prevedel, A., and Harper, F. R.: A method of preventing peptic esophagitis following esophagogastrostomy: experimental and clinical study. J. Thorac. Surg., *28:* 367, 1954.

21. Allison, P. R.: Reflux esophagitis, sliding hiatal hernia, and the anatomy of repair, Surg. Gynecol. Obstet., *92:* 419, 1951.

22. Henderson, R. D., Boszko, A., Mugashe, F., Szczepanski, M. M., and Marryatt, G.: Oesophageal replacement by a gastric tube: an experimental study of the properties of the gastric tube. Br. J. Surg., *61:* 533, 1974.

23. DeMeester, T. R., Johnson, L. F., and Kent, A. H.: Evaluation of current operations for the prevention of gastroesophageal reflux. Ann. Surg., *180:* 511, 1974.

24. Hill, L. D., Gelfand, M., and Peters, W. R.: Intraoperative measurement of lower esophageal sphincter pressure (Abstract). Gastroenterology, *66:* 711, 1974.

25. Sabiston, D. C., and Spencer, F. C.: Technique of Hill, in *Gibbon's Surgery of the Chest,* 3rd Ed. W. B. Saunders, Philadelphia, 1976.

26. Christie, D. L., Mack, D. V., Parker, A. F., Hall, D. G., and Cahill, J. L.: Use of intraoperative esophageal manometrics in surgical treatment of gastroesophageal reflux in pediatric patients. J. Pediatr. Surg., *13:* 648, 1978.

27. Hill, L. D.: Intraoperative measurement of lower esophageal sphincter pressure. J. Thorac. Cadiovasc. Surg., *75:* 378, 1978.

28. Orringer, M. B., Schneider, R., Williams, G., and Sloan, H.: Intraoperative esophageal manometry; is it valid? Presented at 16th Annual Meeting, Society of Thoracic Surgeons, Jan. 1980.

29. Cooper, J. C.: Personal communication.

30. Hill, L. D.: An effective operation for hiatal hernia; an eight-year appraisal. Ann. Surg., *166:* 681, 1967.

31. Hill, L. D., Gelfand, M., and Bauermeister, D.: Simplified management of reflux esophagitis with stricture. Ann. Surg., *172:* 638, 1970.

32. Chappell, J. S.: The surgical management of chalasia of the esophagus. S. Afr. Med. J., *53:* 17, 1978.

33. Maher, J. W., Hollenbeck, J. I., and Woodward, E. R.: An analysis of recurrent esophagitis following posterior gastropexy. Ann. Surg., *187:* 227, 1978.

34. Polk, H. C., and Zeppa, R.: Fundoplication for complicated hiatal hernia; rationale and results. Ann. Thorac. Surg., *7:* 202, 1969.

35. Euler, A. R., Funkalsrud, E. W., and Ament, M. E.: Effect of Nissen fundoplication on the lower esophageal pressure of children with gastroesophageal reflux. Gastroenterology, *72:* 260, 1977.

36. Bushkin, F. L., Neustein, C. L., Parker, T. H., and Woodward, E. R.: Nissen fundoplication for reflux peptic esophagitis. Ann. Surg., *185:* 672, 1977.

37. Bremner, C. G.: Gastric ulcer after the Nissen fundoplication; a complication of alkaline reflux. S. Afr. Med. J., *51:* 791, 1977.

38. Bremner, C. G.: Gastric ulceration after a fundoplication operation for gastroesophageal reflux. Surg. Gynecol. Obstet., *148:* 62, 1979.

39. Henderson, R. D.: Hiatal hernia repair; problems of recurrence and continued symptoms. Ann. Thorac. Surg., *28:* 587, 1979.

40. Saik, R. P., Greenburg, A. G., and Peskin, G. W.: A study of fundoplication disruption and deformity. Am. J. Surg., *134:* 19, 1977.

41. Mullen, T. J., Burke, E. L., and Diamond, A. B.: Esophagogastric fistula. A complication of combined operations for esophageal disease. Arch. Surg., *110:* 826, 1975.

42. Menguy, R.: A modified fundoplication which preserves the ability to belch. Surgery, *84:* 301, 1978.
43. Mustard, R. A.: A survey of techniques and results of hiatus hernia repair. Surg. Gynecol. Obstet., *130:* 131, 1970.
44. Mustard, R. A.: The surgical treatment of esophageal hiatus hernia. Am. J. Surg., *119:* 674, 1970.
45. Ziperman, H. H., Mathewson, C., Jr., Stanek, R. G., and Brugger, A. M.: Hiatal hernia repair by intraperitoneal gastric fixation. Surg. Gynecol. Obstet., *116:* 608, 1963.
46. Zeifer, H. D.: Gastropexy-gastrostomy; use in poor risk elderly patients with symptomatic esophageal hiatus hernia. Am. J. Surg., *116:* 472, 1968.
47. Ziperman, H. H., and Lau, B. M. K.: A four-year reappraisal of hiatus hernia repair by intraperitoneal gastric fixation. Am. J. Surg., *110:* 903, 1965.
48. Mathewson, C., and Lindyberg, K. R.: Further experience with anterior gastric fixation in the management of hiatal hernia. Am. J. Surg., *134:* 102, 1977.
49. Boerema, I.: Hiatus hernia; repair by right-sided subhepatic gastropexy. Surgery, *65:* 884, 1969.

CHAPTER 10

Reducible Hiatal Hernia: Transthoracic Repair

Current judgments concerning the techniques and results expected from an operative procedure depend to a large degree upon the quality of the follow-up reported by the surgeons who developed the operation. In this respect the best reported hiatal hernia repair is the Belsey procedure, and as such it is the criterion against which all others are measured. Belsey has developed his operation, carried out a large series of repairs and carefully refrained from reporting his results until several years had elapsed and the technique could be fully evaluated.

Operative Technique (Belsey Mark IV)

A left thoracotomy gives excellent exposure of the whole length of the intrathoracic esophagus (1–3). The esophagus is mobilized by dividing the inferior pulmonary ligament to the level of the inferior pulmonary vein, which is marked by a constant lymph node at its inferior margin. The pleural margins of the ligament are separated and lifted forward to develop a relatively avascular plane through which it is possible to lift the esophagus and vagi from the pericardium and pleura medially, and the aorta laterally. Once the surgeon has dissected around the esophagus and has preserved the pleura, he can mobilize the esophagus on its pericardial and right pleural surfaces as high as the aortic arch. The blood supply to the esophagus can be preserved along its aortic attachments from the level of the inferior pulmonary vein proximally; however, more extensive mobilization is recommended by Belsey.

The fundus of the stomach is now mobilized in the following simple steps. (This technique is simple once fully understood, but always presents difficulties to the trainee.)

The esophagus is gently pulled proximally, using a sponge and hand control with a Babcock on the diaphragmatic crural rim. This movement exposes the pleural and peritoneal surfaces anteriorly, which can be divided by sharp dissection. The surgeon often opens directly on the anterior esophagogastric fat pad, but can avoid this by opening slightly more to the medial (pericardial) side, allowing more direct access to the abdominal cavity.

Once the peritoneum is open, the left middle finger is inserted into the abdominal cavity and, with the index finger in the thoracic cavity, the vagal nerve is palpated above and below the diaphragm and its course traced down the lesser curvature of the stomach. Holding the vagus to the esophagus, the surgeon by sharp dissection opens the pericardial aspect of the phrenoesophageal ligament and enters the lesser sac posteriorly. Once appreciated, this maneuver is simple to carry out and avoids all risk to the vagus.

The fundus of the stomach is now drawn into the chest. The vagus on the greater curvature can be readily palpated and a finger can be passed across the vagus to lift forward the fatty tissue and the short gastric vessels which run to the lower esophagus and the esophagogastric fat pad. This tissue is divided between clamps and ligated (Fig. 10.1).

Using this technique, both vagi can be carefully preserved and the entire esophagus can be mobilized in a few minutes. After mobilization the anterior esophagogastric fat pad is removed.

Start the repair by placing through the posterior crural heavy silk sutures which will be tied at the end of the procedure. These sutures should be placed deeply in muscle and tied so as to give approximation only; this avoids the temptation to tie the sutures tightly and thus produce tissue necrosis. The

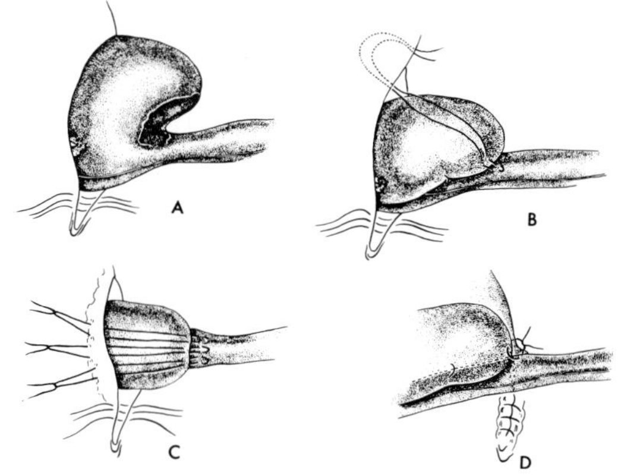

Figure 10.1. Belsey Repair
The Belsey hiatal hernia repair consists of mobilization, repair and fundoplication. The fundus of stomach is brought up into the chest (A), with preservation of the vagi and removal of the gastric fat pad. Posterior crural sutures are placed to be tied later. Fundus is now sutured to the distal 4 to 5 cm of esophagus in two layers, and the proximal sutures are passed through the diaphragm (B and C). Following reduction, the diaphragmatic sutures and the esophagogastro-diaphragmatic sutures are tied to hold the distal esophagus below the diaphragm and narrow the esophageal hiatus (D).

fundus is now wrapped carefully around the distal 5 cm of esophagus by two layers of interrupted mattress sutures. The proximal sutures pass from esophagus to stomach and then pass through the anterior crural rim. The hernia is reduced, the anterior and posterior crural sutures are tied, and the repair is complete.

Although various modifications of the Belsey repair have been described, none has had adequate follow-up, and, until we have such evaluation, the results of these procedures must be measured against the success of the original Belsely Mark IV repair.

In 1967, Belsey reported his follow-up on 632 patients (1) after the Mark IV hernia repair, with 85 per cent having relief of symptoms and anatomic correction. Symptomatic and anatomic recurrence occurred in 5.6 per cent and asymptomatic anatomic recurrence in 1.4 per cent. Four per cent had a poor symptomatic result but no recurrence, and seven patients died during or immediately after the repair (1.2 per cent).

In 1972, Belsey's experience had grown to 848 patients (4–6); by this time the mortality rate was 1 per cent and the recurrence rate

was 11.5 per cent. This increase in recurrences is disappointing, but since his original 632 patients now have a follow-up of more than 5 years and 272 of these patients have been followed up more than 10 years, this new level (11.5 per cent) may represent the recurrence rate to be anticipated in other major studies when they reach maturity.

Hiebert and O'Mara (7) report a 20-year follow-up of 282 patients treated by Belsey Mark IV. Their evaluation is by history and patient written response with 95 per cent follow-up. Their operative mortality was 0.8 per cent. Eighty per cent of patients were satisfied with the operative result, 15 per cent reported fair results and 5 per cent poor results. In those with 20 years follow-up optimum results were achieved in only 70.8 per cent.

This method of follow-up does not review the incidence of anatomic recurrence; however, it is a good method of evaluating patient response.

Nissen Repair

The other major transthoracic procedure, the Nissen repair (8–10), was described earlier as an abdominal repair. The Nissen fundoplication can be used both in reducible and irreducible hiatal hernias (Fig. 10.2).

The basic approach and mobilization is identical to that used for the Belsey repair. Mobilization preserves the vagi, and the anterior fat pad may or may not be removed. The fundus of the stomach is now rolled completely around the esophagus and fixed by three sutures, which go from seromuscular stomach, through muscular esophagus to seromuscular stomach. Mobilization must be adequate and a #50 Fr. bougie is placed in the esophageal lumen to prevent too tight a repair. An excessively tight repair is a surgical disaster, because unlike scar tissue muscle cannot be stretched permanently by bouginage. The dysphagia which accompanies a too tight repair can usually be corrected only by reoperation.

Following fundoplication the hernia is reduced and the posterior crural sutures, previously placed, are tied to approximate the crural margins.

The Nissen repair has been shown to be the most effective in reflux control (11–13). It's major problems are related to gas bloat, which has been reported in up to 13 per cent

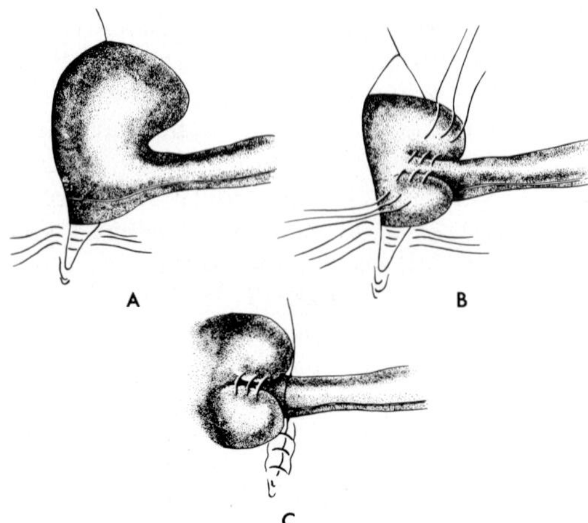

Figure 10.2. Nissen Repair
The Nissen repair requires full fundal mobilization (A). Crural sutures are placed to be tied later. The fundus is wrapped around the distal 4 or 5 cm of esophagus by three sutures which incorporate both gastric and esophageal wall (B). Following hernia reduction, the crural sutures are tied, narrowing the esophageal hiatus in the diaphragm (C).

(14), dysphagia and occasional difficulty in burping and vomiting.

Anatomic recurrence has been discussed in Chapter 9. The difficulty in recognizing anatomic recurrence can be a major problem and may result in long-term disability. Recurrence rates range from 7 to 10 per cent (15) in expert hands and certainly in my experience, judging from the referral pattern, recurrence rates can be much higher. Again judging from referral patterns I believe that the Belsey, Hill and Nissen procedures are all effective operations, however, all carry significant and similar problems of anatomic recurrence.

With the Nissen procedure an intact intrathoracic fundoplication may be effective in reflux control and this method will be discussed in Chapter 11.

Allison Hernia Repair

This procedure was a major advance in surgery of the esophagus when it was introduced in 1951 (16). The basic technique involves mobilization as previously described. Crural sutures are placed posteriorly. The esophagogastric fat pad can be removed, and the firm fibers of the phrenoesophageal liga-

ment are exposed. Sutures are now placed from the esophagus and phrenoesophageal ligament though the anterior crural margin. The esophagus is reduced and the sutures are tied anteriorly and posteriorly (17, 18) (Fig. 10.3).

This procedure produces an anatomic reduction; however, it does not create a long intra-abdominal segment of esophagus and does not create a flap valve mechanism.

Long-term follow-up is available. Allison reports 82 per cent complete symptomatic relief, 5 per cent improved and 13 per cent with poor results. Anatomic recurrence of herniation using very strict radiologic criteria was 49 per cent. Others (19) have reported on the Allison repair indicating that the procedure is still widely in use 28 years after its original description.

Thoracoabdominal Hernia Repair

Collis (20) described the repair of an uncomplicated hiatal hernia through a thoracoabdominal incision. This incision gives optimal exposure of the gastroesophageal junction and allows extension of the procedure to the thorax or abdomen as required, (20) (Fig. 10.4). With the exposure obtained, the surgeon can carry out gastric, duodenal and cholecystic procedures concurrently with ease

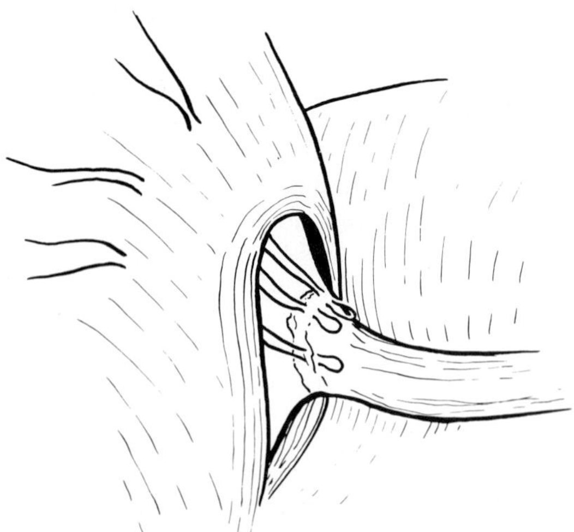

Figure 10.3. Allison Repair
The Allison repair closes the diaphragmatic crura, then sutures phrenoesophageal ligament to diaphragm. This was one of the earlier repairs described.

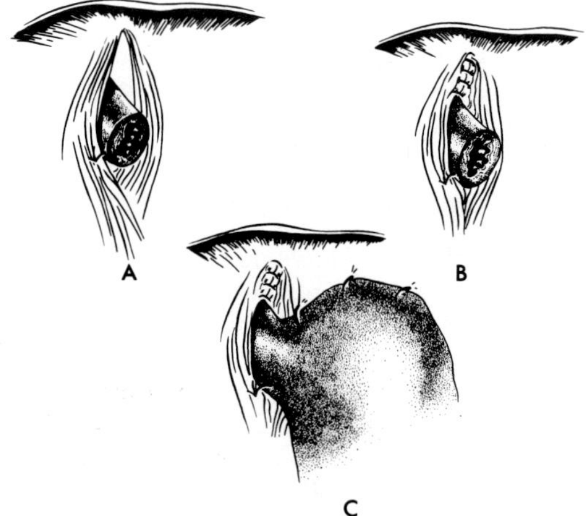

Figure 10.4. Collis Repair
In the Collis repair, a thoracoabdominal incision is used. The esophagogastric junction is sutured to the crura at the level of the arcuate ligament (A). The crura are approximated anteriorly using interrupted sutures (B) and the esophagogastric angle is reconstituted (C).

and can do an esophagogastrectomy or a bowel interposition procedure if necessary.

With the patient on his side inclined at 75 degrees, the incision is made along the line from the umbilicus to the midaxilla and is carried across the costal margin to approximately the 7th interspace. The rectus and the oblique muscles are divided. A 1-cm segment of costal cartilage is removed and the incision extended into the thorax by dividing the intercostal muscles. The diaphragm is divided peripherally, leaving a cuff of tissue on the costal margin and preserving the phrenic nerve. This incision gives extensive exposure and allows careful dissection of the gastroesophageal junction under full vision. Esophageal dissection can be carried to the aortic arch. The fundus of stomach and gastroesophageal junction are fully mobilized, preserving the peritoneal coverings of the crura.

The first stitch uses the phrenoesophageal ligament, stitching it to the decusation of the crura at the arcuate ligament level. The diaphragmatic crura are now closed with interrupted stitches, drawing the crura together in front of the esophagus and sinking the esophagus back into the crural bed. When the diaphragmatic opening is effectively closed, the fundus is sutured to the diaphragm, restoring it to its natural position with two or

three interrupted sutures. The diaphragmatic incision is approximated and the chest and abdomen closed without drainage.

Collis has done this operation, with a few minor adjustments, since 1953 and reported results as recently as 1968 (21). At that time he had a follow-up of at least 4 years on 200 of 230 patients. Results in 76 per cent of these patients were reported as "good" and in 21 per cent as "improved." Anatomic recurrence was reported in 2.5 per cent of patients and 10 per cent had recurrent free reflux.

These results are excellent. This series, because it has been carefully documented, can be compared directly with comparable operative techniques, e.g., the Belsey Mark IV repair (22).

Thoracoabdominal Approach for Hiatal Hernia Recurrence in Patients with Previous Gastric Surgery

In the past 4½ years I have used the thoracoabdominal approach for repair of a recurrent hiatal hernia. The operative technique of repair has been total fundoplication gastroplasty (Nissen gastroplasty: TFG) and this technique is described in the following chapter.

Using the thoracoabdominal approach both the intrathoracic esophagus and the stomach can be dissected under direct vision which minimizes the risk of opening lumen or devascularizing the wall. With this direct vision approach after completion of mobilization both esophagus and stomach appear healthy with minimal damage from scar tissue dissection.

A short thoracoabdominal incision is used and the diaphragm taken down circumferentially. Initial dissection is commenced in the chest freeing the inferior pulmonary ligament and dissecting lung from aorta, pericardium and esophagus. The degree of difficulty varies depending on the routes and number of previous repairs. The esophagus is mobilized medially and along the pericardial surface using a relatively avascular plain as far as the aortic arch. Along the aortic surface, mobilization is to the inferior pulmonary vein. Early dissection is begun at the hiatus, freeing the hernia sac and esophagus; however, only easy dissection is done at this stage and most of the hiatal dissection is completed from the abdomen.

Having mobilized the esophagus, the diaphragm is temporarily sewn to the upper wound margin giving optimal exposure of the fundus of stomach, left lobe of liver and spleen. The surgeon is operating directly over the esophagogastric junction and crura.

The densest scar is usually from liver to stomach. This must be carefully dissected to fully mobilize the left lobe of liver. The lesser sac is entered along its hepatic margin and the right crus of diaphragm clearly visualized.

Along the greater curvature the stomach is mobilized and four or five short gastric vessels are divided. The spleen is vulnerable at this time and must be carefully protected. Once the lesser and greater curvatures are mobile, the hiatal dissection is completed and the esophagus, unless shortened by scar, can be reduced into the abodmen.

The left gastric artery must be carefully protected at all times as division of this artery is one of the reasons for infarction of stomach or esophageal wall in the surgery of recurrent hiatal hernia.

Following mobilization crural sutures are placed to be tied at completion of the operation. My operative technique at this stage would be to do a TFG as the risk of further recurrence with TFG is less than 1 per cent. In this type of repeat hernia repair, the risk of further recurrence must be minimized.

Using a thoracoabdominal approach and TFG over the past 1 to 4½ years, I have done 121 recurrent hiatal hernias, 22 per cent of these had had more than one previous repair. A further 22 per cent had had previous gastric surgery including radical Billroth II resections. Eight of these patients (6.6 per cent) required splenectomy for tears of the capsule because of scar fixation of spleen to stomach, liver or diaphragm. Eleven patients had added surgery including gastrectomy, vagotomy and pyloroplasty, enteroenterostomy and cholecystectomy.

There was no operative or postoperative mortality; two developed wound infections which healed spontaneously. One patient had a postoperative bowel obstruction from a hematobezoar in small bowel. Three patients developed a fistula (2.48 per cent). This is a higher incidence of fistula than in primary repair by TFG (0.84 per cent) and relates to the difficulty of dissecting scar tissue and the risks of devascularization. All of the fistulae healed spontaneously with no long-term disability. In follow-up evaluation 1 to 4½ years following surgery, there were no recurrences and none of these patients had symptomatic or radiologic reflux.

Postgastrectomy Hiatal Hernia Repair

Various authors have advocated Roux-en-Y (23, 24) procedures for reflux following gastric surgery. Certainly bile is an important component of the refluxed bolus; however, food and acid will continue to reflux if the gastroesophageal junction remains incompetent. I have used the thoracoabdominal incision (25) as described with TFG and, where indicated, the previous gastric procedure has been modified. With Billroth II resections, an enteroenterostomy is used for bile diversion rather than a Roux-en-Y as I am concerned about the possibility of fistula with too much surgery at the gastrojejunal anastomosis. Reflux control is difficult to achieve in these patients and experience with the standard Belsey and with partial fundoplication gastroplasty (Belsey gastroplasty) indicates that these methods are ineffective in patients with gastric resection. TFG has reliably controlled reflux in all of these patients.

These series were reported by surgeons who have devoted years to improving techniques for the management of hiatal hernias. All have a significant percentage of failures, and, because of this, surgeons continue to devise new operations. Only by continuous accumulation of data from large series will we be able to select the most reliable techniques. At present, the Belsey, Hill, Nissen and Collis repairs seem to give the best results, and these repairs merit further long-term study and evaluation. We have seen a rising incidence of recurrence in the Belsey repair when evaluated at 10 years. Other repairs will require this long-term study to determine whether they too fail after 10 years.

References

1. Skinner, D. B., and Belsey, R. H.: Surgical management of esophageal reflux and hiatus hernia; long term results with 1030 patients. J. Thorac. Cardiovasc. Surg., *53:* 33, 1967.
2. Baue, A. E., and Belsey, R. H. R.: The treatment of sliding hiatus hernia and reflux esophagitis by the Mark IV technique. Surgery, *62:* 396, 1967.
3. Urschel, H. C., Jr., and Paulson, D. L.: Gastroesophageal reflux and hiatal hernia: complications and

therapy. J. Thorac. Cardiovasc. Surg., *53:* 21, 1967.
4. Orringer, M. B., Skinner, D. B., and Belsey, R. H. R.: Long term results of the Mark IV operation for hiatal hernia and analyses of recurrences and their treatment. J. Thorac. Cardiovasc. Surg., In press.
5. Belsey, R.: Surgical treatment of hiatus hernia and reflux esophagitis—introduction (Editorial). World J. Surg., *1:* 421, 1977.
6. Hiebert, C. A.: The recognition and management of gastroesophageal reflux without hiatal hernia. World J. Surg., *1:* 445, 1977.
7. Hiebert, C. A. and O'Mara, C. S.: The Belsey operation for hiatal hernia; twenty year experience. Am. J. Surg., *137:* 532, 1979.
8. Polk, H. C., Jr., and Zeppa, R.: Fundoplication for complicated hiatal hernia; rationale and results. Ann. Thorac. Surg., *7:* 202, 1969.
9. Moran, J. M., Pihl, C. O., Norton, R. A., and Rheinlander, H. F.: The hiatal hernia-reflux complex; current approaches to correction and evaluation of results. Am. J. Surg., *121:* 403, 1971.
10. Bettex, M., and Stillhart, H.: Operation for hiatus hernia and cardioesophageal achalasia by fundoplication after Nissen. Surgery, *55:* 451, 1964.
11. Dilling, E. W., Peyton, M. D., Cannon, J. P., Kanaly, P. J., and Elkins, R. C.: Comparison of Nissen fundoplication and Belsey Mark IV in the management of gastroesophageal reflux. Am. J. Surg., *134:* 730, 1977.
12. Mokka, R. E., Punto, L., Kairaluoma, M. I., Laitinen, S., and Larmi, T. K.: Surgical treatment of axial hiatal hernia—reflux complex by Nissen fundoplication. A cineradiologic and manometric study. Acta Chir. Scand., *143:* 265, 1977.
13. DeMeester, T. R., Johnson, L. F., and Kent, A. H.: Evaluation of current operations for the prevention of gastroesophageal reflux. Ann. Surg., *180:* 511, 1974.
14. Bushkin, F. L., Neustein, C. L., Parker, T. H., and Woodward, E. R.: Nissen fundoplication for reflux peptic esophagitis. Ann. Surg., *185:* 672, 1977.
15. Woodward, E. R., Rayl, J. E., and Clarke, J. M.: Esophageal hiatus hernia. Curr. Probl. Surg., *1:* 62, 1970.
16. Allison, P. R.: Reflux esophagitis, sliding hiatal hernia and the anatomy of repair. Surg. Gynecol. Obstet., *92:* 419, 1951.
17. Allison, P. R.: Reflux oesophagitis. Its pathology and treatment. Scand. J. Thorac. Cardiovasc. Surg., *6:* 318, 1972.
18. Allison, P. R.: Hiatus hernia; a 20 year retrospective survey. Ann. Surg., *178:* 273, 1973.
19. Gardner, R. J., Bonnabeau, R. C., and Warden, H. E.: Surgical repair of gastroesophageal reflux with sliding hiatal hernia. Am. J. Surg., *133:* 554, 1977.
20. Collis, J. L.: A review of surgical results in hiatus hernia. Thorax, *16:* 114, 1961.
21. Collis, J. L.: Surgical control of reflux in hiatus hernia. Am. J. Surg., *115:* 465, 1968.
22. Moghissi, K.: Conservative surgery in reflux stricture of the oesophagus associated with hiatal hernia. Br. J. Surg., *66:* 221, 1979.
23. Himal, H. S.: Alkaline gastritis and alkaline esophagitis; a review. Can. J. Surg., *20:* 403, 1977.
24. Henderson, R. D., Mugashe, F., Jeejeebhoy, K. N., et al: The motor defect of esophagitis. Can. J. Surg., *17:* 112, 1974.
25. Henderson, R. D.: Gastroesophageal reflux following gastric operation. Ann. Thorac. Surg., *26:* 563, 1978.

CHAPTER 11

Management of the Irreducible Hiatal Hernia

Peptic esophagitis produces a mucosal and submucosal inflammatory change which, if it progresses, will result in panmural esophagitis involving the whole thickness of the esophageal wall. The esophageal wall thickens and its vascularity increases, as in any inflammatory response. As this process continues, circumferential scar formation may produce a peptic stricture; alternately, londitudinal scar formation will result in esophageal shortening. At this stage the hiatal hernia becomes surgically irreducible (1). In its advanced stage panmural peptic esophagitis is obvious and has been well described for many years. In its earlier stages this process is harder to recognize and may receive serious consideration only when the surgeon realizes that wall thickening, fibrosis and shortening may have produced an irreducible hiatal hernia.

It is now widely recognized that severe ulceration and stricture produce major changes in the esophageal wall, and it is becoming evident that these changes may develop without clinical evidence of mucosal ulceration. In patients treated by standard repair, Skinner, Belsey and colleagues (2) reported a recurrence rate of 45 per cent when panmural esophagitis was present. The esophageal shortening in this group of patients exerted considerable tension on the Belsey Mark IV repair. Tension cannot be tolerated in reconstructive surgery, and the high recurrence rate in Belsey's expert hands indicates the limitation of this type of repair in the presence of panmural esophagitis. As the esophagitis progresses, the esophagus shortens to a point where reduction is impossible even under tension. This condition is referred to as "a surgically irreducible hiatal hernia."

Management of the irreducible hernia is much more complex than that of the reducible hiatal hernia because, with shortening, the surgeon cannot create an intra-abdominal esophageal segment and must seek alternate methods of achieving gastroesophageal competence. Many approaches to this problem have been described, and this in itself indicates the severity of the problem. The techniques recommended include gastric resection, bowel replacement and various procedures such as the Thal, the Nissen and the Collis gastroplasty. Each of these methods will be described to give some indication of its relative merits (Table 11.1). However, the reader, if he is to understand the various operative approaches, must have some appreciation of the theories of reflux prevention which underlie each method.

Reflux Control Following Esophageal Resection—Theoretical Considerations

Esophagogastrectomy

Resection of the distal esophagus and esophagogastric anastomosis have been used to manage severe peptic strictures. However, an end-to-end esophagogastric anastomosis provides no effective barrier to reflux (Fig. 11.1) and a 27 per cent incidence of secondary peptic stricture has been reported within 6 months following this procedure (3). Thus, the lesion for which the operation was performed has not been cured; indeed it may become more severe.

The esophagogastric anastomosis can be modified to prevent reflux. Clinically (4) and experimentally (5) it can be shown that complete esophagogastric competence can be

Table 11.1
Surgical Treatment of Irreducible Hernia and Peptic Stricture*

Principle	Technique
1. Alter reflux bolus	Distal gastrectomy
	Payne procedure
	Roux-en-Y or enteroenterostomy
2. Resection and replacement	Stomach
	Large bowel
	Small bowel
3. Plastic reconstruction	Intrathoracic fundoplication (Nissen)
	Thal
	Gastroplasty with partial or total fundoplication

* The presence of an irreducible hiatal hernia makes necessary alternate methods of reflux control, such as altering the refluxed bolus by gastrectomy. However, the surgeon usually elects some form of plastic repair or replacement of the esophagus with bowel.

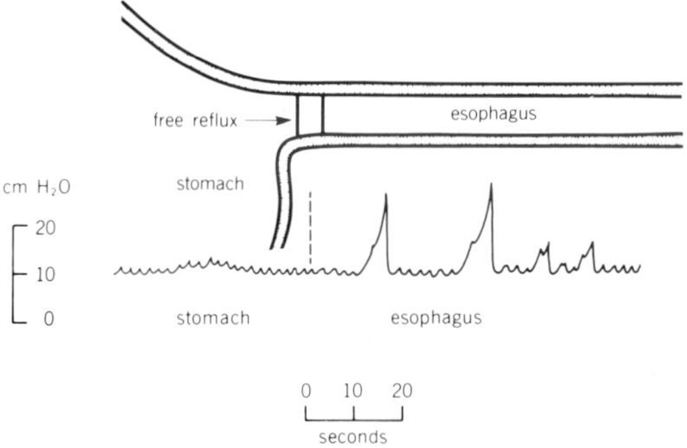

Figure 11.1. End-to-End Esophagogastric Anastomosis
An end-to-end esophagogastric anastomosis is accompanied by free reflux. Manometric studies show no evidence of a high pressure zone. The distal esophageal pressure is elevated and there is usually secondary disordered motor activity from reflux.

achieved by invaginating the esophagus into the stomach for a distance of 4 to 5 cm. We conducted experimental studies in dogs using end-to-end anastomosis and anastomosis plus invagination of the esophagus into the stomach. Free reflux occurred with end-to-end anastomosis, and competence was achieved only when 4 to 5 cm of esophagus were

invaginated into the stomach (Fig. 11.2). Radiologic studies with abdominal pressure showed the invaginated esophagus was compressed by the surrounding stomach. Manometrically the surrounding compression maintained the intraluminal pressure in the distal esophagus at the gastric level, with the esophageal pressure falling to normal levels at the upper end of the invagination (Fig. 11.2).

Human studies have shown that invagination esophagogastrectomy effectively controls reflux. The results of radiologic and manometric studies in these patients are identical to those in the dog, indicating that this procedure has created an effective flap valve mechanism.

Plastic Procedures—Fundoplication

The intrathoracic Nissen operation wraps the distal esophagus with stomach and the Woodward modification of the Thal operation (6) uses the same fundoplication technique. These methods of reflux control, which are the same as that used in the invagination esophagogastrectomy, use transmitted intra-

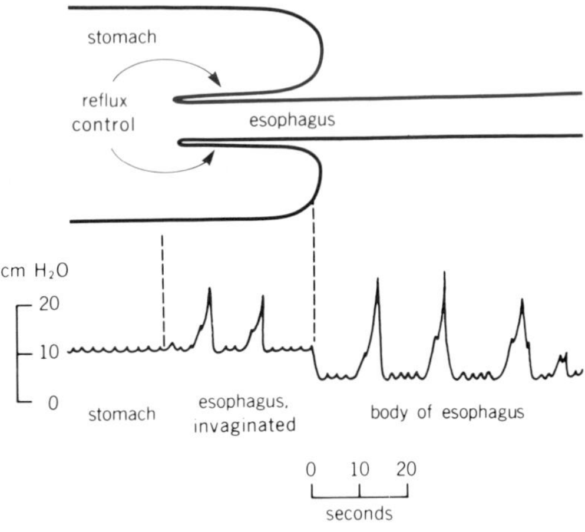

Figure 11.2. Invagination Esophagogastrectomy
Invagination of the lower esophagus for a distance of 4 to 5 cm prevents reflux. After this procedure, manometric studies show that the transmission of pressure around the lower esophagus maintains the pressure in the invaginated lower esophagus at gastric levels. At the upper margin of the invaginated esophagus the pressure abruptly falls to normal esophageal pressure. Clinically and in the experimental animal there is no evidence of reflux.

gastric pressure to close the distal esophagus and create a flap valve.

Esophageal Replacement—Bowel

Replacement of the esophagus by colon in man does not seem to be attended by reflux and, although there are occasional reports of ulceration and stricture following colonic interposition, these are rare (7, 8). We have investigated colonic interposition in dogs and have shown that free reflux occurs when a 6-cm segment of colon is maintained below or above the diaphragm (Fig. 11.3) (9). If the length of subdiaphragmatic colon is increased to 12 cm, reflux control becomes effective; however, similar colonic segments above the diaphragm do not prevent reflux. Myotomy of a subdiaphragmatic 12-cm segment of colon results in free reflux. Manometric studies show that basal tone in the colonic segment is 2 cm of water, which acts as a weak pressure barrier to reflux. Following myotomy the colonic tone falls to 0 cm of water and free reflux occurs.

From this study we have proposed that a 12-cm segment of colon has sufficient basal tone to prevent reflux when maintained below the diaphragm. Jones and colleagues (10), who have reported peristalsis in the transplanted colon, believe that this motor activity keeps the colonic segment clear of refluxed material and prevents damage from the refluxed bolus. The peristaltic motor wave they describe is weak and intermittent, and does not seem to be sufficient for adequate colonic protection. We found no evidence of peristaltic activity in colonic segments despite prolonged motor studies.

In the human it is necessary to leave a 10- to 15-cm segment of colon below the diaphragm because this organ is tethered by its blood supply. This length of colon below the diaphragm is forced upon the surgeon by local anatomy and may explain the effectiveness of colon interposition in preventing reflux.

These same principles probably apply to replacement of the esophagus by small bowel, but no one has yet determined the length of bowel necessary for reflux control.

Gastric Tubes

Heimlich (11) has replaced excised esophagus with gastric tubes (Fig. 11.4), and we have studied gastric tubes in the experimental animal (12). The gastroesophageal junction can be excised and the lower esophagus replaced by a tubed segment of stomach (#50 Fr size). This segment, if maintained in the chest, permits free reflux; however, a 2.5- to 6-cm segment of stomach tube, maintained below the diaphragm, controls reflux. The segment of tubed stomach has a constant tone (10 cm of water) which is much higher than in the colon, and this probably accounts for the ability of the shorter segment to prevent reflux. Myotomy of the gastric tube reduces its tone to 0 cm of water and allows free reflux.

This same principle is used in the gastro-

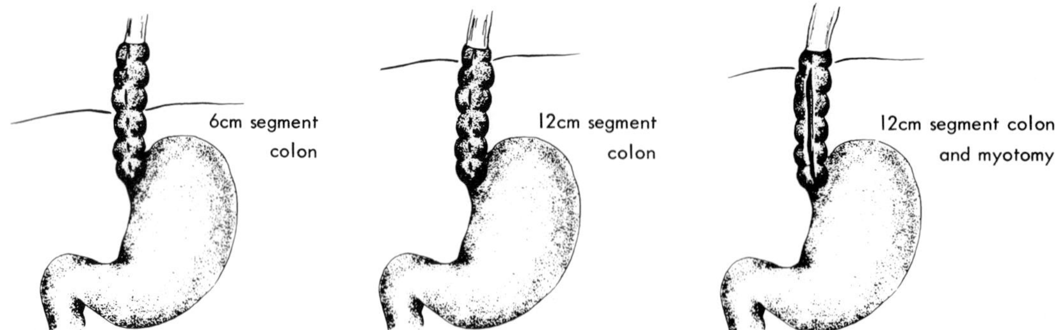

Figure 11.3
In the experimental animal, one can study the ability of the colon to prevent reflux by resecting the gastroesophageal junction and replacing it by a segment of colon . The colon has an average tone of 2 cm of water. A 6-cm segment of subdiaphragmatic colon does not prevent reflux, but reflux can be controlled if the length of the subdiaphragmatic segment is increased to 12 cm. Myotomy of the subdiaphragmatic segment, which lowers the manometric tone to 0 cm of water, permits free reflux again.

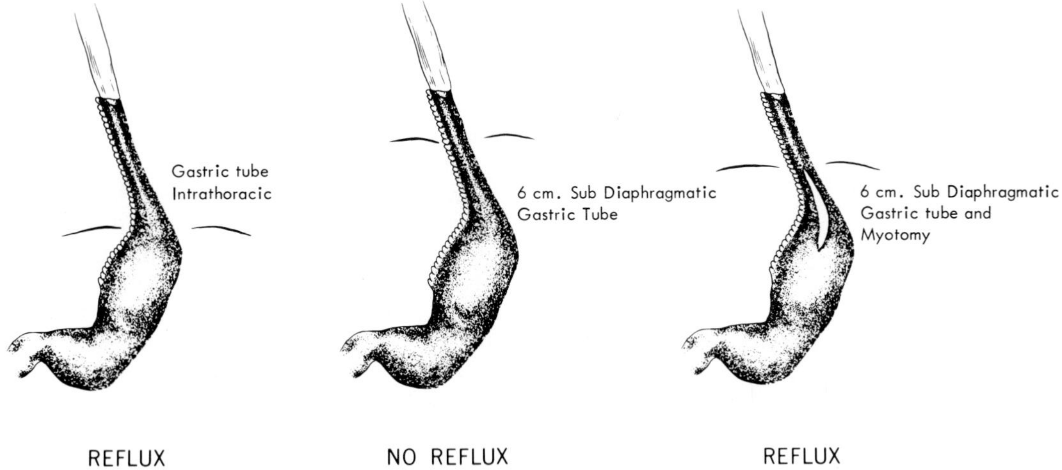

Figure 11.4
In this figure the lower esophagus and gastroesophageal junction have been excised and replaced by a tubed segment taken from the greater curvature of stomach. When the gastric tube, which has a tone of 10 to 15 cm of water, is maintained entirely within the thorax, free reflux occurs. However, a 2.5- to 6-cm segment of colon maintained below the diaphragm prevents reflux. Myotomy of the gastric tube lowers the tone to 0 cm of water and permits free reflux again.

plasty in which a tubed segment of stomach achieves reflux control. Radiologic studies after gastroplasty demonstrate that these patients did achieve effective reflux control. Manometric studies confirm that the gastric tube component of the gastroplasty has a constant tone. (It is lower in the human than in dogs and averages 4 cm of water.) This tubal tone appears to be adequate for reflux control.

These principles have been applied to the design of operations to prevent reflux associated with an irreducible hiatal hernia.

Treatment—Surgically Irreducible Hiatal Hernia

Distal Gastrectomy

Tanner and Westerholm (13) recommend distal Polya gastrectomy instead of bowel replacement in patients with peptic stricture of the esophagus and an associated irreducible hiatal hernia. Their 16-year follow-up includes 16 of the 22 patients operated upon up to 1950. One patient died after operation (4.5 per cent), 4 died from unrelated disease during follow-up and 1 was lost to follow-up. Five patients became symptom-free, but 11 had some degree of residual dysphagia. Subsequent radiologic studies showed that the

stenosis had resolved to varying degrees. Although this study suggests that distal gastrectomy produces some resolution of peptic stricture, Tanner and Westerholm's results are not as good as those reported after bowel replacement.

Some patients with hiatal hernias develop severe symptoms following gastrectomy, and indeed the bile gastritis and esophagitis associated with this operation may produce rapidly progressive esophageal disease. Thirty-six of my own patients who required surgical correction of a hiatal hernia had had previous gastric surgery. Their symptoms were more severe than those in the average group of symptomatic hiatal hernia patients and severe peptic esophagitis was much more frequent. My findings, which are contrary to those reported by Tanner, suggest that bile reflux following gastrectomy increases the severity of the symptoms (14–16).

Case 1. This 65-year-old man had a gastroenterostomy for a duodenal ulcer in 1938. In 1965 he had a Billroth II gastrectomy and hiatal hernia repair. For 5 years he had had severe heartburn, reflux into the throat, night aspiration and moderate pharyngoesophageal and gastroesophageal dysphagia. A recurrent hiatal hernia was demonstrated radiologically with free reflux. Manometrically he had a normal tone at the gastroesophageal junction, but had a severe disorder of motor activity (75 per cent) in his lower esophagus. Endoscopically he had a Stage I chronic esophagitis and a severe bile gastritis.

His esophagus, which was exposed in a thoracoabdominal approach, was thickened and shortened. A modified Collis gastroplasty was done to correct the hernia and an enteroenterostomy was made to decrease bile flow to his stomach. Three years after operation he remains free of symptoms.

This case demonstrates the severe symptoms and the esophageal pathology characteristic of the 36 patients who had a hiatal hernia and previous gastric surgery.

Case 2. Mrs. M., a 35-year-old woman, had a tragic past history of misdiagnosis with two intercostal neurectomies for left chest pain before she was recognized as having a large gastric ulcer. She was treated by 80 per cent Billroth II resection with Roux-en-Y anastomosis. She was first seen because of intractable reflux and severe aspiration with episodes of cyanosis.

Treatment was by thoracoabdominal total fundoplication gastroplasty. This gave effective relief to her symptoms and she remains well and off medication 2 years after surgery.

Severe reflux symptoms were present despite a Roux-en-Y bile diversion. Reflux is of gastric content and certainly in this patient with only a small stomach remnant her symptoms were severe.

Payne Procedure

Payne and Olsen (17) have extended the principles outlined by Tanner. He has devised a very extensive operation, dividing vagi, resecting distal stenosed esophagus, removing distal stomach and performing a Roux-en-Y jejunal anastomosis.

While he reports good results, he emphasizes that his procedure is restricted to extreme cases where other methods have failed (see Fig. 18.3).

Essentially he is removing the stricture but also destroying the antireflux mechanism. He then depends upon gastrectomy and Roux-en-Y anastomosis to alter the quality of the refluxed bolus (18, 19).

Reflux Control and Bile Diversion

Having seen many patients in severe reflux difficulty following distal gastrectomy, I do not believe that bile diversion is the procedure of choice. Case 2, Mrs. M., is an example where reflux and aspiration complicated a radical gastrectomy (80 per cent) and Roux-en-Y anastomosis. Essentially this patient had had the treatment recommended by Tanner and Payne.

My approach has been to use a thoracoabdominal incision (Chapter 10), mobilize intrathoracic esophagus and esophagogastric junction and correct reflux by total fundoplication gastroplasty (TFG: Nissen gastroplasty). Bile diversion, if necessary, in a Billroth II gastrectomy has been by enteroenterostomy. I have avoided the Roux-en-Y procedure, particularly in radical gastrectomies, because of the gastrojejunal anastomosis lying too close to the gastroplasty. Partial fundoplication gastroplasty (PFG: Belsey gastroplasty) is ineffective in reflux control in patients with previous gastrectomies, particularly in patients with radical gastrectomies and previous hiatal hernia repair.

The results achieved in 22 of these patients have been excellent with no evidence of continued reflux and an immediate return to a more satisfactory diet (20).

Esophageal Resection and Replacement

Esophagogastrectomy

Most surgeons have abandoned esophagogastrectomy because of the severe reflux which follows this procedure and the high incidence of peptic esophagitis and stricture after operation. Occasionally, however, patients with benign strictures require this operation and, when it is done, reflux can be controlled by invaginating 5 cm of esophagus into the stomach. This procedure cannot be recommended for the relief of peptic stricture, but in unusual circumstances may be done and can give effective control of reflux.

To perform the invagination procedure, I resect the distal esophagus, sparing as much stomach as possible. The site for the anastomosis is selected, but before anastomosis the gastric fundus is rolled behind the esophagus to form the posterior portion of the invagination. An end-to-end anastomosis is now performed and it is gently flipped down into the stomach and the anterior surface of stomach rolled over the esophagus and sutured in position. Invaginated in this manner, a 5-cm segment of esophagus will prevent reflux (Fig. 11.5) (21).

Case 3. Mrs. J, age 65, had had multiple pre-

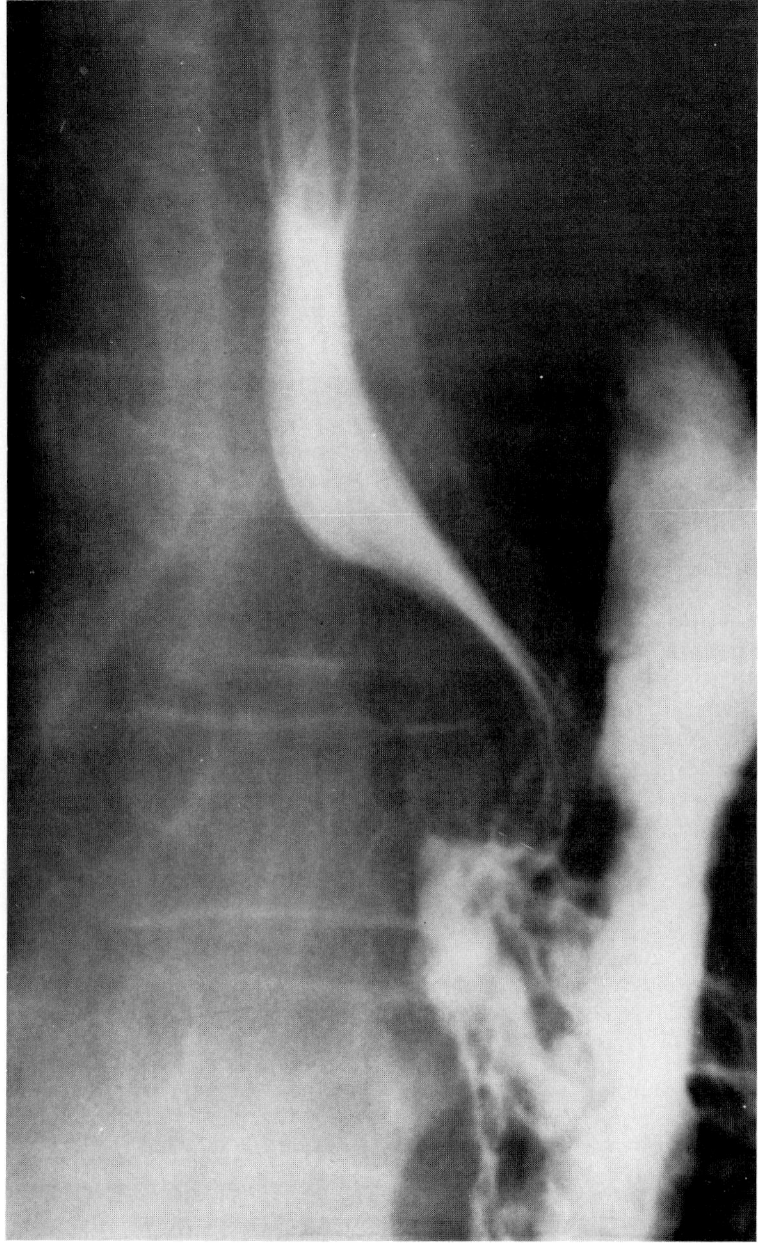

Figure 11.5
The patient (Mrs. D.) had an invagination esophagogastrectomy for cancer of the lower esophagus. Stomach was wrapped circumferentially for a distance of 5 cm. Follow-up studies indicated no radiologic evidence of reflux. This figure shows the stomach compressing the distal esophagus and preventing reflux.

vious operations including a Billroth I gastrectomy and two hiatal hernia repairs. She had advanced rheumatoid arthritis and was confined to bed or a chair. A severe peptic stricture had been present for 10 years and had become undilatable. She could swallow only liquids of a watery consistency, and her weight was reduced to 65 pounds.

Before surgery she had 1 month of intravenous alimentation. At operation the stricture was undilatable and had to be resected. An end-to-end esophagogastric anastomosis without invagination was necessary because of the stomach size and massive scar.

She has been maintained on antacids postoperatively and has required dilatation twice in 18 months; however, she tolerates a solid diet and is very much improved.

This type of surgery is rarely indicated for a benign stricture; however, it was considered life saving in this particular patient.

Heimlich-Gavrialu Tube

These authors (11) have described a gastric tube reconstruction which effectively replaces long esophageal segments, but this tube has been used only occasionally to manage peptic stricture (21). The long-term results of such tube replacements remain to be determined because they have been employed chiefly in the presence of carcinoma of the esophagus (Fig. 11.6).

Reflux and peptic ulceration have been described after the insertion of these gastric tube segments (22–24). However, in the experimental animal, maintenance of a 6-cm gastric tube below the diaphragm controls reflux. In two such resections I have done for benign disease, the patients had no clinical or radiologic evidence of reflux when a 6-cm segment was maintained below the diaphragm. The tubes used in these patients were taken to the level of the aortic arch only.

Case 4. Mrs. H., age 73, had had pancreatitis 2 years earlier and had nasogastric intubation for 6 weeks. She developed severe peptic stenosis and an undilatable stricture. Attempted dilatation following surgical mobilization split the esophagus. The fundus of the stomach was then mobilized into the left chest and a tube of stomach, prepared from the greater curvature, was anastomosed to the esophagus at the level of the aortic arch. Six centimeters of stomach tube were maintained be-

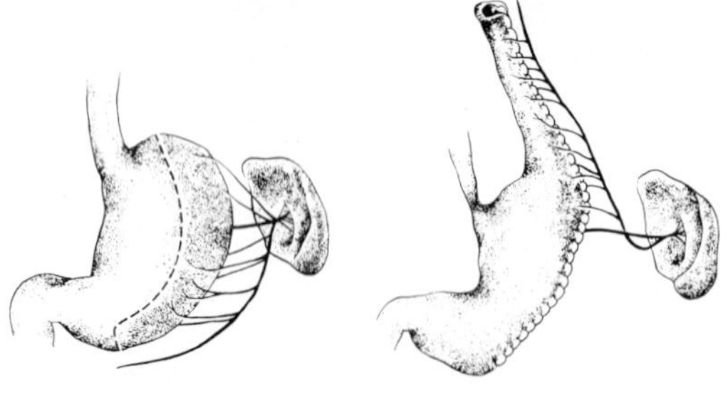

Figure 11.6. Heimlich-Gavrialu Tube
The Heimlich-Gavrialu tube is prepared from the greater curvature of stomach and, with its splenic blood supply, it can be used to replace the entire esophagus.

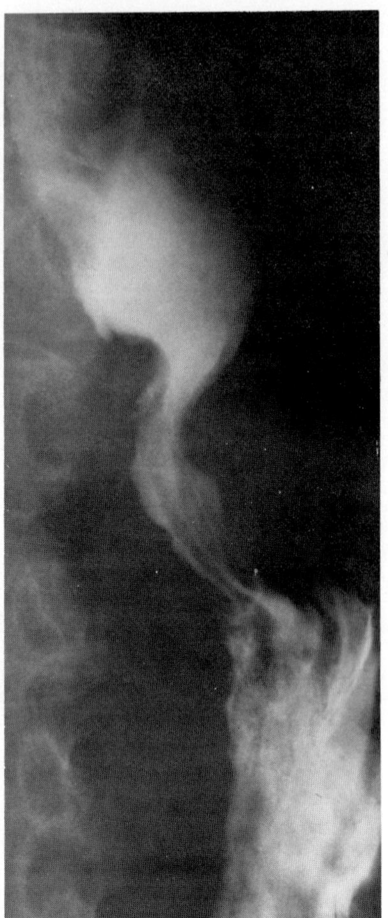

Figure 11.7
The patient (Mrs. H.) had a resection of the distal esophagus and replacement by a tube of stomach fashioned from the greater curvature and vascularized by the short gastric arteries. Six centimeters of stomach are maintained below the diaphragm and the fundus of the stomach is wrapped around this tube segment. Clinically and radiologically there is no evidence of reflux.

low the diaphragm and wrapped with gastric fundus in a manner similar to that used for a Belsey repair. Subsequent radiologic studies showed a satisfactory functioning tube with no evidence of reflux (Fig. 11.7).

Colon Replacement of Lower Esophagus

This technique, which has been used extensively, is highly effective in the management of peptic stricture (25, 26). The operative field is approached usually via a short thoracoabdominal incision. Colon is mobilized from the sigmoid to the hepatic flexure. The trans-

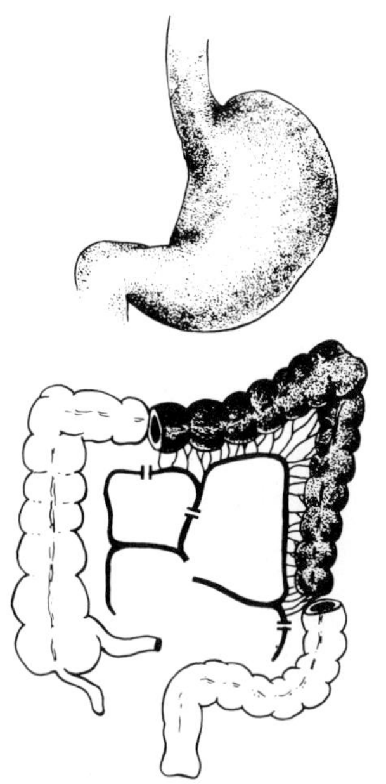

Figure 11.8. Colonic Blood Supply for Segmental Replacement of Lower Esophagus
The left colon can be used to replace the entire esophagus. The colon is pedicled on the ascending branch of the left colic artery, the marginal artery of the colon and the distal divisions of the middle colic artery.

plant has an ideal blood supply which is derived from the ascending branch of the left colic artery, the colonic marginal artery and the branches of the middle colic artery (Fig. 11.8). Careful mobilization is necessary to avoid arterial and venous damage during dissection. The middle colic artery is isolated at its origin because its branches, which come off early, must be preserved if this segment of colon is to be used. For short segment replacement, the middle colic artery can often be preserved. Once the segment is mobilized, its vascularity can be checked by clamping the arteries for division with bulldog clamps. The bowel segment chosen for transplantation should then be checked carefully for edema, discoloration and pulsatile blood flow. If the segment is satisfactory, the vessels can be divided and the bowel divided and wrapped in a moist saline sponge. Colonic continuity is restored by end-to-end anastomosis and the colonic mesentery closed.

The diseased segment of esophagus is resected back to healthy esophageal wall. Only

a small rim of stomach is removed at the cardia, taking care to leave no squamous epithelium, because, if left in contact with gastric juice, this type of mucosa can ulcerate later. A pyloroplasty or pyloromyotomy is now performed because the vagal nerves almost always are sacrificed at the time of esophageal resection.

The colonic segment and pedicle can be passed behind the gastric antrum and brought through the lesser sac (Fig. 11.9). Distal colon is anastomosed to the antrum anteriorly and an end-to-end coloesophageal anastomosis is performed in the chest after passing the colonic segment through the diaphragmatic hiatus. The operation is a major undertaking but, in experienced hands, can be accomplished with a low mortality.

In 1965 Belsey (3) described a series of 92

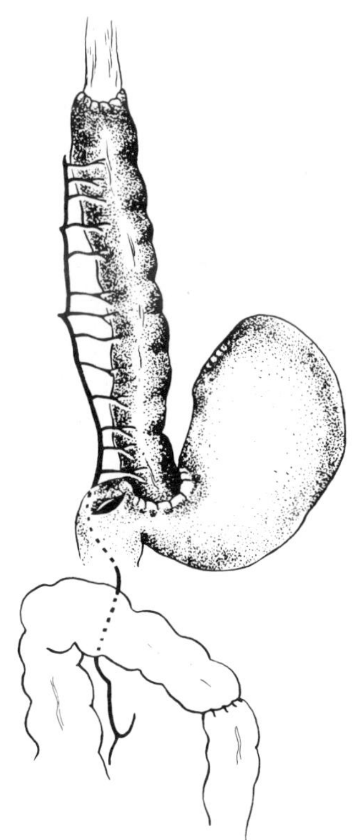

Figure 11.9 Colonic Replacement of Lower Esophagus
Here a segment of colon, based on the ascending branch of colic artery, has been used to replace the distal esophagus. The esophagus and the vagal nerves have been resected and a pyloroplasty performed.

colon transplants. At follow-up, 81 of these patients were without symptoms and 11 had mild residual symptoms. Parenthetically, he added some interesting observations on colonic function. Radiologic studies in the prone position showed barium pooling in the colonic segments, and did not show any active colonic motility—findings which are contrary to the results of more recent motor studies (3, 10, 27). He did not report reflux, probably because of the long intra-abdominal segment tethered by its blood supply. Subsequent colonic ulceration has been reported but these incidents are relatively uncommon.

Case 5. Mrs. R., age 55, had a total esophagectomy and colon interposition for an esophageal carcinoma. Initially she progressed well but 6 months after operation developed major dysphagia to solids and on endoscopy and radiologic examination was shown to have a gastrocolonic stricture. The stricture was resected and the colon was reanastomosed to the fundus of stomach at

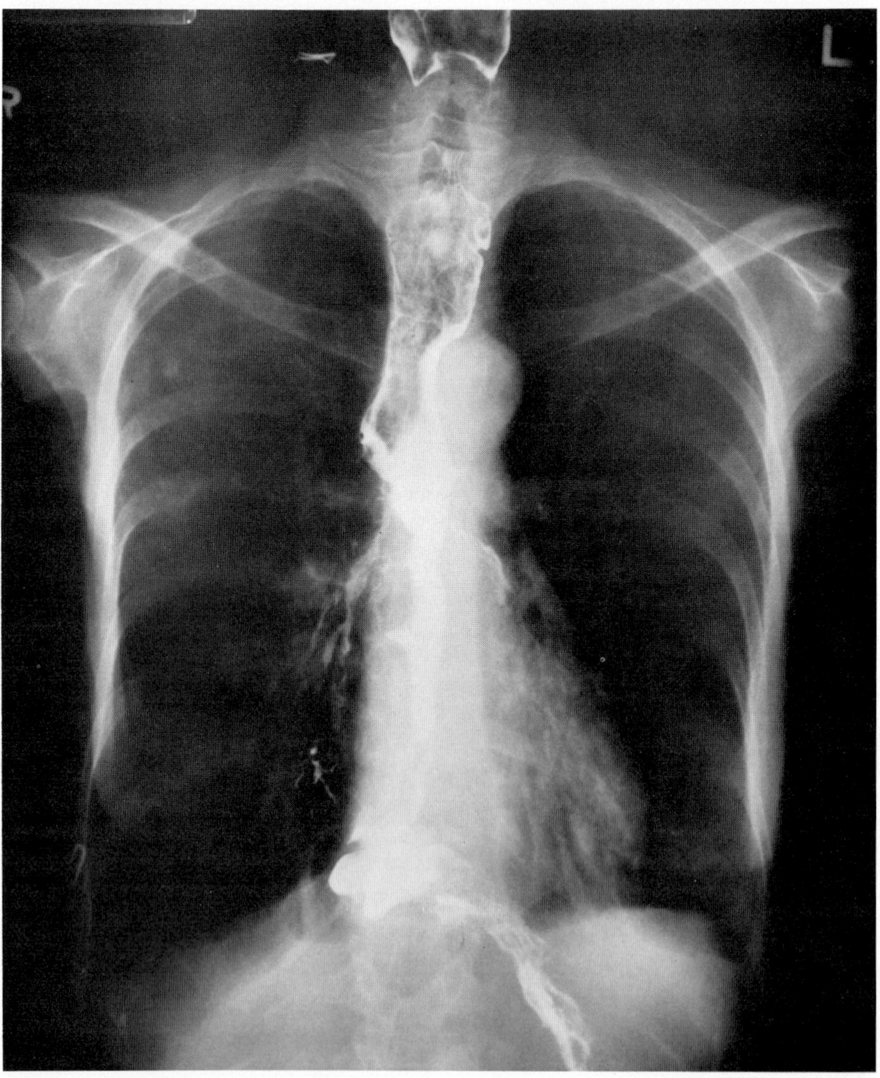

Figure 11.10
Anteroposterior view of chest showing a segment of colon replacing the esophagus and its anastomosis to the gastric antrum. This patient showed no clinical or radiologic evidence of reflux. Subsequently, the subdiaphragmatic segment of colon had to be excised because of stenosis at the cologastric anastomosis (Fig. 11.11) and, following this, free reflux developed.

the diaphragmatic level. Although swallowing was immediately improved, she developed free clinical and radiologic reflux. She continued to have reflux over the following 6 months until she died from metastatic malignancy. During this time, despite clinically significant reflux, she did not develop a stricture.

The case illustrates the value of the intra-abdominal segment of colon in preventing reflux (Figs. 11.10 and 11.11).

The right colon and transverse colon have also been used for colonic interposition (28). A higher incidence of regurgitation is reported with transverse colon in which an antiperistalti   ment is

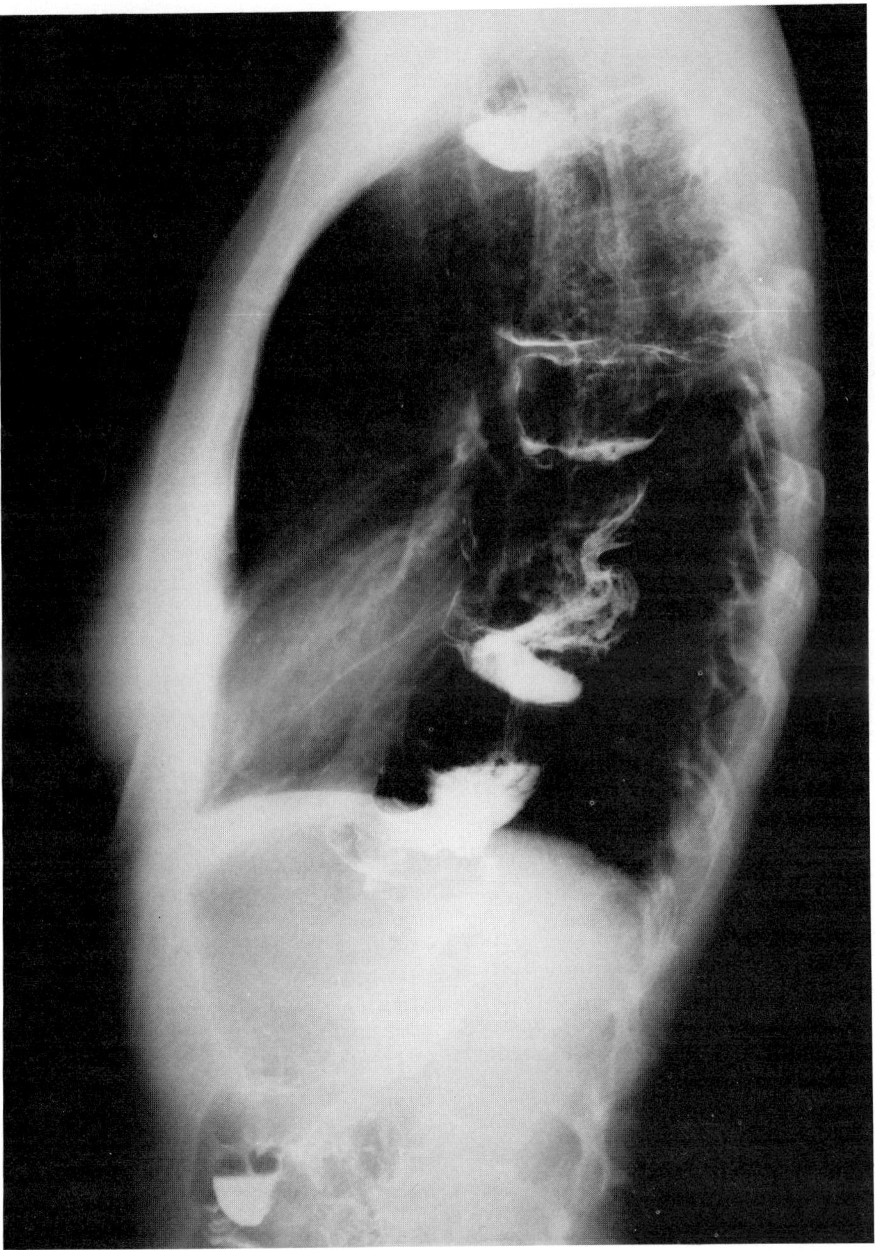

Figure 11.11
Lateral view of colonic replacement segment, now anastomosed to the fundus of stomach. There was clinical and radiologic reflux, because resection of the intra-abdominal segment removed the reflux control mechanism.

used. More recently, an operation has been devised in children which uses right colon to replace esophagus while preserving the gastroesophageal junction (29). This approach has seen limited use to date and no long-term follow-up studies have been done.

Small Bowel Replacement of Esophagus

Jejunal replacement of the esophagus for peptic stricture, as described by Merendino and colleagues (30, 31), has also proved effective. This operation can be performed using the thoracoabdominal approach described previously. The mobilized bowel can be used to replace the distal esophagus and, if necessary, the replacement can be carried into the neck. In expert hands the operative mortality can be held to 4 per cent (32).

The small bowel, which retains its peristaltic function, should be used in an isoperistaltic manner (33). Because it retains motor function, the bowel empties effectively and does not show the barium pooling seen in colonic transplants. If a segment of bowel is maintained below the diaphragm, these patients do not complain of reflux.

It is difficult to compare the relative merits of colon and small bowel in replacement surgery. Various authors have described advantages that one has over the other, but in general I find little to choose between them. For long segment replacement I have used colon because of its ease of mobilization.

Plastic Procedures for Peptic Stricture of Esophagus

Each of the three procedures now in common use aims at preserving the intact esophagus, and each has its own advocates. The Thal and Nissen procedures secure cardioesophageal competence by intrathoracic fundoplication, whereas the Collis gastroplasty prevents reflux by lengthening the esophagus and doing an intra-abdominal fundoplication around a gastric tube. The Thal procedure splits the peptic stricture while the Nissen and Collis procedures dilate the stricture and allow healing after control of the reflux.

Thal Operation

The Thal procedure can be done through a standard left thoracotomy. The fundus of the stomach is mobilized, as previously described, and brought into the chest. An inci-

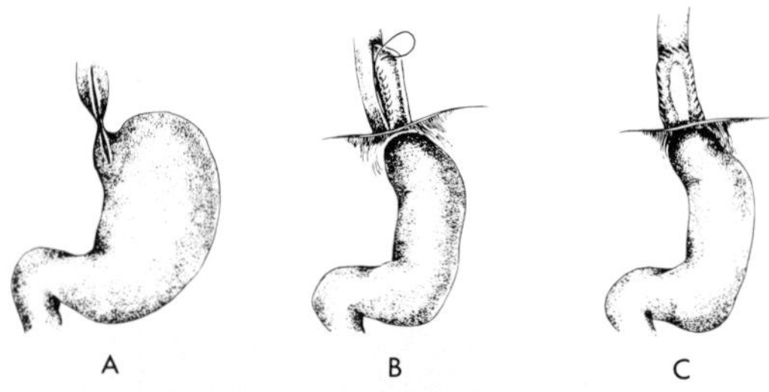

Figure 11.12. Thal Procedure
In the Thal procedure, a peptic stricture of the esophagus is opened by a longitudinal incision. A portion of gastric wall is used to close the esophageal defect. This procedure maintains a portion of gastric fundus in the thoracic cavity, but does not control reflux.

sion is now made along the full length of stricture, laying it open from stomach to healthy esophagus (Fig. 11.12). The opening may be modified by closing its lateral margins as in the Mikulicz pyloroplasty. Fundus of stomach is now anchored to the lower margin of the defect, and a continuous suture is used to anastomose the fundus of stomach to the margins of the defect. This simple fundic patch opens the esophageal lumen and immediately relieves the mechanical dysphagia. The operation has been modified by adding a skin graft to the fundic patch, giving protection to the serosal covering.

Thal's initial report of this procedure described 16 patients, 2 with achalasia, 3 with peptic stricture and 11 with hiatal hernia. One patient died after operation from leakage. In 1968 Thal reviewed 22 patients with a peptic stricture treated by his technique. Of these, 1 died and 3 of the remaining 21 developed recurrent peptic stricture within 6 weeks. His follow-up in 1968 was from 4 months to 3 years.

Adverse reports which have continued to appear concerning this procedure indicate that the major hazards are continued reflux and stricture formation.

Ashcraft et al. (36) have recently reported 100 patients with a Thal procedure and the gastroesophageal junction maintained below the diaphragm. There were 8 deaths unrelated to the operation and 4 recurrences. They feel that this is a good and safe procedure.

Woodward and colleagues (6, 37, 38) modified the Thal procedure by adding a Nissen fundoplication (Fig. 11.13) and achieved

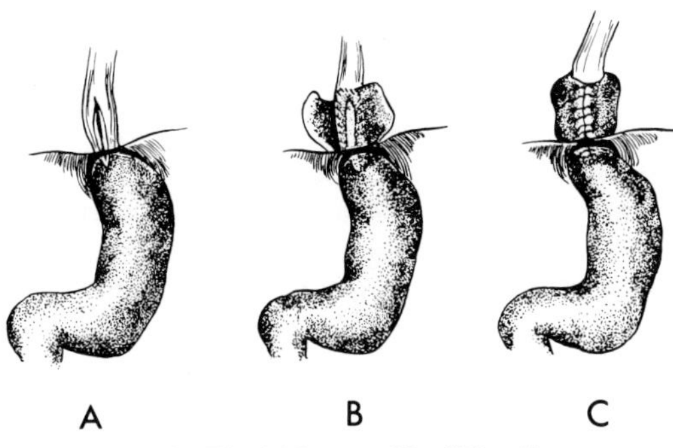

Figure 11.13. Thal-Nissen Modification
Thal-Nissen modification—patch and fundoplication (Woodward). Because of the potential for reflux in the Thal operation, Woodward added a circumferential wrapping of stomach around the lower esophagus. This complete fundoplication, like the invagination esophagogastrectomy (Fig. 11.2), prevents reflux.

more effective reflux control. Of 28 patients treated by the Thal operation with Nissen fundoplication, they have described good results in 21, fair results in 5, and poor results in 2. Their poor results were in those patients who did not have a complete fundoplication.

The modification by Woodward et al. (39–42) of the Thal procedure does appear to improve the surgical result. The numbers of patients so far reported are small and the follow-up is not yet long enough to permit adequate assessment. Woodward et al. have had some difficulties with the development of paraesophageal hernias at the site where stomach passes through diaphragm.

Intrathoracic Nissen Fundoplication

This operative procedure was described earlier (Chapter 9) as a potential transabdominal hernia repair. The surgical technique is identical, but in this instance the fundoplication is left in the chest (Fig. 11.14).

Several workers have reported that this procedure is effective in the control of reflux (43, 44). The intrathoracic fundoplication transmits intra-abdominal pressure to the lower esophagus and, by so doing, maintains constant closure of the invaginated segment of esophagus.

Both the Nissen and Thal procedures carry potential hazards. These operations employ a circumferential fundoplication which, if wrapped too tightly, may produce dysphagia. Unlike scar tissue, a wrap of healthy muscle

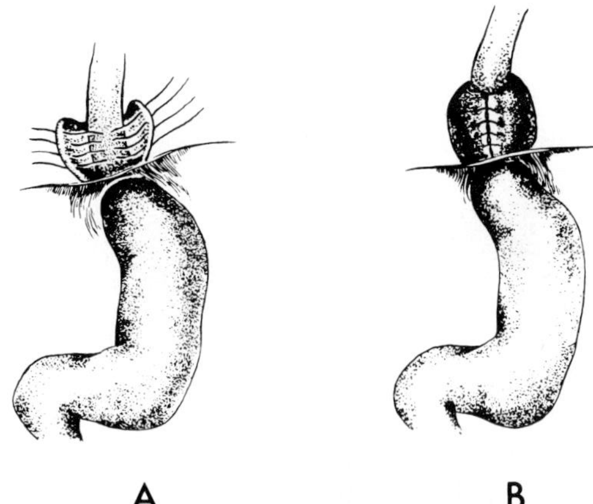

Figure 11.14. Nissen Fundoplication
The intrathoracic Nissen fundoplication wraps the lower esophagus circumferentially with fundus of stomach. Abdominal pressure transmitted to the lower esophagus maintains closure of this segment and supports the gastroesophageal junction. This procedure provides effective reflux control.

does not dilate and the dysphagia may be permanent. A second hazard that has not yet been fully evaluated is that of ulceration in the gastric fundus. Drainage from the fundus is not always effective, and pooling of food and gastric acid may produce secondary ulceration in the intrathoracic pouch of stomach with the hazard of hemorrhage or perforation. This complication is associated with large incarcerated hiatal hernias—the situation which these operations produce. Early reports indicate that this theoretical hazard may be clinically significant (45).

Case 6. Mr. H., age 72, had had two previous hiatal hernia repairs and had developed a further recurrence. He was known to have an ulcer at the esophagogastric junction. Two days following prostatectomy this ulcer perforated into his left chest and he went into profound shock. In the operating room we found that his esophagus was thickened and edematous and that he had a large perforation through the base of his esophagogastric ulcer. The perforation was closed and fundus of stomach mobilized (as a Nissen fundoplication) to patch the distal esophagus and to control reflux (Fig. 11.15). Here the stomach was used to patch the esophageal perforation, because in this situation gastroplasty was considered too dangerous and the risk of further leakage was too great. This patient has remained well and has no clinical or radiologic evidence of reflux 3 years after his Nissen fundoplication.

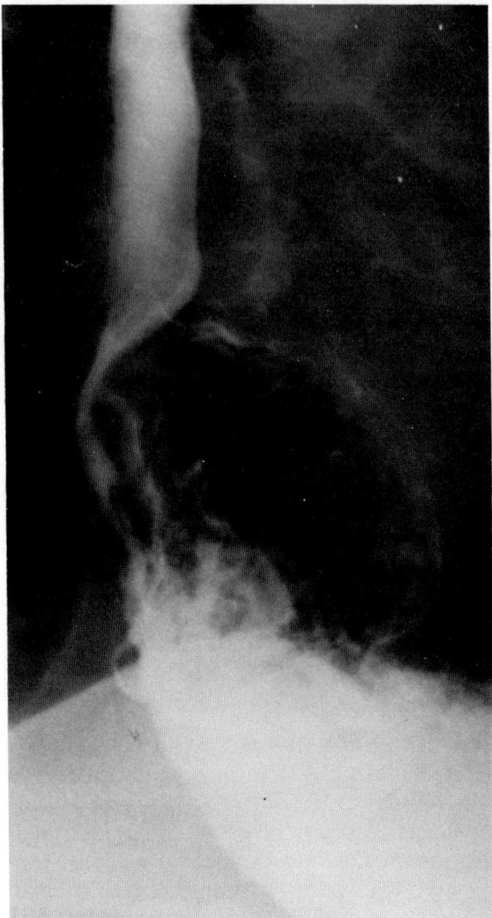

Figure 11.15
In this patient (Mr. H.) a spontaneous perforation of an esophagogastric ulcer complicating a hiatal hernia was treated by direct suture and patching of the perforation by a Nissen fundoplication. The radiograph shows the fundus of stomach in an intrathoracic position. There is no clinical or radiologic evidence of reflux.

Case 7. Mrs. H, age 48, had had three hernia repairs, the last being 1½ years before admission. This latter procedure was an intrathoracic Nissen fundoplication. She presented with a history of three major upper gastrointestinal bleeds. Endoscopically the intrathoracic stomach was inflamed and ulcerated. Because of continued bleeding she was reoperated on and a TFG was performed. Now 1 year postoperatively she is asymptomatic with no further bleeding or anaemia.

Intrathoracic fundoplications can be complicated by ulceration and for this reason I avoid this approach where possible.

Gastroplasty

Collis in 1957 (46) originally described his gastroplasty as a method of reflux control in patients with a short esophagus. He cut a tube from the lesser curvature of stomach and used his method of hernia repair sewing stomach along the lateral margin of the tube as a method of anchoring the gastroplasty below the diaphragm. Pearson and Henderson in 1971 and 1973 (47, 48) described a similar operation but used a modified Belsey fundoplication for fixation of the gastroplasty tube. In 1977 Henderson (49) described failures of the Belsey gastroplasty (partial fundoplication gastroplasty: PFG) and described the new operative approach of total fundoplication gastroplasty (TFG) which was more effective in reflux control. Variations of this operative approach were published by Bingham in 1977 (50) and by Evangelist et al. in 1978 (51) in which instead of cutting a gastroplasty tube they used staples without division. A similar variation on PFG has been published by Langer in 1973 (52) for management of moderate degrees of esophageal shortening.

Several variations on the gastroplasty procedure are available and for the purpose of discussion they will be divided into partial and total fundoplication gastroplasties.

Partial Fundoplication Gastroplasty

Collis (46) designed the gastroplasty tube for management of reflux in the scarred and shortened esophagus. The method was introduced to avoid the necessity of resection and replacement which was the recommended method of treating advanced peptic disease.

The procedure is performed using a short thoracoabdominal incision with mobilization of esophagus and proximal stomach. His gastroplasty tube was cut over a small bougie (approximately #20 Fr) and with the tube prepared he then approximated the crura anteriorly. Fundus of stomach was sewn along the lateral border of the gastroplasty restoring its normal anatomic position but not attempting to create any flap valve mechanism.

In follow-up studies he reports 59 per cent of patients with moderate to severe radiologic reflux and 50 per cent with reflux symptoms. Patients with stricture were dilated postoper-

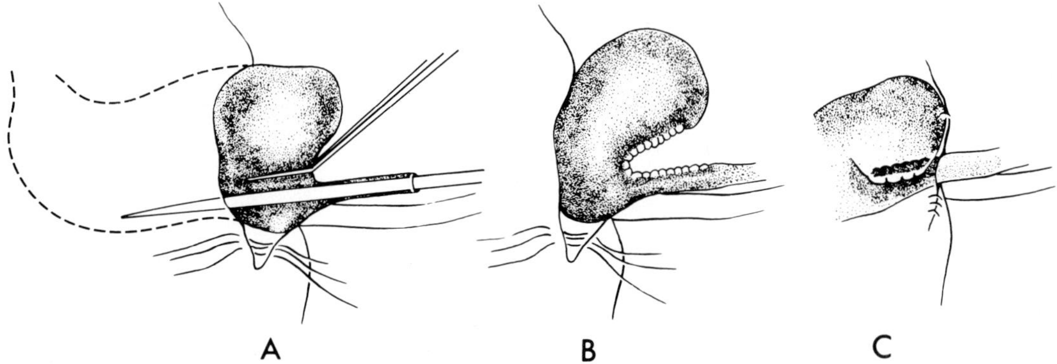

Figure 11.16
The partial fundoplication gastroplasty is performed by fully mobilizing the fundus of stomach and drawing the esophagogastric junction into the chest. A stricture, if it is present, is dilated and clamps are placed flush with a #46 to #50 Malloney bougie (A). The gastric tube is cut and closed in two layers (B). The hiatal hernia repair is completed around the gastric tube by a modified Belsey technique (C).

atively as necessary; however, he used a general anaesthetic and the rigid esophagoscope for direct bougienage. This limited bougienage to #26 to #30 Fr.

Belsey Type (Fig. 11.16)

This procedure can be performed as a thoracoabdominal or pure thoracic operation. I use a thoracic approach and reserve the thoracoabdominal for the management of recurrent hiatal hernias. The gastroplasty tube is fashioned over a #50 Fr bougie and the tube is 5 cm in length. A two-thirds fundoplication of the Belsey type is used to anchor the gastroplasty below the diaphragm and for the purpose of reflux control.

Between 1969 and June 1975 I performed 137 PFG procedures and at review had follow-up of 135 patients. In only two patients was there anatomic recurrence radiologically (1.5 per cent). The incidence of continued reflux was high at 44.6 per cent; however, only 26.7 per cent of these had significant reflux symptomatology. This incidence of radiologic reflux is high; however, it is comparable with that reported by DeMeester et al. (53) in evaluation of patients with the standard Belsey fundoplication. All patients with reflux, including reflux with the water syphon test, are included in the report.

Symptomatic reflux occurred in 26.7 per cent, and this is a more important statistic. The incidence of persistent or recurrent reflux

symptoms is similar to that reported by Hiebert and O'Mara (54) in reviewing their 20-year experience with the standard Belsey fundoplication.

In the group of 36 patients (26.7 per cent) with symptomatic and radiologic reflux, 10 (7.4 per cent) have required conversion to a total fundoplication gastroplasty because of the severity of symptoms.

The reflux problem seen with PFG is most severe in patients with previous myotomy of the esophagus or scleroderma. Poor results were also obtained in patients with previous gastric surgery. Moderately good results were obtained in patients with peptic stricture.

These results are comparable to those reported by Orringer and Sloan (55, 56). In his series of 83 patients he had several operative problems including 2 deaths, 2 necrotic gastroplasty tubes and 2 leaks. This complication rate may be related to his method of fundoplication which differs considerably from that originally reported. In follow-up at 12 months he has 19 per cent with symptomatic reflux and 30 per cent by pH testing. One would anticipate a further increase in reflux with a longer follow-up.

Pearson and colleagues (57, 58) continue to report good results with PFG; however, they have 13.4 per cent moderate to severe reflux and 6.5 per cent symptomatic reflux. They do not report their total incidence of reflux. Eleven per cent of patients have persistent and troublesome dysphagia.

Ellis et al. (59) and Childress and Martel (60) have used both PFG and TFG and report better results with TFG as a method of managing the short esophagus.

Clearly further evaluation of these patients is necessary; however, in my hands I have discontinued the use of PFG and now use TFG with much more satisfactory results.

PFG with Uncut Tube

Langer (52) has reported a small series of patients with PFG and a stapled but uncut gastroplasty tube. The numbers of patients are too small for adequate assessment of the results.

Total Fundoplication Gastroplasty

This has been my operation of choice in the management of gastroesophageal reflux for the past 4½ years (61, 62). In the first year the procedure was used only on patients with complex problems of recurrence, stricture, myotomy, scleroderma or previous gastric surgery; however, the results achieved were better than those achieved by standard Nissen procedure in uncomplicated patients, and for this reason it is now used as the elective procedure for reflux control. In the past 3 years I have used a standard Nissen 5 times and have had to resect esophagus for stricture only twice. Three hundred and fifty-nine patients are available with a 6-month to 4½-year follow-up.

Two methods of fundoplication are being used. For uncomplicated cases I use a left 7th interspace thoracotomy and for recurrence or previous gastric surgery I use a short thoracoabdominal incision.

Using the left thoracotomy, the inferior pulmonary ligament is divided and the esophagus mobilized medially and on its pericardial surface to the aortic arch. Laterally I mobilize to the level of the inferior pulmo-

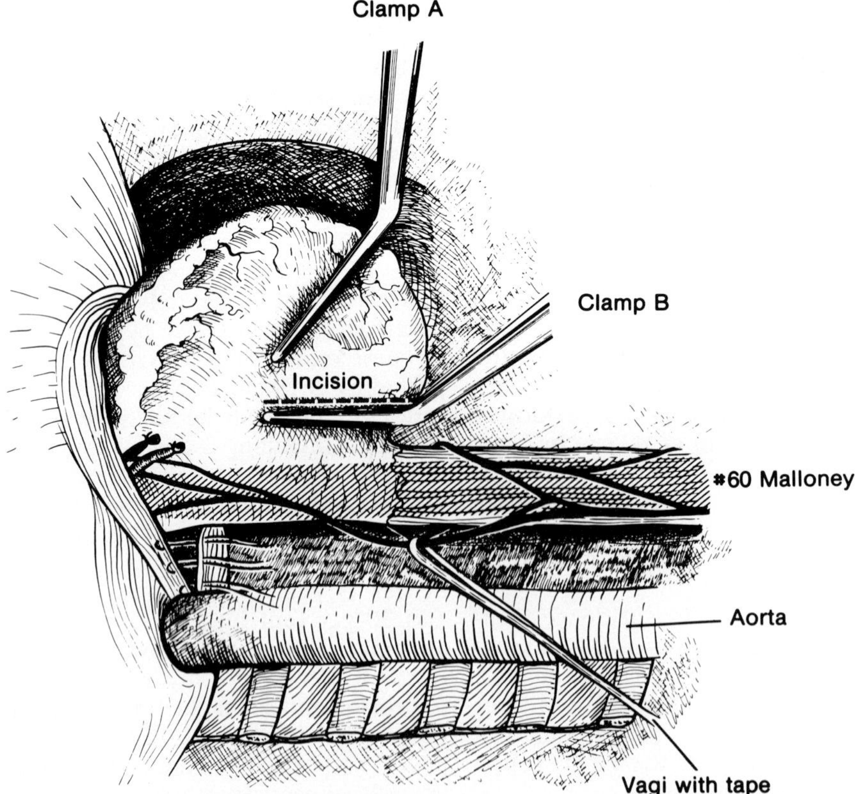

Figure 11.17. Transthoracic Preparation of Gastroplasty Tube
Using the transthoracic approach, the fundus of stomach is mobilized. The gastroplasty tube cut over a #60 Fr Malloney bougie and then closed in two layers using catgut and silk.

nary vein. The esophagogastric junction is fully mobilized and often one to two short gastric arteries have to be divided. The esophagogastric fat pad is removed. Posterior crural sutures are placed deeply in the crural muscle to be tied following hernia reduction. At this Stage I often place a #1 silk thread around the vagi to hold them clear of the gastroplasty and to avoid injury.

A #60 Malloney bougie is passed and right angled deBakey clamps placed snugly along the bougie with one angled into fundus to prevent spillage. Scalpel dissection is used to cut a 5 cm tube leaving a 2 mm cuff of stomach for closure. The bougie is pulled back into the esophagus. A full thickness continuous 00 chromic suture is used to close the gastroplasty and fundus and the clamps removed. A second layer of 000 silk with careful invagination is now placed as a continuous suture. Upon completion of the gastroplasty tube the #60 Fr bougie is again passed and the tube is carefully inspected to ensure that it is 5 cm long and snugly fits throughout its length over the bougie.

With the gastroplasty tube completed the fundoplication is begun and the method of fundoplication varies from the thoracic to the thoracoabdominal position.

Using the thoracic approach (Fig. 11.17), the gastroplasty tube and fundus are sewn together using 00 silk mattress sutures and 2 cm of distal esophagus is incorporated in the fundoplication. With this solid fixation the fundus is then rotated around the esophagus and sewn together with 000 silk mattress sutures to complete the fundoplication (Fig. 11.18).

Using the thoracoabdominal approach a loose fundoplication cannot be achieved by this method and instead the fundus is rotated behind the esophagus in a clockwise manner (Figs. 11.19 and 11.20). With the fundus lying as for its completion wrap it is then sewn to the distal 2 cm of esophagus and gastroplasty suture line with five interrupted 00 silk mattress sutures. The fundoplication is now completed by sewing stomach to stomach. The wrap is competed without the use of a bougie; however, it is very loose and allows a finger to be placed easily between the fundoplication and gastroplasy tube.

In the TFG the length of the gastroplasty tube should be 5 cm, and 2 cm of distal esophagus is incorporated if the esophageal length is adequate. The fundoplication must not exceed 2 cm in completion wrap. These lengths have been learned by trial and error, however, if strictly adhered to, they avoid problems of dysphagia and in most instances allow the patient to burp and if necessary vomit. In early experience with TFG too long a wrap led to dysphagia.

Results of Surgery

Three hundred and fifty-nine patients have been treated by TFG with a follow-up of from 1 to 4½ years (average 28.4 months). Three hundred and fifty-five are available for evaluation by history (98.9 per cent), 319 by radiology (88.9 per cent) and 240 by manometry (66.9 per cent).

Their preoperative symptoms are summarized in Tables 11.2, 11.3, and 11.4. One hundred and seventy-seven (49.3 per cent) patients had one or more complicating factors of previous surgery, scleroderma, ulcerative esophagitis or stricture (Table 11.5).

In follow-up there was no mortality and 3.7 per cent had major morbidity (Table

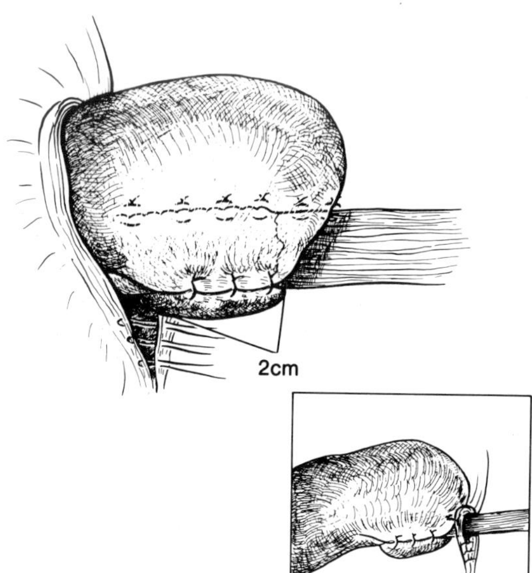
Figure 11.18. Transthoracic Total Fundoplication Gastroplasty
Fundus of stomach is sewn directly to the gastroplasty suture line and distal 2 cm of esophagus for firm fixation. Total fundoplication is completed over a distance of 2 cm.

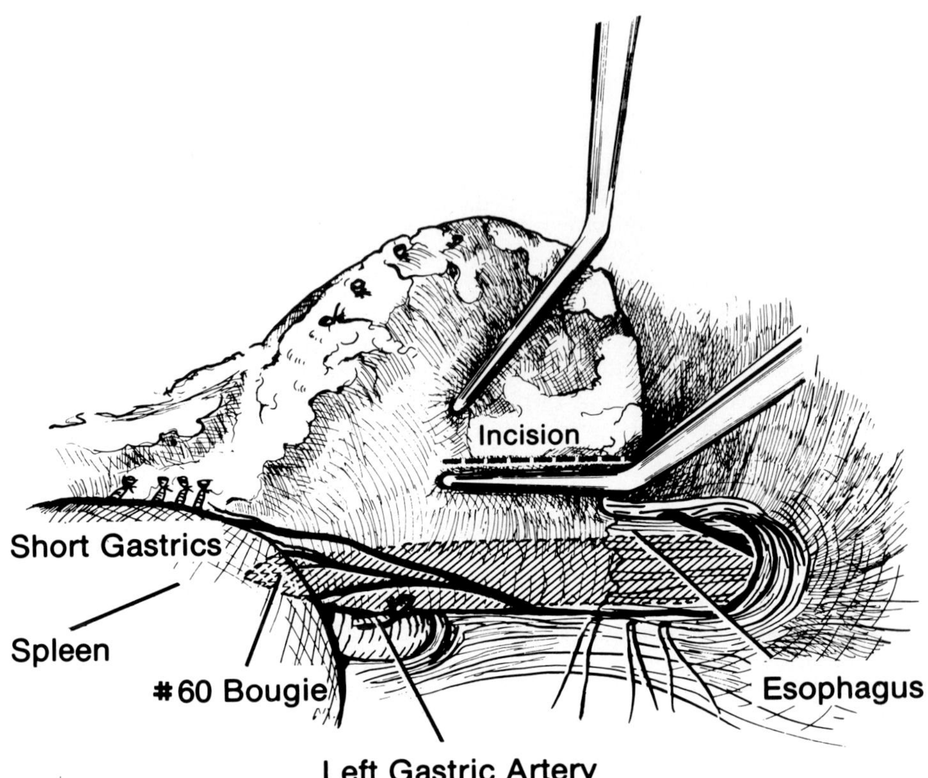

Figure 11.19. Thoracoabdominal Preparation of Gastroplasty Tube
Using the thoracoabdominal approach in patients with recurrent hiatal hernias, the gastroplasty tube is prepared. The left gastric artery is carefully preserved. Before sewing fundus to the gastroplasty tube, the fundus is rotated in a clockwise manner to position it for final suturing.

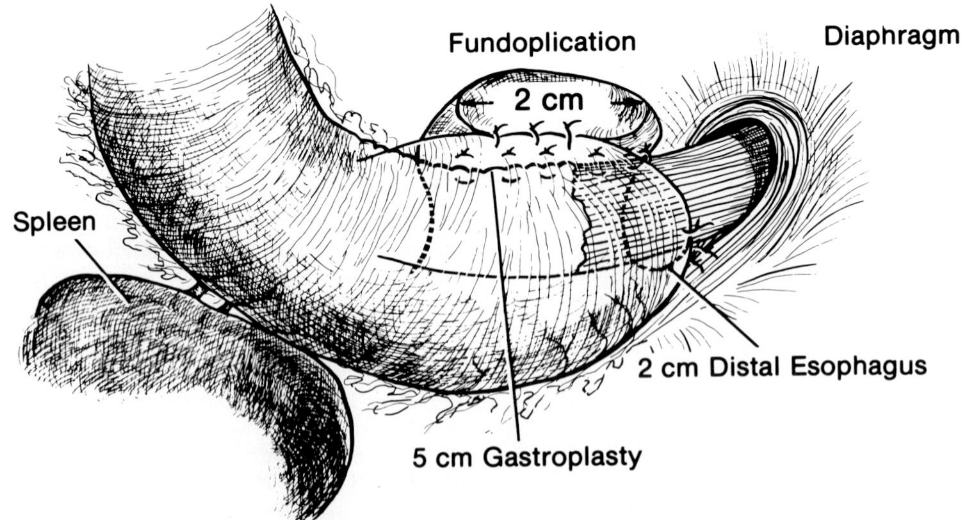

Figure 11.20. Thoracoabdominal Total Fundoplication Gastroplasty
With the fundus rotated in position it is sewn directly to the gastroplasty suture line and distal 2 cm of esophagus. The fundoplication is completed over a distance of 2 cm.

Table 11.2
359 Patients with TFG—Preoperative Symptoms*

	No.	%
Heartburn	359	100
Reflux	304	86.7
Aspiration	147	41
Hiccoughs	99	27.6
Eructation	254	70.6
Water brash	85	23.7
Nausea	251	70
Vomiting	56	15.6
Motor dysphagia		
Total	258	71.9
Gastroesophageal	205	57.1
Pharyngoesophageal	152	42.3
Mechanical dysphagia	26	7.2

* Heartburn, recognizable reflux, dysphagia and nausea are the most common symptoms of gastroesophageal reflux.

Table 11.3
Precipitating Factors (359 TFG)*

	No.	%
Food		
Quality	351	97.8
Quantity	344	95.8
Posture	263	73.3
Exercise	53	14.8
Hunger	63	17.6

* In patients with reflux eating is the most common cause of heartburn; however, posture, exercise and hunger may produce pain and in some these factors are dominant.

Table 11.4
Presenting Symptoms (359 TFG)*

	No.	%
Pain	307	85.6
Pharyngoesophageal dysphagia	18	5
Gastroesophageal dysphagia	29	8
Nausea	3	0.8
Bleeding	1	0.3
Aspiration	1	0.3

* Almost all patients have a single, or presenting, symptom which is dominant. In patients with reflux, pain was by far the most common presenting symptom.

Table 11.5
Complicating Factors*

	No.	%
Previous esophageal surgery	124	34.5
Previous gastric surgery	54	15.0
Scleroderma	2	0.6
Ulcerative esophagitis	36	10.0
Stricture	26	7.2
Total Patients with Complicated Surgery	177	49.2

* The factors listed in this table all add to the technical difficulty of surgical reflux control.

Table 11.6
Results*

	No.	%
Mortality	0	0
Morbidity		
Fistulae	5	1.4
Wound infection	4	1.1
Evisceration	1	0.3
Bowel obstruction	1	0.3
Empyema and subphrenic abscess	2	0.6

* The operative mortality and morbidity are low and are similar to those found with standard hiatal hernia repair.

Table 11.7
Follow-up Assessment*

	No.	%
I No recurrence no reflux	351	98.8
III(A) Revision for dysphagia	3	0.9
III(B) Anatomic recurrence	1	0.3

* Using the gastroplasty tube the incidence of anatomic recurrence is low. This has been confirmed by published reports of the gastroplasty.

11.6). Three hundred and fifty-one (98.9 per cent) have no recurrence or reflux by history, radiology, manometry and pH testing. Three (0.9 per cent) have required revision for dysphagia and one patient (0.3 per cent) has developed anatomic recurrence (Table 11.7).

Evaluation of the Function of TFG

There are two factors of importance in understanding the rationale of TFG. The first is its low anatomic recurrence rate and the second its effectiveness in reflux control.

Anatomic recurrence is rare in all reported series of TFG and PFG. There are two possible explanations, one being that with esophageal lengthening this is a repair without tension. The second factor which I believe is very important is that the lower end of the gastroplasty tube is anchored by the left gastric artery. Using a normal anatomic structure to anchor the repair is of importance in preventing recurrence. I have not yet seen a breakdown of the fundoplication and this I believe is due to the firmness of the anchoring sutures through full thickness of gastroplasty tube suture line and stomach.

Reflux Control (62–64)

The two factors possibly responsible for reflux control are the gastroplasty tube and the method of fundoplication. Contrary to some reports in the 240 manometric studies conducted postoperatively and in the postoperative studies in patients with PFG, the maximum gastroplasty tone is 8 cm H_2O and the average 2 cm H_2O. This tone is unlikely to be of importance in reflux control.

We have studied the response of the gastroplasty tube to an ingested meal. Serum gastrin levels increase in response to the meal; however, there is no corresponding tone increase in the gastroplasty tube or HPZ. When abdominal compression is applied pressures in the gastroplasty increase in a 1/1 ratio, but it shows no evidence of an augmented neurogenic response.

Since the gastroplasty tube is of low tone with no evidence of a hormonally stimulated tone response and no augmented neurogenic response, it seems unlikely that this is the source of reflux control. HPZ tone has been shown to increase from a preoperative level of 12.04 to a postoperative level of 18.35 (6.31 cm of water increase (52.4 per cent). The HPZ tone increase is considered to be the effect of reflux control and while the fundoplication may further augment tone, it is not the prime factor in initiating the tone increase.

The fundoplication is critical. A gastroplasty tube without a fundoplication is ineffective in reflux control. Collis reports 59 per cent moderate to severe reflux. With the addition of 270 degrees of fundoplication the reported incidence of reflux falls to 13 to 44.6 per cent. Now adding total fundoplication reflux is irradicated.

With total fundoplication the gastroplasty tube and usually also the HPZ are surrounded by transmitted gastric pressure. Any intraluminal or extraluminal pressure increase is equally distributed to the 5-cm gastroplasty tube giving effective compression and prevention of reflux. Two cases illustrate the effectiveness of the Nissen total fundoplication for reflux control in the absence of the HPZ.

Case 8. Mrs. G, age 76, presented with a history

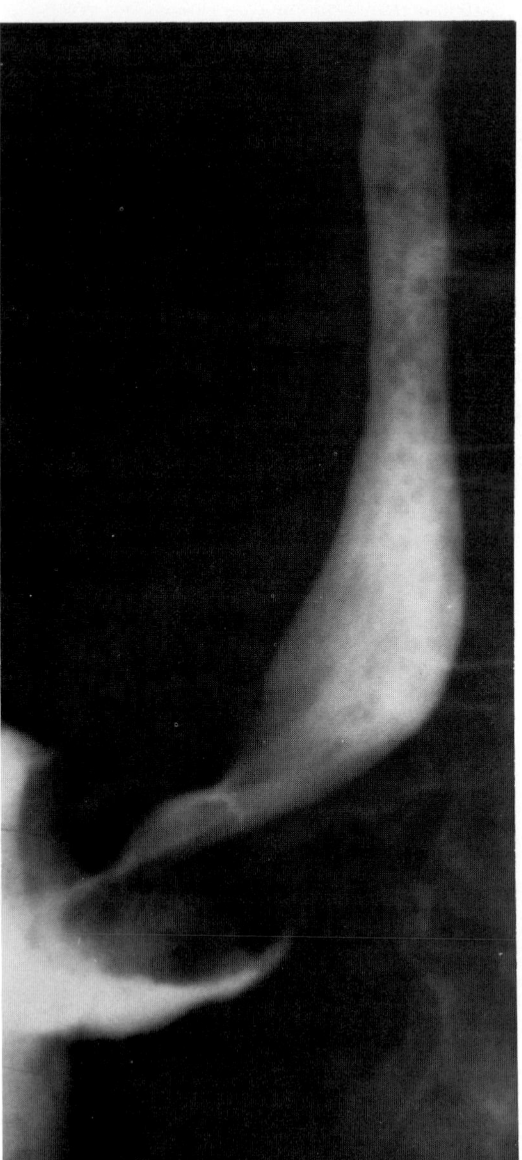

Figure 11.21
Mrs. G., Case 8. This patient has effective reflux control. Radiologically, the total fundoplication is clearly demonstrated and the lower esophagus is compressed by gastric pressure in the surrounding fundus. Solids passed without recognizable obstruction.

of early satiety and epigastric fullness. On examination she had a 20-cm epigastric mass. Radiologic examination showed gastric compression and angiography demonstrated a very vascular mass with its blood supply derived from the coeliac axis. Endoscopically, apart from compression, the stomach was normal.

At operation a 3½-kg leiomyosarcoma was excised from the gastric fundus. The HPZ and proximal stomach were resected, and an end-to-end anastomosis with invagination was constructed below the diaphragm.

This patient now depends for reflux control on her invagination anastomosis. Clinically, radiologically (Fig. 11.21), manometrically (Fig. 11.22) and by pH studies, there is no evidence of reflux. She is now eating well without indigestion or heartburn 2 years after her surgery.

Case 9. Mrs. E, age 56, had had three previous hiatal hernia repairs followed by a bypass side-to-side esophagogastrostomy, 15 years before evaluation. She presented with severe heartburn and mechanical dysphagia from a stricture at the site of the esophagogastrostomy.

Radiologically the esophagogastric bypass was patent and her normal esophagogastric junction was replaced by a 2-mm fibrosed tube. At operation the esophagogastric junction was destroyed by her previous surgery. The esophagogastric bypass was tubular and a #60 Fr bougie could be passed, stretching the stricture. The esophagogastric tube was used as a gastroplasty tube and fundus of stomach wrapped to produce a total fundoplication. Essentially this patient had a TFG with resection of her atrophied HPZ.

Now 2 years after surgery she eats normally and has clinical and radiologic reflux control.

These two patients demonstrate clearly that a subdiaphragmatic total fundoplication is effective in reflux control. Neither the HPZ nor a gastroplasty tube is necessary for reflux control. In my opinion the role of the gastroplasty tube is to prevent anatomic recurrence.

Uncut Total Fundoplication Gastroplasty Tubes

These are now being reported by Bingham (50) and more recently by Evangelist et al. (51). The reported results are satisfactory and again show the value of total fundoplication as a method of reflux control. Bingham doc-

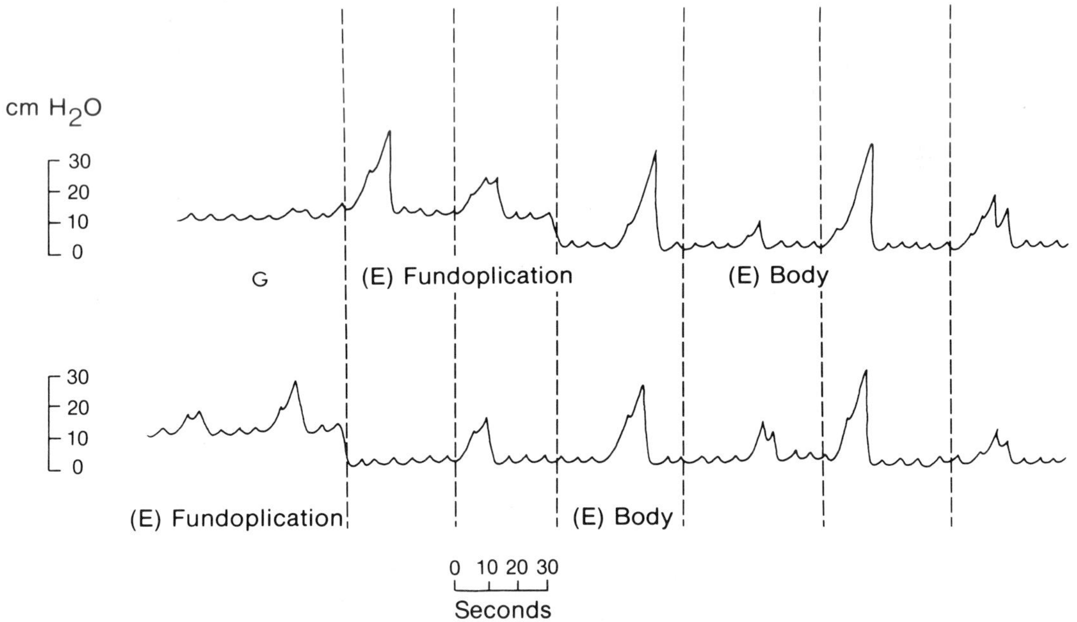

Figure 11.22. Resected HPZ and Nissen Fundoplication
Manometric studies in Mrs. G., Case 8, show a normal stomach (G). The HPZ has been resected and the lower esophagus ((E) fundoplication) is elevated to gastric pressure. There is a sharp fall in esophageal pressure ((E) body) at the upper margin of the fundoplication. These findings are similar to the manometric pattern present with intrathoracic fundoplication following esophageal resection (Fig. 11.2) and indicate the presence of an effective flap valve mechanism controlling reflux.

uments a significant incidence of recurrent reflux following breakdown of the staple division. I have used an uncut tube in conjunction with highly selective vagotomy in 3 patients. All have done well in early follow-up; however, I did not feel that the method of fundoplication was as adequate and have discontinued this method.

Several procedures have been described which are suitable for management of the short esophagus and are equally adaptable to the management of any complex esophageal problem. The optimum choice of procedure has not yet been unanimously selected, and considerable thought and experience are necessary by the individual surgeon before making an appropriate choice.

References

1. Paulson, D. L., Shaw, R. R., and Kee, J. L.: Esophageal hiatal diaphragmatic hernia and its complications. Ann. Surg., *155:* 957, 1962.
2. Skinner, D. B., Belsey, R. H. R., Hendrix, T. R., and Zuidema, G. D. (Editors): *Gastroesophageal Reflux and Hiatal Hernia.* Little, Brown & Co., Boston, 1972.
3. Belsey, R. H.: Reconstruction of the esophagus with left colon. J. Thorac. Cardiovasc. Surg., *49:* 33, 1965.
4. Pearson, F. G., Henderson, R. D., and Parrish, R. M.: An operative technique for control of reflux following esophagogastrostomy. J. Thorac. Cardiovasc. Surg., *58:* 668, 1969.
5. Henderson, R. D., Lind, J. F., and Feaver, B.: Invagination for control of reflux after esophagogastric anastomosis. Can. J. Surg., *14:* 195, 1971.
6. Woodward, E. R., Rayl, J. E., and Clarke, J. M.: Esophageal hiatus hernia. Curr. Probl. Surg., *1:* 62, 1970.
7. Higton, D. I. R., and Lord, I. J.: Dysphagia following colon pedicle grafts. Br. J. Surg., *57:* 825, 1970.
8. Lores, M. E., Ortiz, V., and Marquez, E.: Massive reflux complicating colon interposition in an infant. Bol. Asoc. Med. PR, *70:* 172, 1978.
9. Henderson, R. D., Fung, K., Dube, P., and Marryatt, G.: Esophageal reconstruction; an experimental approach to the control of reflux after esophageal resection. Can. J. Surg., *18:* 165, 1975.
10. Jones, E. L., Skinner, D. B., Demeester, T. R., Elkins, R. C., and Zuidema, G. D.: Response of the interposed human colonic segment to an acid challenge. Ann. Surg., *177:* 75, 1973.
11. Heimlich, H. J.: Reconstruction of entire esophagus and restoration of swallowing with reversed gastric tube. N.Y. State J. Med., *61:* 2478, 1961.
12. Henderson, R. D., Boszko, A., Mugashe, F., Szczepanski, M. M., and Marryatt, G.: Oesophageal replacement by gastric tube; an experimental study of the properties of the gastric tube. Br. J. Surg., *61:* 533, 1974.
13. Tanner, N. C., and Westerholm, P.: Partial gastrectomy in the treatment of esophageal stricture after hiatal hernia. Am. J. Surg., *115:* 449, 1968.
14. Himal, H. S., and MacLean, L. D.: Bile esophagitis. Can. J. Surg., *16:* 17, 1973.
15. Gillson, E. W., De Castro, V. A. M., Nyhus, L. M., Kusakari, K., and Bombeck, C. T.: The significance of bile in reflux esophagitis. Surg. Gynecol. Obstet., *134:* 419, 1972.
16. Ottosen, P., Behrendt, F., and Sondergaard, T.: Treatment of carcinoma of esophagus and cardia; description of a new operative technique. Acta Chir. Scand., *117:* 181, 1959.
17. Payne, W. S., and Olsen, A. M.: *The Esophagus.* Lea & Febiger, Philadelphia, 1974.
18. Coppinger, W. R., Job, H., and DeLauro, J. E.: Surgical treatment of reflux gastritis and esophagitis. Arch. Surg., *106:* 463, 1973.
19. Windsor, C. W.: Gastroesophageal reflux after partial gastrectomy. Br. Med. J., *2:* 1233, 1964.
20. Henderson, R. D.: Gastroesophageal reflux following gastric operation. Ann. Thorac. Surg., *26:* 563, 1978.
21. Burrington, J. D., and Stephens, C. A.: Esophageal replacement with a gastric tube in infants and children. J. Pediatr. Surg., *3:* 24, 1968.
22. Anderson, K. D., and Randolph, J. G.: Gastric tube for esophageal replacement in children. J. Thorac. Cardiovasc. Surg., *61:* 50, 1971.
23. Heimlich, H. J.: Esophagoplasty with reversed gastric tube. Review of fifty-three cases. Am. J. Surg., *123:* 80, 1972.
24. Lam, K. H., Lim, T. K., Wong, J., and Ong, G. B.: Changes in metabolism of major food components in patients with intrathoracic replacement of the oesophagus with the stomach. Br. J. Surg., *65:* 489, 1978.
25. May, I. A., and Samson, P. C.: Esophageal reconstruction and replacements. Ann. Thorac. Surg., *7:* 249, 1969.
26. El-Domeiri, A., Martini, N., and Beattie, E. J., Jr.: Esophageal reconstruction by colon interposition. Arch. Surg., *100:* 358, 1970.
27. Jones, E. L., Booth, D. J., Cameron, J. L., Zuidema, G. D., and Skinner, D. B.: Functional evaluation of esophageal reconstruction. Ann. Thorac. Surg., *12:* 331, 1971.
28. Scanlon, E. F., and Staley, C. J.: The use of the ascending and right half of the transverse colon in esophagoplasty. Surg. Gynecol. Obstet., *107:* 99, 1958.
29. Waterston, D.: Long term clinical state after resection with colon replacement in children. In *Surgery of the Esophagus; The Coventry Conference,* edited by R. A. Smith and R. E. Smith. Butterworths, London, 1972.
30. Merendino, K. A., and Dillard, D. H.: Concept of sphincter substitution by an interposed jejunal segment for anatomic and physiologic abnormalities at esophagogastric junction; with special reference to reflux esophagitis, cardiospasm and esophageal varices. Ann. Surg., *142:* 486, 1955.
31. Merendino, K. A., and Thomas, G. I.: The jejunal interposition operation for substitution of the esophagogastric sphincter; present status. Surgery, *44:* 1112, 1958.

32. Allison, P. R.: Peptic oesophagitis and oesophageal stricture. Lancet, *2:* 199, 1970.
33. Hanna, E. A., Harrison, A. W., and Derrick, J. R.: Long-term results of visceral esophageal substitutes. Ann. Thorac. Surg., *3:* 111, 1967.
34. Thal, A. P., Hatafuku, T., and Kurtzman, R.: New operation for distal esophageal stricture. Arch. Surg., *90:* 464, 1965.
35. Thal, A. P.: A unified approach to surgical problems of the esophagogastric junction. Ann. Surg., *168:* 542, 1968.
36. Ashcraft, K. W., Goodwin, C. D., Amoury, R. W., McGill, C. W., and Holder, T. M.: Thal fundoplication: a simple and safe operative treatment for gastroesophageal reflux. J. Pediatr. Surg., *13:* 643, 1978.
37. Clarke, J. M., Rayl, J. E., and Woodward, E. R.: Experience with the Thal and Nissen operations in the treatment of reflux esophagitis with stricture; a preliminary report. Am. Surg., *35:* 89, 1969.
38. Thomas, H. F., Clarke, J. M., Rayl, J. E., and Woodward, E. R.: Results of the combined fundic patch-fundoplication operation in the treatment of reflux esophagitis with stricture. Surg. Gynecol. Obstet., *135:* 241, 1972.
39. Woodward, E. R.: Surgical treatment of gastroesophageal reflux and its complications. World J. Surg., *1:* 453, 1977.
40. Woodward, E. R.: Surgical treatment of reflux esophagitis and stricture. Postgrad. Med., *61:* 143, 1977.
41. Hollenbeck, J. I., and Woodward, E. R.: Treatment of peptic esophageal stricture with combined fundic patch-fundoplication. Ann. Surg., *182:* 472, 1975.
42. O'Leary, J. P., Hollenbeck, J. I., and Woodward, E. R.: Surgical treatment of esophageal stricture in patients with scleroderma. Am. Surg., *41:* 131, 1975.
43. Nyhus, L. M., and Harkins, H. N.: The treatment of hiatal hernia and esophageal reflux by fundoplication. In *Hernia,* edited by L. M. Nyhus and H. N. Harkins. J. B. Lippincott Co., Philadelphia, 1964.
44. Nissen, R., Rossetti, M., and Siewert, R.: 20 years in the management of reflux disease using fundoplication. Chirurg, *48:* 634, 1977.
45. Megerand, R.: Personal communication, 1972.
46. Collis, J. L.: Gastroplasty. Thorax, *16:* 197, 1961.
47. Pearson, F. G., and Henderson, R. D.: Experimental and clinical studies of gastroplasty in the management of acquired short esophagus. Surg. Gynecol. Obstet., *136:* 737, 1973.
48. Pearson, F. G., Langer, B., and Henderson, R. D.: Gastroplasty and Belsey hiatus hernia repair; an operation for the management of peptic stricture with acquired short esophagus. J. Thorac. Cardiovasc. Surg., *61:* 50, 1971.
50. Bingham, J. A.: Hiatus hernia repair combined with the construction of an anti-reflux valve in the stomach. Br. J. Surg., *64:* 460, 1977.
51. Evangelist, F. A., Taylor, F. H., and Alford, J. D.: The modified Collis-Nissen operation for control of gastroesophageal reflux. Ann. Thorac. Surg., *26:* 107, 1978.
52. Langer, B.: Modified gastroplasty; A simple operation for reflux esophagitis with moderate degrees of shortening. Can. J. Surg., *16:* 84, 1973.
53. DeMeester, T. R., Johnson, L. F., and Kent, A. H.: Evaluation of current operations for the prevention of gatroesophageal reflux. Ann. Surg., *180:* 511, 1974.
54. Hiebert, C. A., and O'Mara, C. S.: The Belsey operation for hiatal hernia; a twenty year experience. Am. J. Surg., *137:* 532, 1979.
55. Orringer, M. B., and Sloan, H.: Complications and failings of the combined Collis-Belsey operation. J. Thorac. Cardiovasc. Surg., *74:* 726, 1977.
56. Orringer, M. B., and Sloan, H.: Collis-Belsey reconstruction of the esophagogastric junction. Indications, physiology and technical considerations. J. Thorac. Cardiovasc. Surg., *71:* 295, 1976.
57. Pearson, F. G.: Surgical management of acquired short esophagus with dilatable peptic stricture. World J. Surg., *1:* 463, 1977.
58. Pearson, F. G., Cooper, J. D., and Nelms, J. M.: Gastroplasty and fundoplication in the management of complex reflux problems. J. Thorac. Cardiovasc. Surg., *76:* 665, 1978.
59. Ellis, F. H., Leonardi, H. K., Dabuzhsky, L., and Crozier, R. E.: Surgery for short esophagus with stricture: an experimental and clinical manometric study. Ann. Surg., *188:* 341, 1978.
60. Childress, M. H., and Martel, W.: Radiologic appearance of the Collis-Belsey fundoplication. J. Can. Assoc. Radiol., *28:* 282, 1977.
61. Henderson, R. D.: The gastroplasty tube as a method of reflux control. Can. J. Surg., *21:* 264, 1978.
62. Henderson, R. D.: Results of total fundoplication gastroplasty in 359 patients. To be published.
63. Orringer, M. B., and Sloan, H.: Combined Collis-Nissen reconstruction of the esophagogastric junction. Ann. Thorac. Surg., *25:* 16, 1978.
64. Cooper, J. D., Gill, S. S., Nelems, J. M., and Pearson, F. G.: Intraoperative and postoperative esophageal manometric findings with Collis gastroplasty and Belsey hiatal hernia repair for gastroesophageal reflux. J. Thorac. Cardiovasc. Surg., *74:* 744, 1977.

Achalasia and Primary Disordered Motor Activity

CHAPTER 12

Achalasia

Etiology

Achalasia of the esophagus is characterized by a failure of relaxation at the gastroesophageal junction and absence of peristalsis from the body of the esophagus. The term, introduced by Hurst in 1913, is derived from the Greek word which denotes lack of relaxation. In the 17th century Willis not only described the symptoms but also devised a simple if heroic treatment; he forced food into his patient's stomach with a whalebone bougie and using this technique was able to keep his patient nourished.

The esophagus responds to the motor obstruction in a manner not seen in other esophageal diseases, because the motor defect in achalasia is quite different. Achalasia has two unique features: first, the failure of relaxation in the gastroesophageal junction is constant and, second, the body of the esophagus dilates progressively in response to motor obstruction.

Food obstruction in hiatal hernia is due to motor spasm in the body of the esophagus, which occurs at variable levels and acts intermittently. Almost all such patients at times eat meals with no recognizable obstruction (Fig. 12.1). When motor spasm is secondary to reflux, the food bolus remains in the esophagus for only a short period and then passes into the stomach or is regurgitated. The obstruction with a peptic stricture is constant, but it is specific for the size of the bolus. If the food particles are small enough or the food is liquid, the feeding passes the obstruction, but if it is too large it is regurgitated. Again, apart from transient episodes where the bolus impacts in the stricture, the esophagus remains empty (Fig. 12.2).

Uncomplicated scleroderma produces an adynamic esophagus, and food descends by gravity drainage. If the disorder is associated with a peptic stricture, obstruction develops.

Despite the combination of a mechanical obstruction and an adynamic esophagus, the esophagus can still empty itself because the food either passes into the stomach or is regurgitated. Although scleroderma may be accompanied by minor degrees of dilatation, this never reaches the extreme seen in achalasia. The failure of gastroesophageal relaxation which characterizes achalasia presents a constant obstruction to both liquids and solids. As the years pass, the body of the esophagus progressively dilates and becomes a reservoir for undigested food; the retained bulk increases with each meal, and between meals some of this content slowly gravitates through into the stomach. In advanced achalasia this esophageal retention is constant and accounts for the unique symptoms and radiologic features encountered in this disorder (Figs. 12.3 and 12.4).

Despite the long history and despite extensive investigation of the disorder, its etiology remains elusive. The various theories advanced to explain it can be divided into three groups.

1. Neurogenic — ganglion deficiency
— vagal nerve degeneration
— central vagal motorneuron disease
2. Myogenic
3. Hormonal — altered sensitivity to gastrin
4. Congenital

These theories are based largely on the analysis of human data, but studies have been done in animals that develop achalasia-like disorders and in those treated to produce a motor defect similar to achalasia.

Animal Studies

Many workers have attempted to reproduce achalasia in animals by damaging the esophagus with cold (1) and with neurotoxins

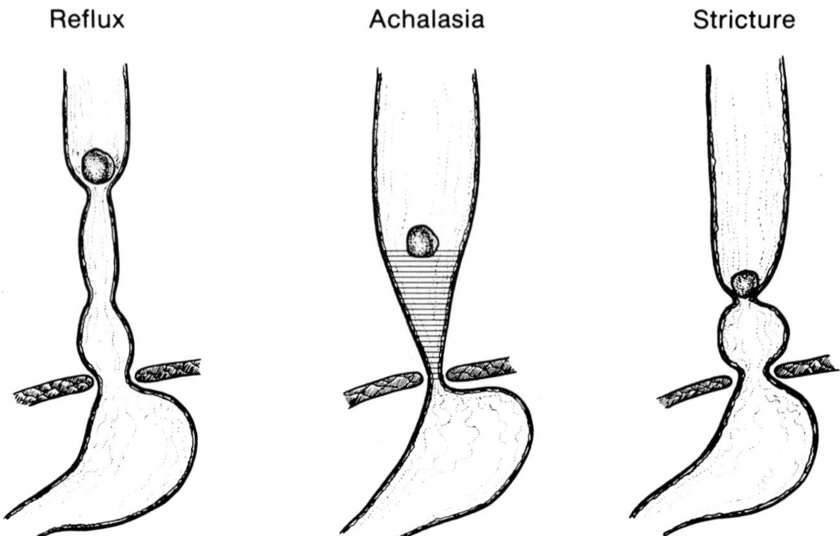

Figure 12.1
In patients with reflux obstruction secondary to motor spasm the obstruction may occur to liquids or solids; however, on occasion food will be swallowed without difficulty. Patients with a stricture have constant food obstruction, occurring whenever the food particle is larger than the stricture lumen size. With achalasia the high pressure zone does not relax; obstruction is constant and occurs to both liquids and solids.

(2). Ischemia has been studied experimentally to determine whether or not it could account for ganglion cell loss in congenital or acquired achalasia (3–7). These methods produce damage in the ganglion cells, and also damage muscle cells. In any event, these changes cannot be compared directly to the human condition. By itself, the added muscle damage may explain some of the motor changes produced (8–10).

Electrolytic lesions (11) in the medulla of dogs and cats produce motor and radiologic changes similar to human achalasia. In dogs direct section of the vagi (12) at a high cervical level blocks esophageal peristalsis and the gastroesophageal junction fails to relax.

In these animal studies progressive esophageal dilatation can be shown radiologically. The changes produced by neurogenic injury certainly mimic human achalasia, but some important differences exist which make it impossible to directly compare the experimental model to the human. Of primary importance is the species difference, and in the dog in addition there is a major structural difference, as the dog's esophagus is composed of striated muscle. Also the denervation in the experimental animal is total and involves the recurrent laryngeal nerves also. In the human we do not see such total denervation, making it very difficult to compare the two situations. Finally, in the experimental animal studies are short-term, unlike the human counterpart where most patients have an established esophageal disorder of many years' duration.

In nature certain animals have achalasia-like conditions; the dog may show progressive esophageal dilatation, food obstruction and regurgitation (13). This process, which is found in certain species, may occur in several dogs, in the same litter, suggesting that the disorder is inherited. At first sight this would seem to offer an ideal experimental model; however, the motor defect here is different from achalasia (14) and occasionally may go on to spontaneous remission.

Human Studies

Neurogenic Theory of Achalasia

The most widely accepted theory is that the achalasia is secondary to ganglion-cell deficiency in Auerbach's plexus (15, 16).

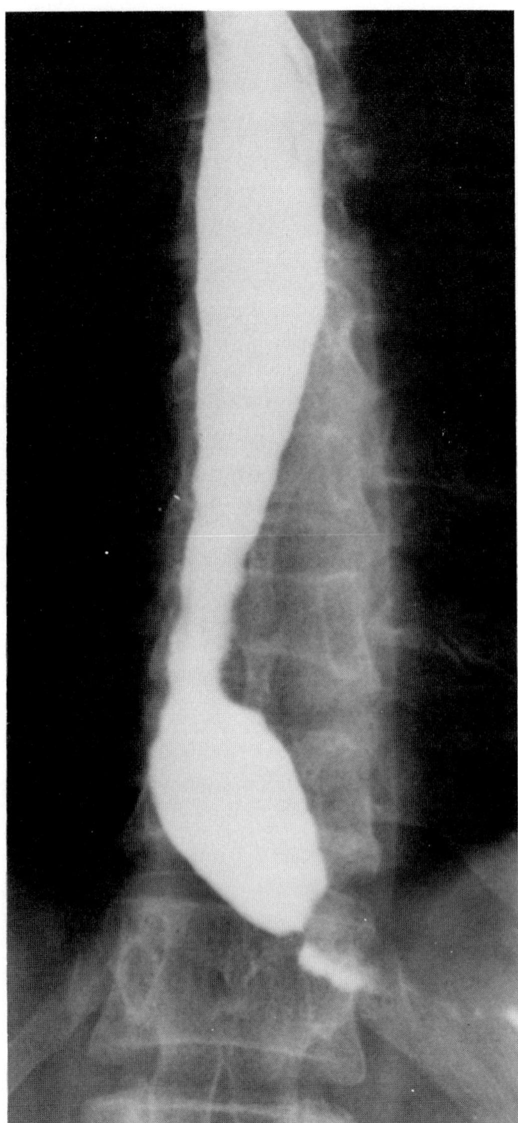

Figure 12.2
This patient has a hiatal hernia and tight peptic stricture. Despite frequent obstruction to solids, there is no food retention and all food either passes to the stomach or is regurgitated.

Hence it has been compared to Hirschsprung's disease, but unlike Hirschsprung's, which is congenital, achalasia usually develops in early adult life. Chagas' disease of the esophagus—a disease largely confined to South America—is similar to achalasia, but is due to the destruction of ganglion cells by *Trypanosoma cruzi* (17–19). In any event, recent studies have challenged early reports of ganglion deficiency and, indeed, although ganglion cells are usually reduced in achalasia, they are seldom absent and their numbers may be normal. Cassella et al. reported that the ganglion cells in the gastroesophageal junction were reduced by an average of 50 per cent (20).

In patients with achalasia, electron microscopic studies of the vagal nerves have demonstrated degenerative changes, of a type similar to Wallerian degeneration (20), which may be responsible for decreased vagal function in the esophagus as well as in other organs. In addition, Woolam and associates (21) have shown that in a proportion of patients with achalasia, gastric acid secretion stimulated through the vagi by the Hollander test is abnormal. This altered gastric acid secretion although not always present provides strong supporting evidence of vagal nerve degeneration.

Autopsy studies occasionally demonstrate changes in the dorsal motor nucleus of the vagus (22, 23)—changes which may be responsible for the distal vagal nerve degeneration and the alteration in ganglion cells of Auerbach's plexus. These reports are based on studies of small numbers of patients and, in themselves, do not justify general acceptance of the neurogenic theory.

Ganglion cell deficiency suggests a neurogenic origin for achalasia. This theory has been tested by using cholinergic drugs to stimulate the esophagus. Cannon's law states that denervated structures become exquisitely sensitive to the chemical mediator which had been their stimulus when the nerves were intact (24). Using this law, esophageal stimulation by cholinergic drugs has been shown to produce a diffuse esophageal spasm (25). This sensitivity to cholinergic drugs is very effective proof that neurogenic injury is present.

Myogenic Theory

Pharmacologic Studies

Several workers have studied the pharmacologic properties of strips of esophageal muscle taken from the gastroesophageal junction at operation in normal subjects and in patients with achalasia (26). Normally both the longitudinal and the circular muscle of

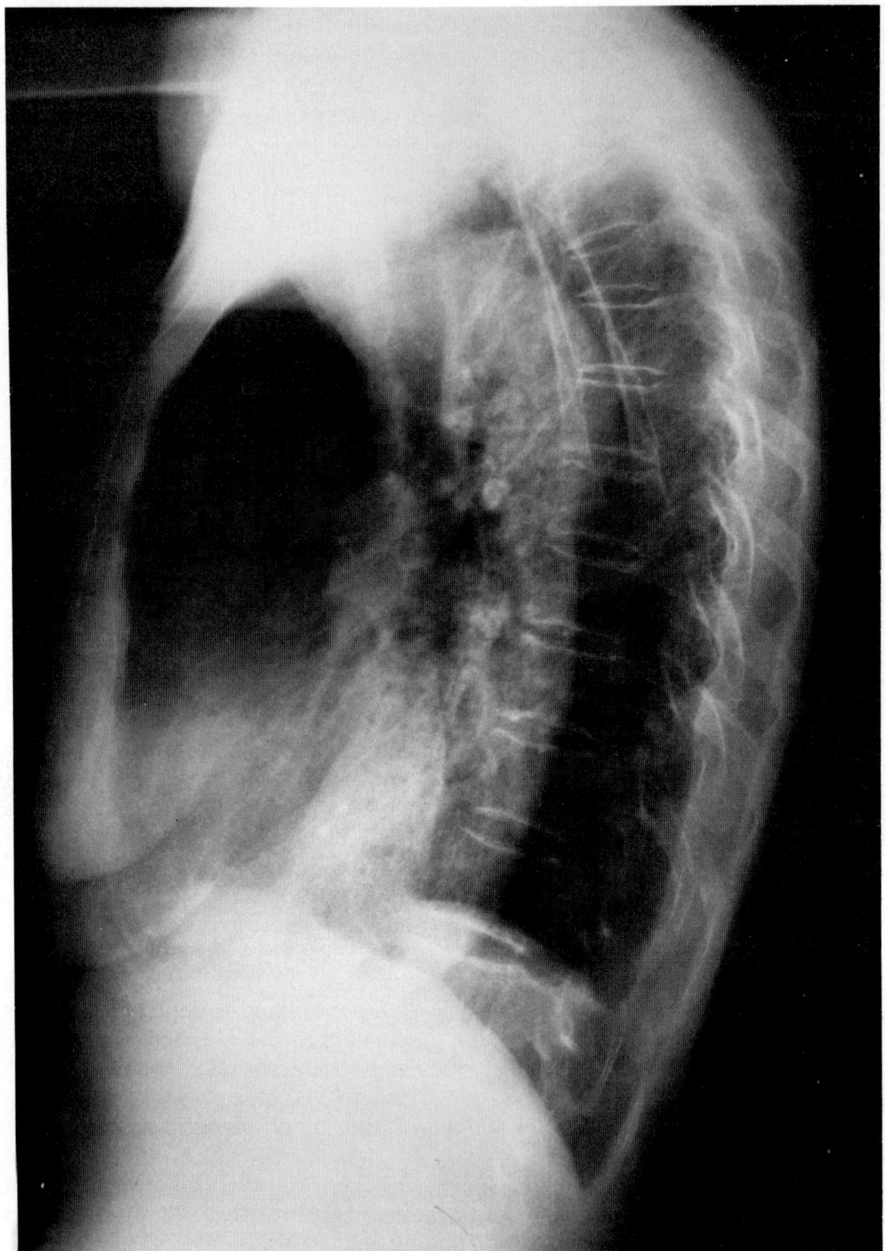

Figure 12.3
In this patient a Stage III achalasia is present. The esophagus is dilated and tortuous. There is massive food retention with an air fluid level in the upper mediastinum.

the esophagus contain α- and β-adrenergic receptors. Muscle taken from patients with achalasia exhibited no β-adrenergic activity, i.e., that which inhibits muscle contraction. Misiewicz and colleagues (27) believe this finding explains the loss of relaxation at the gastroesophageal junction.

Ganglion cell counts in these same groups of patients showed a marked deficiency in those with achalasia.

Muscle Cell Changes

Muscle cell changes have been demonstrated using the electron microscope. These

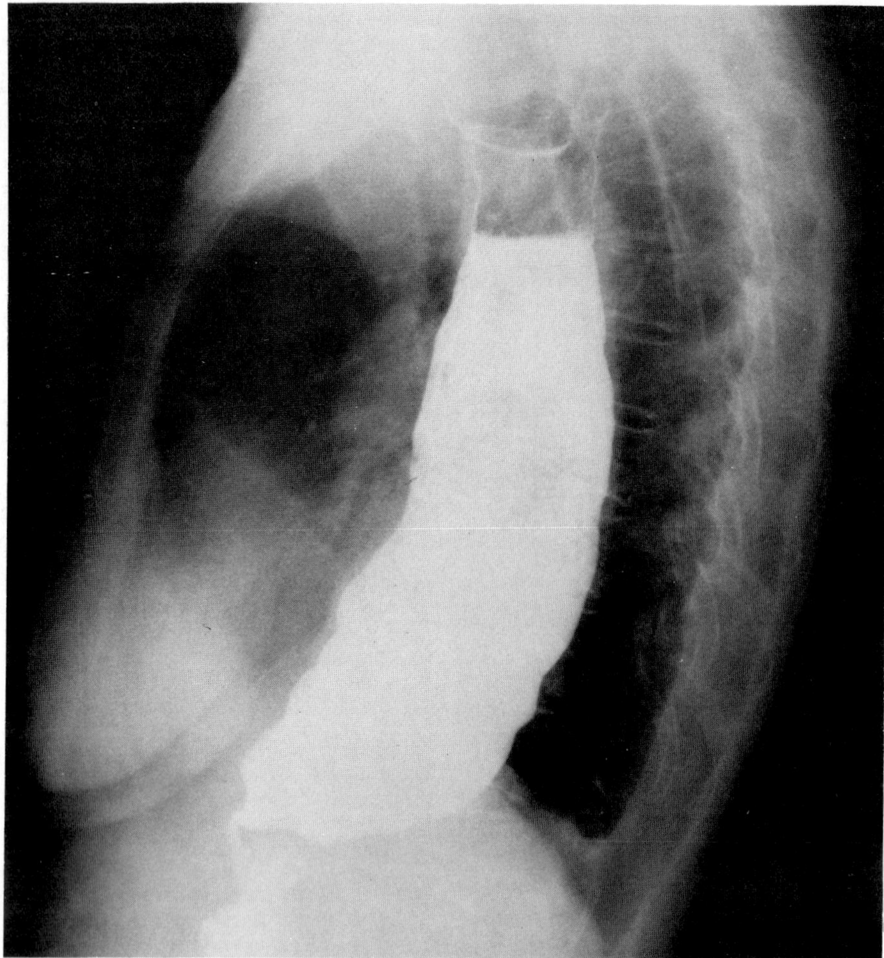

Figure 12.4
The same patient as illustrated in Figure 12.3. In this case contrast material is used to better display the low fluid retention and upper mediastinal air fluid level.

changes, which were most marked at the junctional zone between the narrow distal segment of esophagus and the proximal dilated esophagus, fit the pattern of cellular autolysis (9, 10, 19).

Hormonal Theory

In manometric studies of the gastroesophageal junction the achalasia patient has a higher average pressure than normal subjects (28, 29). In the normal subject, when the stomach is acidified, gastrin release is suppressed and the gastroesophageal junctional pressure falls; however, in achalasia this fall in pressure is more marked. In achalasia patients also the gastroesophageal junction is supersensitive to exogenous gastrin injection.

This is not an unexpected finding as gastrin acts through cholinergic fibers and should stimulate the esophagus in the presence of nerve degeneration.

Congenital Theory

Achalasia does occur in the newborn although this is much rarer than in adults (30). There are also rare reports of achalasia occurring in siblings suggesting a congenital autosomol recessive disorder (31, 32). A syndrome of deafness and short stature, vitiligo, muscle wasting and achalasia has been described (33). The rarity of these reports suggests that although congenital achalasia does occur it is rare and cannot be considered as the prime etiology.

Most of the substantial body of data bearing on the etiology of achalasia suggests that it is a neurogenic disorder secondary to vagal nerve degeneration. Anatomically the available evidence locates the major pathologic changes in the vagal nerves. However, the cause of the vagal degeneration and its exact site have not been defined. Sensitivity to gastrin in achalasia, although it suggests an alternate etiology, may be explained in terms of an increased sensitivity of the gastroesophageal junction secondary to nerve degeneration.

Many etiologic factors may produce vagal degeneration, and achalasia may represent an end process reflecting a major esophageal response to neurogenic deficiency.

Although basic and clinical investigations have not yet assigned a cause to achalasia, they have produced much information that is of diagnostic value and in future may have therapeutic value.

Diagnostically vagal degeneration can be recognized and used to support the clinical diagnosis. In such patients the gastric acidity is low, and they do not respond to insulin stimulation during the Hollander test (34, 35). On manometry, cholinergic drugs produce an increase in esophageal tone (25) and this is of some diagnostic value. Both of these investigations are now applied clinically in the assessment of the achalasia patient.

The response of the esophagus to gastrin and the reduction in tone of the gastroesophageal junction following gastrin inhibition by gastric acidification suggest that gastrin inhibition may produce the chemical "myotomy" of the gastroesophageal junction. Although this mechanism is still theoretical, it is a promising first step toward the medical management of achalasia.

References

 1. Alnor, P.: On the pathogenesis of cardiospasm: an experimental study. J. Thorac. Cardiovasc. Surg., *36:* 141, 1958.
 2. Deloyers, L., Cordier, R., and Dupres, H.: A new approach to the physiology of so-called cardiospasm; experimental production of cardiospasm in cats after destruction of Auerbach's plexus. Ann. Surg., *146:* 167, 1957.
 3. Earlam, R. J.: Ganglion cell changes in experimental stenosis of the gut. Gut, *12:* 393, 1971.
 4. Earlam, R. J.: A vascular cause for aganglionic bowel. A new hypothesis. Am. J. Dig. Dis., *17:* 225, 1972.
 5. Earlam, R. J., Schlegel, J. F., and Ellis, F. H., Jr.: Effects of ischemia of lower esophagus and esophagogastric junction on canine esophageal motor function. J. Thorac. Cardiov. Surg., *54:* 822, 1967.
 6. Louw, J. H.: Congenital intestinal atresia and stenosis in the newborn. Observations on its pathogenesis and treatment. Ann. R. Coll. Surg. Engl., *25:* 209, 1959.
 7. Barnard, C. N.: The genesis of intestinal atresia. Surg. Forum, *7:* 393, 1956.
 8. Harrison, G. K., and Melcher, D. H.: Oesophageal-muscle changes in achalasia. Lancet, *1:* 530, 1969.
 9. Alnor, P.: On the pathogenesis of cardiospasm; an experimental study. J. Thorac. Surg., *36:* 141, 1958.
10. Haman, J. W., O'Hagarty, M. T., and Byrnes, C. K.: The ultrastructure of human smooth muscle: 1. Studies of all surface and connections in normal achalasia esophageal smooth muscle. Exp. Mol. Path., *1:* 204, 1962.
11. Higgs, B., Kerr, F. W., and Ellis, F. H., Jr.: The experimental production of esophageal achalasia by electrolytic lesions in the medulla. J. Thorac. Cardiovasc. Surg., *50:* 613, 1965.
12. Carveth, S. W., Schlegel, J. F., Code, C. F., and Ellis, F. H.: Esophageal motility after vagotomy, phrenectomy, myotomy and myomectomy in dogs. Surg. Gynecol. Obstet., *114:* 31, 1962.
13. Hoffer, R. E., Valdes-Dapena, A., and Baue, A. E.: A comparative study of naturally occurring canine achalasia. Arch. Surg., *95:* 83, 1967.
14. Diamant, N., Szczepanski, M., and Mui, H.: Manometric characteristics of idiopathic megaesophagus in the dog; an unsuitable animal model for achalasia in man. Gastroenterology, *65:* 216, 1973.
15. Rake, G. W.: Pathology of achalasia of cardia. Guy's Hosp. Rep., *77:* 141, 1927.
16. Adams, C. W., Brain, R. H., and Trounce, J. R.: Ganglion cells in achalasia of the cardia. Virchows Arch. Pathol. Anat., *372:* 75, 1976.
17. Etzel, E.: Megaoesophagus and its neuropathology; clinical and anatomo-pathological research. Guy's Hosp. Rep., *87:* 158, 1937.
18. Koberle, F.: Chagas' disease and Chagas' syndromes; the pathology of American typanosomiasis. Adv. Parasitol., *6:* 63, 1968.
19. Earlam, R. J.: Gastrointestinal aspects of Chagas' disease. Am. J. Dig. Dis., *17:* 559, 1972.
20. Cassella, R. R., Ellis, F. H., Jr., and Brown, A. L. Jr.: Fine-structure changes in achalasia of the esophagus; 1. Vagus nerves. Am. J. Pathol., *46:* 279, 1965.
21. Woolam, G. L., Maher, F. T., and Ellis, F. H., Jr.: Vagal nerve function in achalasia of the esophagus. Surg. Forum, *18:* 362, 1967.
22. Elder, J. B., and Gillespie, G.: The vagus and achalasia. Gut, *10:* 1045, 1969.
23. Kimura, K.: The nature of idiopathic esophagus dilatation. Jap. J. Gastroenterol., *1:* 199, 1929.
24. Davenport, H. W.: *Physiology of the Digestive Tract: An Introductory Text.* Year Book Medical Publishers, Chicago, 1961.
25. Kramer, P., and Ingelfinger, F. J.: Esophageal sensitivity to mecholyl in cardiospasm. Gastroenterology, *19:* 242, 1951.
26. Trounce, J. R., Deuchar, D. C., Kauntze, R., and Thomas, G. A.: Studies in achalasia of the cardia. Q. J. Med., *26:* 433, 1957.
27. Misiewicz, J. J., Waller, S. L., Anthony, P. P., and Gummer, J. W. P.: Achalasia of the cardia; pharmacology and histopathology of isolated cardiac

sphincteric muscle from patients with and without achalasia. Q. J. Med., *38:* 17, 1969.

28. Cohen, S., Lipshutz, W., and Hughes, W.: Role of gastrin supersensitivity in the pathogenesis of lower esophageal sphincter hypertension in achalasia. J. Clin. Invest., *50:* 1241, 1971.

29. Editorial: Gastrin and the gastroesophageal sphincter. J.A.M.A., *217:* 1098, 1971.

30. Muralidharan, S., Jairaj, P. S., Periyanayagam, W. J., and John, S.: Achalasia cardia; a review of 100 cases. Aust. N.Z. J. Surg., *48:* 167, 1978.

31. Westley, C. R., Herbst, J. J., Goldman, S., and Wiser, W. C.: Infantile achalasia; inherited as an autosomal recessive disorder. J. Pediatr., *87:* 243, 1975.

32. London, F. A., Raab, D. E., and Fuller, J.: Achalasia in three siblings; a rare occurrence. Mayo Clin. Proc., *52:* 97, 1977.

33. Rozychi, D. L., Ruben, R. J., Rapin, I., and Sprio, A. J.: Autosomal recessive deafness associated with short stature, vitiligo, muscle wasting and achalasia. Arch. Otolaryngol., *93:* 194, 1971.

34. Hollander, F.: Insulin test for presence of intact nerve fibers after vagal operations for peptic ulcer. Gastroenterology, *7:* 607, 1946.

35. Perey, B. J. F.: Recent advances in the physiology of gastric acid secretion. Can. Med. Assoc. J., *89:* 1183, 1963.

CHAPTER 13

Achalasia: Investigation

Often the symptoms of achalasia are non-specific, and the physician must depend upon investigative procedures to establish the diagnosis. However, taken in conjunction with the various investigations, the symptoms help to stage the disease, assess its progression and establish the priorities of therapy.

Although Willis described this disorder in the 17th century, very few cases were reported until this century. Mikulicz could collect only 100 cases from the world literature in 1904 (1, 2). This paucity of case material almost certainly reflects the absence of specific diagnostic tools up to the time when radiology and esophageal manometry were introduced.

Achalasia can occur at any age from infancy to the end of life. There is no particular sex distribution. The major symptoms are dysphagia, regurgitation and pain; less common symptoms include respiratory symptoms secondary to aspiration, late-stage weight loss, vitamin deficiency, hemorrhage and arthritis (3). Secondary carcinoma is sufficiently frequent that it should be considered a complication of this disorder (4).

The symptoms can be understood best by considering the radiologic staging of the disease. To some extent, the symptoms change as the esophagus progressively dilates. Radiologically Stage I is when the largest diameter of the esophagus is less than 4 cm; Stage II when the diameter is more than 4 but less than 6 cm and Stage III when the diameter is greater than 6 cm (5).

Stage I (Fig. 13.1)

Radiologically and chronologically, this usually represents an early phase of the disease in which the esophagus still retains its motor power. These patients have marked dysphagia and often pain, which is associated with spastic obstruction to the passage of food. Some patients may regurgitate, but all manage to pass some food into the stomach. This stage includes those with "vigorous" achalasia who have more marked esophageal motor activity and more prominent pain.

In children achalasia presents as failure to thrive, frequent regurgitation and occasionally, recurrent aspiration and respiratory infections (6, 7).

Stage II (Fig. 13.2)

This phase is characterized by a gradual lessening of symptoms as the esophagus begins to dilate and to retain food. Pain and regurgitation are clearly less frequent and recognizable food obstruction may be intermittent. These patients often describe retrosternal fullness and discomfort, and may note sensitivity to cold liquids or even occasional total obstruction. In general, they may ignore their difficulties for years because their symptoms have abated.

Stage III (Fig. 13.3)

This marks the end stage of achalasia. The esophagus assumes a sigmoid shape, and food retention is massive. The only distress these patients describe is a full retrosternal discomfort. Regurgitation, night aspiration and respiratory symptoms are more common, and these patients may develop respiratory symptoms from aspiration. Weight loss tends to be slowly progressive, and only rarely do these patients develop hemorrhages and vitamin deficiency. The arthritis described in these patients is probably secondary to suppuration of the lung, and patients in this group are subject to esophageal carcinoma.

Pain

The pain described by patients with achalasia arises in the esophagus and generally cannot be distinguished from other forms of esophageal pain (8). Most typically, these patients describe a retrosternal fullness and

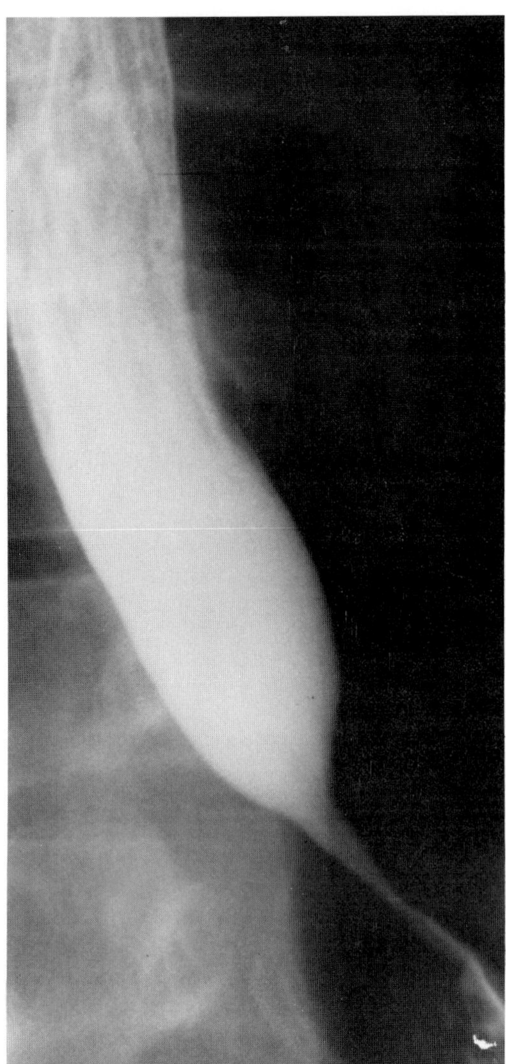

Figure 13.1. Stage I Achalasia
Stage I achalasia is defined radiologically as an esophageal diameter of less than 4 cm. The other typical radiologic feature illustrated here is the "bird beak" gastroesophageal junction.

discomfort associated with eating, which is relieved when the food is regurgitated or passes into the stomach by gravity. The patient with vigorous achalasia may complain of spontaneous pain unrelated to eating or to other activities. This pain can be sufficiently severe and frequent that it becomes the patient's major symptom, and may so resemble heartburn that it cannot be distinguished from the distress of hiatal hernia.

Spontaneous pain is an important symptom to recognize as it is often refractory to dilatation or surgical myotomy. In a series of 102 patients treated by Heller myotomy only 37 per cent were pain-free postoperatively (9).

Dysphagia

The difficulty in swallowing is secondary to motor spasm. In patients with hiatal hernias or diffuse spasm, even when dysphagia is severe it will fluctuate and occasionally food is eaten without recognizable obstruction. Although patients with achalasia exhibit similar variability, the dysphagia becomes constant as the disease progresses and then there are no periods of remission. The constancy of this obstruction can be confirmed radiologically; the dilated esophagus shows a constant air-fluid level, which indicates persistent obstruction (Fig. 13.3). This characteristic feature is related to the failure of the gastroesophageal junction to relax.

Regurgitation

Regurgitation is common; 60 per cent (8) of achalasia patients complain of it. The quality of the regurgitated bolus has important diagnostic implications. In hiatal hernia, the patient describes refluxed material as sour, bitter or burning; in mechanical stricture, the regurgitant tastes like the food he swallowed earlier. Patients with achalasia complain that the taste has altered, but do not describe the burning so characteristic of gastric reflux. In some patients this specific taste change may point to the diagnosis (Fig. 13.4).

Weight Loss

Weight loss is a feature of advanced disease and is associated with massive retention (3). It is occasionally seen in those with very acute and frequent regurgitation. Weight loss is not common in most nonmalignant esophageal disease because with mechanical obstruction milk and other nutritious foods can still be taken fairly well. In achalasia weight loss can be profound owing to the constancy of the obstruction, and if the process is not reversed can lead on to general debility and death.

Respiratory Symptoms

Respiratory symptoms are frequent and tend to be severe (10–12). These symptoms present in 33 percent of patients with achalasia and are usually more severe than in

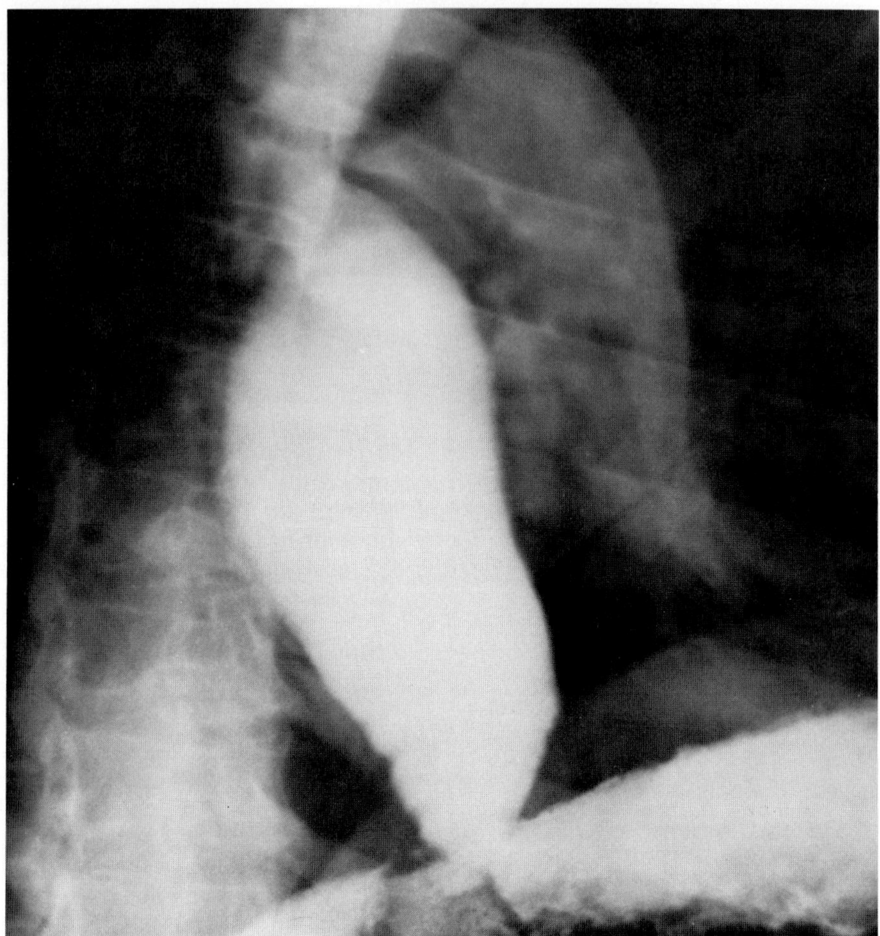

Figure 13.2. Stage II Achalasia
Stage II achalasia is defined radiologically as an esophageal diameter of 4 to 6 cm. Esophageal retention is present, but the esophagus has not developed the sigmoid configuration of a late-stage achalasia.

patients with a hiatal hernia. In general, respiratory symptoms reflect the quality, frequency and quantity of the aspirate and, in addition, may reflect the condition of the lung parenchyma and tracheobronchial tree. In achalasia the main variant is the quality of the aspirate, which tends to be pooled and contaminated bolus. This specific problem (infection) is unique in achalasia because few other esophageal diseases are associated with prolonged esophageal retention of food (Fig. 13.5).

Carcinoma of Esophagus in Achalasia

Esophageal carcinoma, which has been reported in 2.7 (13) to 19 percent (14) of patients with achalasia, must be rigorously excluded by endoscopy and radiology in all patients. This cancer usually develops in Stage III achalasia in the presence of massive distention of the esophagus and longstanding stasis; here the malignancy is secondary to chronic mucosal irritation. In the presence of dilatation, symptoms of obstruction may be long delayed, and often these patients present with far advanced cancer.

If the carcinoma is due to chronic irritation from esophageal pooling, the most effective prevention would be improvement in drainage by dilatation or by surgery. Unfortunately reports suggest that despite adequate surgical drainage as many as 8.5 percent (15) of patients go on to develop carcinoma (16). This late complication has only recently been

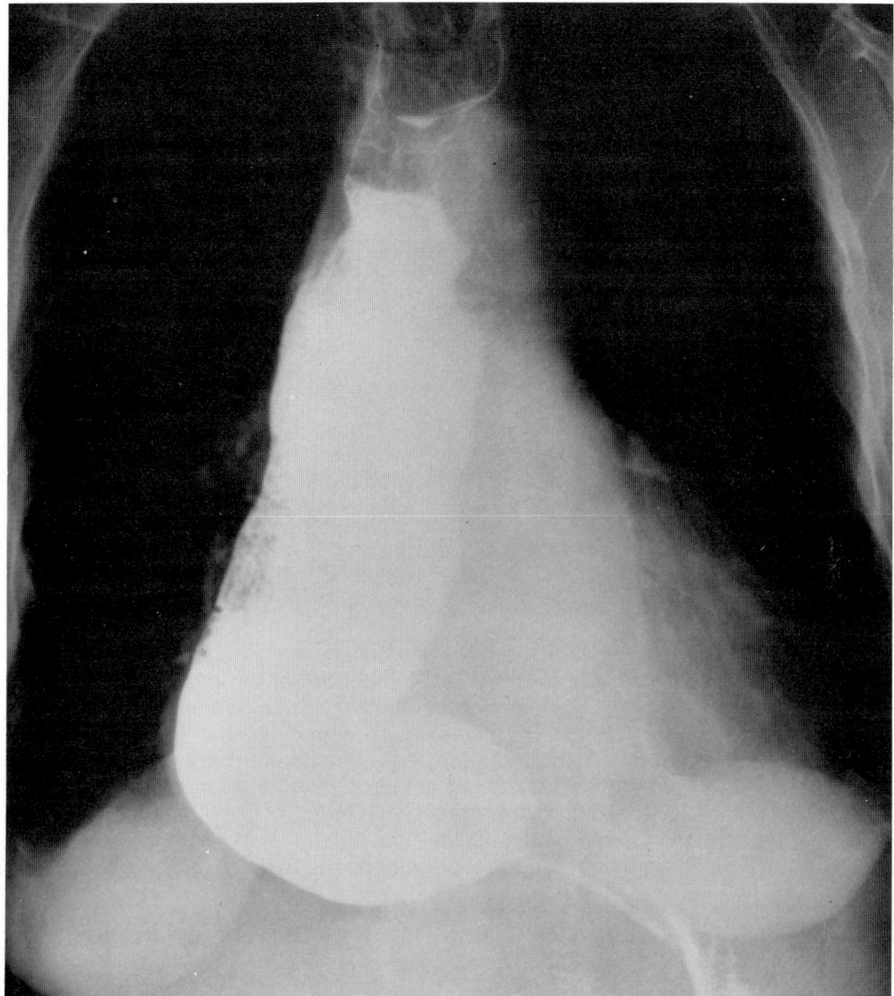

Figure 13.3. Stage III Achalasia
Stage III achalasia is characterized by massive (greater than 6 cm) dilatation of the esophagus and food retention. The air-fluid level is often of a high level in the mediastinum. The constancy of the air-fluid level indicates that the obstruction is continuous and unremitting.

recognized, but its presence clearly indicates the necessity of long-term follow-up of these patients. Although the symptoms of achalasia are described and related to each other in terms of the stage of the disease, this concordance is not always clear. Each patient is individual and in each the dominant symptom may vary. Many patients describe the progression of their illness in a way that resembles a slow progression from stage to stage, but exceptions are frequent; e.g., a young patient may present with Stage III achalasia without a preceding history.

Case 1. Mr. C., age 23, presented with a history of severe dysphagia. Immediately following each meal he developed retrosternal fullness, usually relieved by regurgitation of altered food content. The symptoms began acutely 6 weeks before and had remained severe. He gave no prior history of esophagal problems.

Radiologic evaluation (Fig. 13.4) showed a Stage III achalasia. The x-ray is typical, showing a tapered gastroesophageal junction and proximal esophageal dilatation and retention. Manometric studies were also typical, with a normal tone gastroesophageal junction, no relaxation and total low amplitude esophageal disordered motor activity.

He was treated by transthoracic Heller myotomy and hernia repair. It is now years since surgical correction and he continues to progress well.

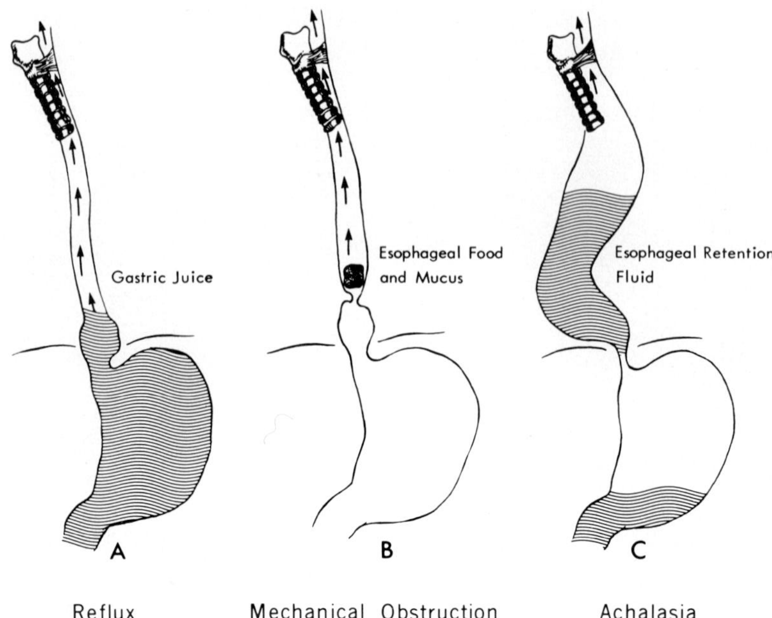

Figure 13.4. Return of Gastrointestinal Content to Throat
Taste and content of a regurgitated bolus vary with the source of the regurgitant. In gastroesophageal reflux, the return is gastric content and contains food, saliva and gastric and possibly duodenal secretions. The taste is bitter, burning or sour. With mechanical or some forms of motor esophageal obstruction, the return is saliva, esophageal mucus and food content. The esophagus usually does not tolerate the presence of an obstructed bolus and regurgitation is early. The taste is that of food. Achalasia is associated with esophageal retention. The esophageal content is food, saliva and mucus, but, because of stagnation and the presence of bacteria, some fermentation may take place and the content is altered in taste often being sweet-tasting.

Patients with achalasia often develop techniques to assist food passage. They may drink fluids to fill their esophagus and use the resultant hydrostatic pressure to push nutrients into the stomach. Some learn to increase intrathoracic pressure by a forced Valsalva maneuver and thus force food through to the stomach. However, most patients find the symptoms so severe that they seek medical advice.

Evaluation of Symptoms

In evaluating the achalasia patient, history, radiology, endoscopy and manometry are all important investigative tools. Each of these supplies a component of information necessary for accuracy in diagnosis. In my experience, of those patients seen with failed Heller myotomy, the majority had never had achalasia and the mistake in diagnosis was a direct result of incomplete preoperative investigation (5).

Radiologic Features of Achalasia

Radiologic changes can be detected in a radiograph of the chest and also by using contrast material (17). A plain chest film usually shows very little until the disorder has progressed to Stage III (Fig. 13.6). These patients may exhibit an air-fluid level in the dilated esophagus at a varible level in the mediastinum. Usually there is no gas in the gastric fundus, because gas gathers above the fluid and does not pass through the gastroesophageal junction. The bulk of the sigmoid esophagus produces a characteristic right upper mediastinal fullness.

Examination with contrast medium has clinical value in assessment and in choice of therapy because it permits a radiologic staging.

| Stage I | —an esophageal diameter of less than 4 cm |
| Stage II | —an esophageal diameter between 4 and 6 cm |

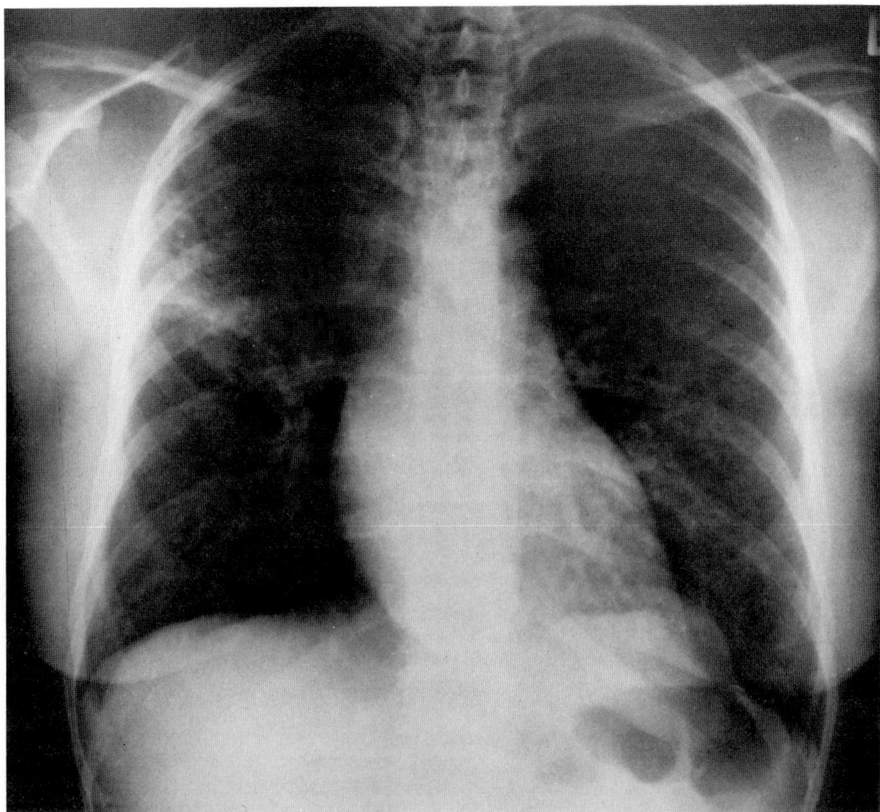

Figure 13.5
Radiograph of the chest (Mrs. A., age 33) showing changes of aspiration pneumonia at both apices. Aspiration pneumonia was her dominant problem. She described frequent night aspiration and multiple major episodes of respiratory infection. Surgical drainage by Heller myotomy has alleviated her esophageal symptoms, and she has had no further episodes of aspiration pneumonia.

Stage III —an esophageal diameter greater than 6 cm

In Stages I and II there is often vigorous disordered motor activity which is manifested as multiple contraction zones (18). In Stage III achalasia the esophagus is a flaccid bag, and shows very little motor activity.

The gastroesophageal junction, because of its failure to relax, imposes a characteristic "bird beak" appearance on the barium column. At fluoroscopy small quantities of contrast material can be seen to pass through, even though the junction does not relax.

Radiology can be used to assess esophageal emptying time. This is a test applicable to any motor obstruction of the esophagus and is particularly useful in achalasia. The patient drinks 400 cc of water as quickly as possible while in a standing position. The time taken for the esophagus to empty is measured by stop watch. This test has been adapted using barium as a method of comparing preoperative and postoperative esophageal emptying and is of value as a method of quantitating esophageal dysfunction (9, 19).

The changes noted in the lung parenchyma, which are secondary to aspiration, are encountered most commonly in patients with Stage III achalasia (20).

In the typical patient, the radiologic features are diagnostic; however, many disorders can mimic achalasia. Every physician who accepts responsibility for such patients should recognize this difficulty in radiologic diagnosis. Incorrect diagnosis and inappropriate treatment not only may fail to cure the disorder and relieve the symptoms but may induce a major exacerbation of symptoms.

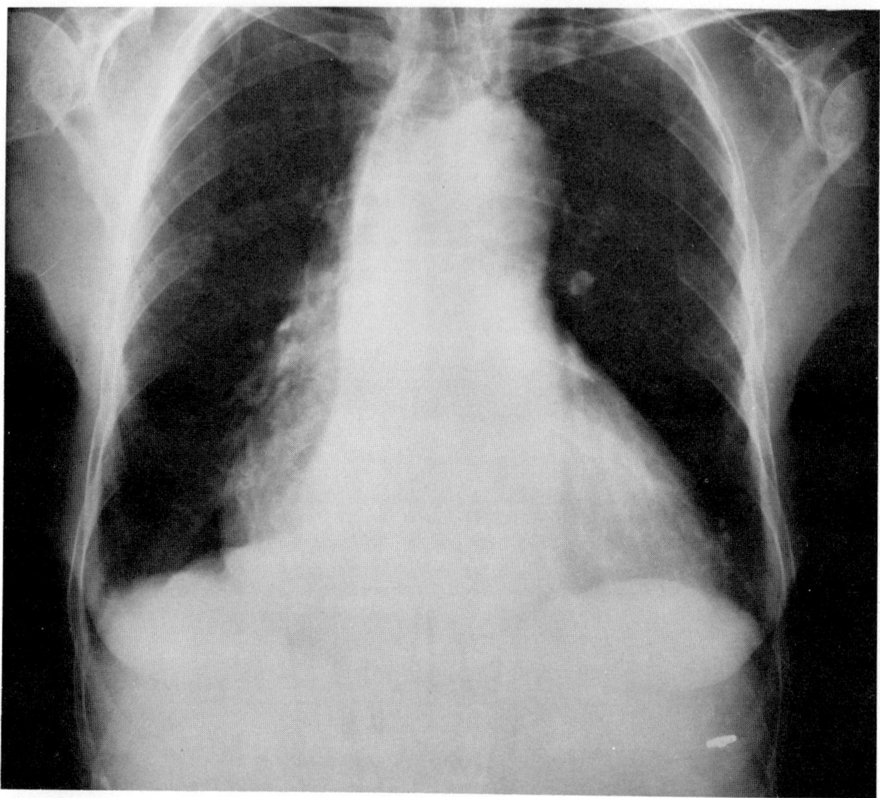

Figure 13.6. Stage III Achalasia
Radiograph shows the presence of a dilated esophagus with fullness in the right upper mediastinum and an air-fluid level at the base of the neck.

Manometric Characteristics

The classic manometric features of achalasia are those of a slightly hypertonic, non-relaxing sphincter which responds to deglutition by premature contraction (Fig. 13.7). In the body of the esophagus all motor waves are simultaneous (21–24). The motor waves have a common manometric appearance due to pressure conduction in a fluid-filled esophagus. This common cavity effect is artificial but gives a mirror image appearance to the waves which is of diagnostic importance. In the upper esophagus the motor waves, although simultaneous are usually of slightly higher amplitude and no longer demonstrate the mirror image appearance. This portion of esophagus is rarely fluid-filled and, in addition, is composed of striated muscle, accounting for the altered appearance of the waves.

This is the pattern of motor change used in the diagnosis of achalasia and in the majority of patients it is clearly recognizable and es-tablishes the diagnosis with a high degree of certainty. Three variations in this motor pattern occur which can make the precise diagnosis of achalasia more complex. Relaxation has been shown to be occasionally present in achalasia (25, 26). When it occurs it is more marked in the lower high pressure zone and is incomplete and of short duration, being interrupted by premature contraction. Peristalsis is also described in achalasia and, although this is rare, it adds considerably to the diagnostic problem. The third variable is the vigorous type of achalasia which is associated with high amplitude motor waves (greater than 50 cm of water) in the body of the esophagus (27–30).

Each of these variations makes the manometric differentiation between achalasia and diffuse spasm very difficult and in some patients quite impossible. In addition, patients have been described in whom the manometric features of diffuse spasm have progressed to those of classic achalasia (31). Similarly, fol-

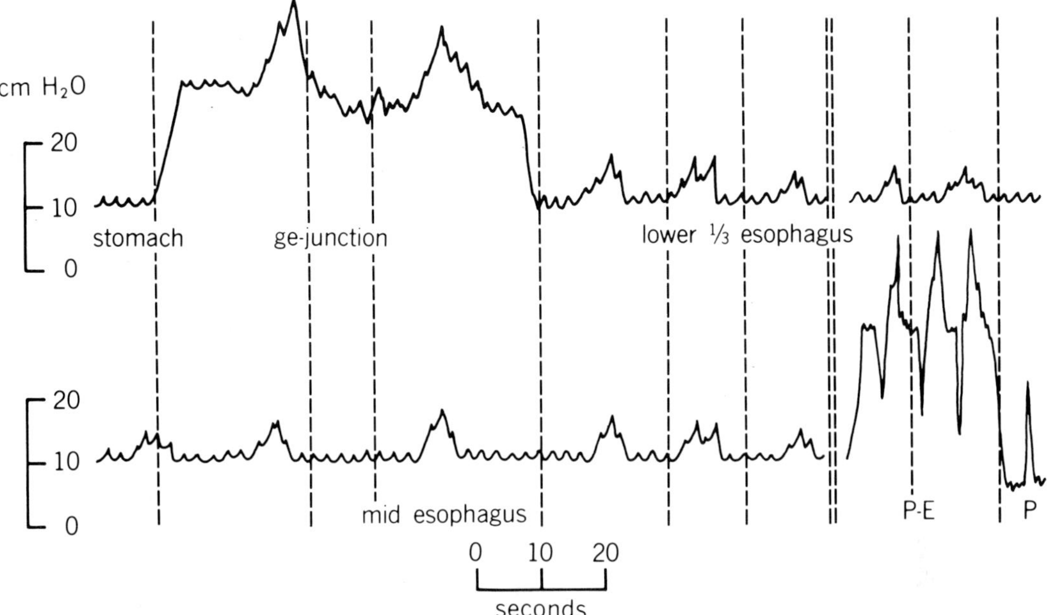

Figure 13.7. Esophageal Manometry in Achalasia
Diagrammatic representation of the esophageal manometry shows two simultaneous pressure recordings with the lower trace 5 cm proximal in the esophagus. Each vertical line indicates a 1-cm proximal move of the manometric catheters. The double line indicates a major move to the proximal esophagus. The gastroesophageal (ge) junction has a tone of 25 cm, which is higher than the normal average tone. There is contraction but no relaxation in response to deglutition. The body of the esophagus has a high pressure due to fluid retention and the disordered motor activity is total and of low amplitude. The pharyngoesophageal (P-E) junction and pharynx (P) are normal.

lowing bag dilatation of the esophagus for achalasia the reappearance of relaxation and peristalsis has been described (25). Based on these manometric features the two diseases, achalasia and diffuse spasm, seem to have features in common. Although in the majority of patients a precise diagnosis can be made, there is a grey area where precise classification is difficult.

Because of these variables in the motor pattern, a new method of manometric classification has been advocated which allows subdivision of the motor features dependant upon the presence of peristalsis, relaxation and vigorous motor waves in the body of the esophagus (25). Using this method the presence of peristalsis in the motor tracing is symbolized as P and absent peristalsis as p. Relaxation is symbolized R and absent relaxation r. Motor waves greater than 50 cm of water are V and low amplitude motor waves v. The eight possible variants are listed in Table 13.1. Classic achalasia would be written as prv; vigorous achalasia as prV and

Table 13.1

Manometric Classification of Achalasia and Diffuse Spasm*

prv	Classic achalasia
pRv	Achalasia with high pressure zone relaxation
prV	Vigorous achalasia
Prv	Peristalsis—rare, if ever, with achalasia
PRV	Standard diffuse spasm
pRV	Diffuse spasm without peristalsis
PRv	Low amplitude diffuse spasm
PrV	Diffuse spasm without relaxation

* In this classification of achalasia and diffuse spasm the symbol p is used for absent peristalsis, P for peristalsis, r for absent relaxation, R for relaxation, v for low amplitude motor waves and V for high amplitude motor waves.

classic diffuse spasm as PRV. This classification recognizes the many variants seen in the spectrum of diffuse spasm and achalasia and allows for manometric classification. With more experience this type of detailed definition may allow for recognition of clinical patterns and more effective therapy.

Although the classification seems simple the technical aspects of manometric evaluation remain complex. Minor degrees of relaxation are difficult to recognize as small decreases in sphincteric pressure may be due to variations in respiratory pattern and may not be due to sphincteric activity. Peristalsis when present is recognizable; however, in achalasia it is very rare. For the purpose of classification vigorous motor activity has been defined as the presence of 20 per cent or more of motor waves with an amplitude of 50 cm of water or greater.

Using this method and reviewing 44 patients with manometric studies diagnosed as achalasia, 38 (86.3 per cent) fall into the group of classic achalasia of the prv type (Table 13.2). Three patients had minor relaxation (pRv—6.8 per cent) (Fig. 13.8); two had vigorous (Fig. 13.9) achalasia with more than 2 per cent of motor waves above 50 cm of water (prV—4.5 per cent) and one patient had minor relaxation and probable rare peristalsis (PRv—2.2 per cent). These patients all had radiologic features of achalasia, presented with dysphagia as their dominant symptom and at operation had the typical appearance of the achalasia esophagus.

Other features of diagnostic value can be obtained from the analysis of the 44 patients with achalasia. The tone of the sphincter varied considerable (Table 13.2). Normal tone is considered to be 15 to 20 cm of water. Thirty-eight patients had good sphincteric studies and the tone varied from 4 to 38 cm of water (average 15.9 cm of water). Eighteen

Table 13.2
Analysis of Manometry in Achalasia (44 Patients)*

High pressure zone 15.6 (range 6–34)
Esophageal pressure 16.6 (range 4–30)
% disordered motor activity 99.8 (range 98–100)
Average tone disordered motor activity 14.5 (range 8–65)
  Classification prv = 38 (86.3%)—standard
                  pRv = 3 (6.8%)—relaxing
                  prV = 2 (4.6%)—vigorous
                  Prv = 1 (2.3%)—peristalsis

* Using the PRV classification classic achalasia is most common, occurring in 86.3 per cent. Although relaxation and vigorous motor activity occurred they were rare. I have seen only one patient with possible esophageal peristalsis.

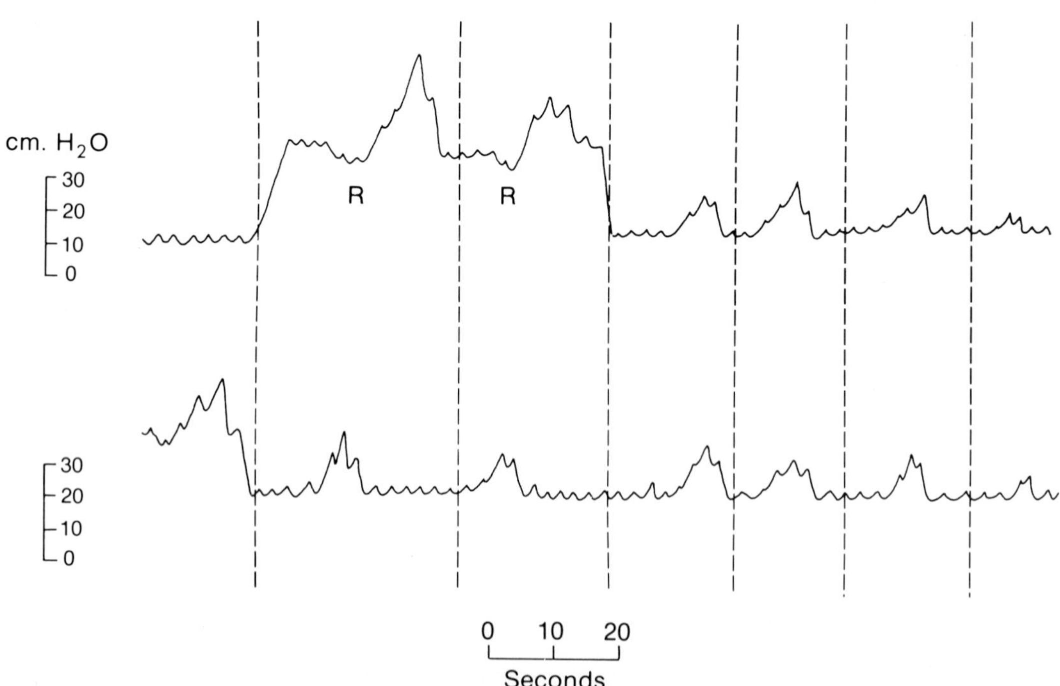

Figure 13.8. Achalasia with Minor Relaxation in High Pressure Zone (HPZ)
The tracing is typical of achalasia with normal gastric pressure, a normal tone HPZ and high esophageal basal pressure with poorly formed simultaneous mirror image motor waves. In the HPZ there are minor relaxations (R) of short duration preceding the motor contraction wave.

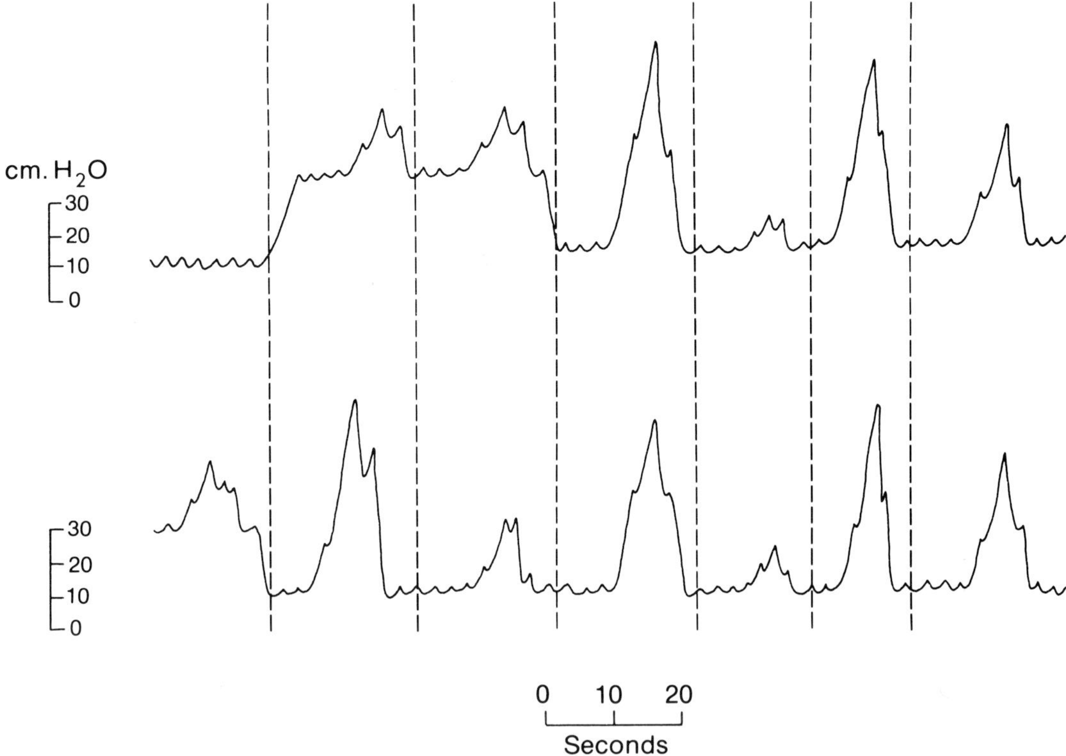

Figure 13.9. Vigorous Achalasia
In vigorous achalasia the esophageal motor waves are of high amplitude (many exceeding 50 cm of water). For the purpose of classification I refers to vigorous achalasia as being present when 20 per cent or more of the motor waves exceed 50cm of water. This is a very rare form of achalasia in the adult.

had a low tone, 10 were in the normal range and 10 were high tone sphincters. The pressure in the body of the esophagus, normally 2 to 6 cm of water, was mostly elevated. Only one patient had a pressure below 6 cm and the average esophageal pressure was 17 cm of water.

Mecholyl Test

The Mecholyl (acetyl-β-methylcholine chloride) test was devised to further characterize the motor features of achalasia. According to Cannon's law, this drug, a cholinergic, should produce a marked reaction in denervated tissue. When administered intramuscularly in a dose of 6 to 10 mg, it produced contractions in the lower esophagus in 11 of 15 patients with achalasia (Fig. 13.10) but no reaction in 10 normal subjects (32, 33). The 4 patients with achalasia who exhibited no motor response had a Stage III achalasia and may have reached the stage at which the

esophagus could no longer respond to stimulation.

Although most patients with achalasia respond to Mecholyl, this type of response is seen occasionally in patients who do not have achalasia; e.g., a positive Mecholyl test may occur in diffuse esophageal spasm. This disorder may also be secondary to neurogenic degeneration, which would account for the positive response. For this reason, a positive Mecholyl test should not be considered an absolute indicator of achalasia.

Endoscopy

The endoscopic features of achalasia are typical only in the late stages of the disease. In the early stages there is often only a mild erythema, but under local anesthesia it may be possible to show that the gastroesophageal junction does not relax. As the disease progresses, dilatation of the esophagus is readily recognized at endoscopy. The closed gastroesophageal junction may be difficult to ne-

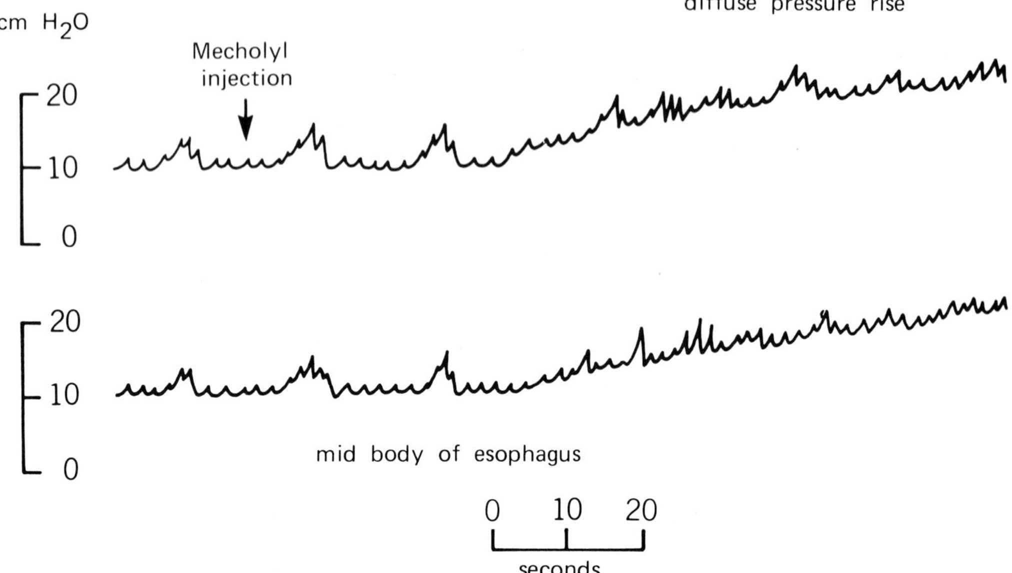

Figure 13.10. Mecholyl Test
In achalasia when Mecholyl is injected there is a diffuse pressure rise in the esophagus. This pressure rise is associated with retrosternal discomfort. The test is of some value in the differential diagnosis of achalasia.

gotiate with the endoscope, and indeed it is easy to perforate the lower esophagus because of the sigmoid curve of the organ. At this stage the mucosa is thickened and has a diffusely pebbled appearance.

In those with advanced disease the esophagus must be carefully cleared out by lavage before proceeding to endoscopy. This is essential to achieve adequate visualization and to avoid aspiration of debris in sedated or anesthetized patients. Only endoscopy can exclude carcinoma of the esophagus. Carcinoma develops in up to 19 per cent (14) of these patients, and hence it must be sought in all patients before treating the achalasia.

The most helpful investigations are the history, radiology, manometry and endoscopy, and if a complete investigation is carried out a specific diagnosis can be made in most patients. However, despite careful investigation these patients present many difficult problems in diagnosis and any "short-cut" in investigation opens the door to misdiagnosis and potential therapeutic disaster.

Differential Diagnosis

Common problems in differential diagnosis center around the interpretation of the esophageal motor changes and the specific radiologic features of achalasia. Manometrically diffuse spasm (5), and scleroderma may both mimic achalasia. Other disorders such as dyschalasia (34) may be separate diseases or may be minor variants of true achalasia. In diffuse esophageal spasm (DES) (30) the motor changes consist of spasm in the lower two-thirds of the esophagus, peristalsis in the upper third and a gastroesophageal junction of normal tone which relaxes in response to deglutition. In most patients this disorder can be distinguished from achalasia, but in some, particularly those with long-standing dysfunction, the esophagus retains fluid in its proximal third and peristalsis is difficult to demonstrate. As noted earlier, the Mecholyl test does not adequately separate DES from achalasia, because it may be positive in either condition. To further compound the difficulty in differential diagnosis some workers have reported that DES occasionally progresses to true achalasia.

Case 2. Mr. J., age 72, was referred with a diagnosis of "carcinoma of the lung" because he had night coughing, progressive dyspnea and radiologic fullness in the right upper mediastinum (Fig. 13.11). Radiologically the lower two-thirds of his esophagus was narrow, spastic and thick-walled, while his upper esophagus was dilated with an air fluid level. Manometric studies were possi-

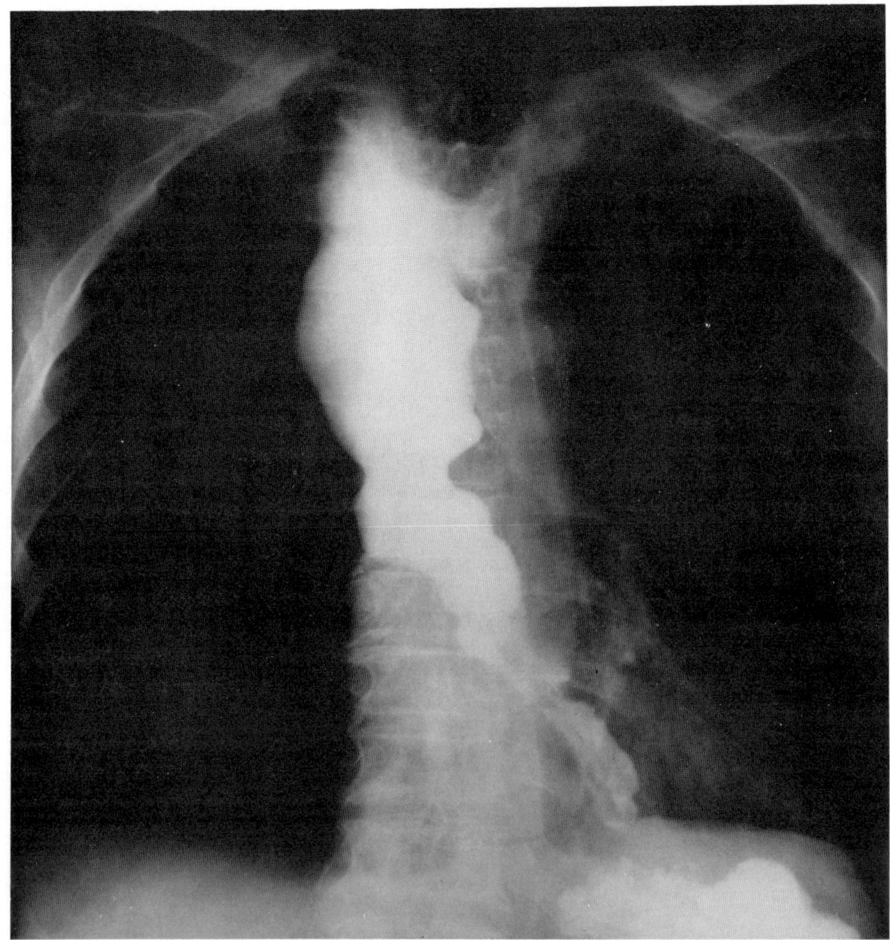

Figure 13.11
Mr. J. (Case 2), age 72. This radiograph shows some features of achalasia, but the esophageal distention is proximal, while the distal esophagus is spastic and thick-walled. Manometrically this patient had diffuse esophageal spasm.

ble only in the body of the esophagus because the tubes would not pass through the gastroesophageal junction. No peristaltic motor activity was demonstrated, but the disordered motor waves were of high amplitude and prolonged duration.

At operation the esophagus was thickwalled and spastic, and a myotomy was done from the stomach to 6 cm above the aortic arch, together with a gastroplasty. The degree of esophageal wall thickening and spasm was considered diagnostic of DES was no evidence of dilatation, and the dilatation noted radiologically began above the level of the aortic arch.

Postoperative manometric studies showed well-formed peristaltic motor waves in the upper third of esophagus above the level of myotomy. Peristalsis does not occur in achalasia and, because of this postoperative study and the findings at operation, a conclusive diagnosis of DES could be made.

Scleroderma is also difficult to distinguish from achalasia on manometry (35). Often these patients show other evidence of systemic collagen disease, e.g., telangiectasia, or Raynaud's phenomenon. The gastroesophageal junctional pressure is reduced and motor activity in the lower two-thirds of the esophagus is absent or markedly reduced. In most of these patients peristalsis can be demonstrated in the upper third of the esophagus, and this will differentiate the adynamic esophagus of scleroderma from achalasia.

Hiatal hernia can usually be distinguished from achalasia. However, if reflux continues after myotomy has been performed, the combination of surgical trauma and reflux can make the differential diagnosis extremely difficult.

Case 3. Mr. K., age 54, developed dysphagia in 1945 and was treated by duodenal feedings for 6 months. Bouginage gave him some clinical improvement. In 1950 a diagnosis of achalasia was made and he had pneumatic bag dilatation. In 1961 a Heller myotomy was performed because of a recurrence of his dysphagia (Fig. 13.12).

In 1971 he was first seen and re-evaluated because of persistent major dysphagia. Esophagoscopy showed a Stage IV esophagitis, and radiologic studies showed a tapered gastroesophageal junction secondary to stricture. Manometry demonstrated that the gastroesophageal junction could relax and it showed definite esophageal peristaltic motor activity (Fig. 13.12). He was dilated to #60 Fr with Maloney bougies and had an excellent symptomatic improvement. This patient remained well for 2 years, but eventually required a gastroplasty for control of reflux.

The patient never did have achalasia, but for a period of 20 years he had treatment which was inappropriate. When first seen in 1945, endoscopy would have confirmed the presence of a stricture and dilatation would have avoided the necessity of duodenal feeding. If he had had manometric evaluation in 1961 he would not have been submitted to a Heller myotomy. Definitive repair of

his hernia could have been performed at that stage. Pneumatic bag dilatation and myotomy compound the problem of reflux by further reducing the tone of the gastroesophageal junction. Properly oriented therapy was first instituted in 1971, at which time a correct diagnosis was based primarily on manometric studies.

I have seen several such patients in whom achalasia could have been excluded but who nevertheless were submitted to unnecessary myotomies. These patients, whose symptoms are usually worse following myotomy, illustrate the importance of accurate diagnosis. Carcinoma of the stomach (4), particularly that type referred to as linitis plastica, can produce a tapered constriction at the gastroesophageal junction, and such patients may develop secondary esophageal dilatation, if the lesion is of long standing.

Case 4. When first seen, Mr. D., age 70, had had severe dysphagia for 2 years and initially had been treated for achalasia by bougienage. When bougienage failed, he had a gastrostomy and for 6 months received his total alimentation by this

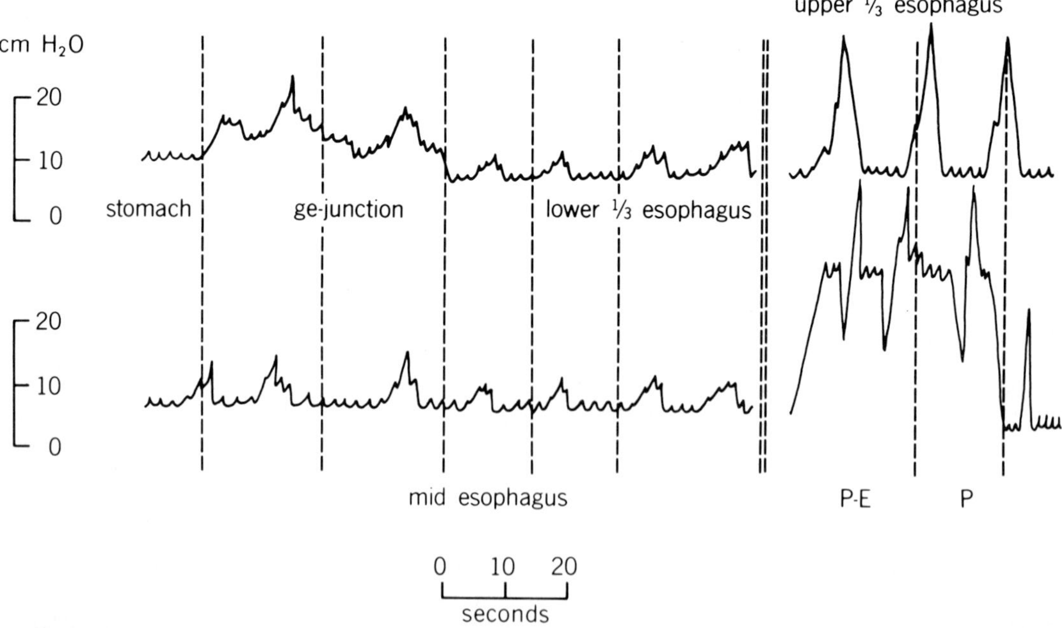

Figure 13.12

Mr. K. (Case 3), age 54, had previous surgical management for a hiatal hernia and stricture which included a Heller myotomy. Manometrically his gastroesophageal (ge) junction is low tone, secondary to the myotomy, but retains relaxation and contraction in response to deglutition. The lower esophagus has a severe low tone disordered motor activity secondary to his previous myotomy. In the proximal esophagus there is normal peristalsis. The cricopharynx (P-E) and pharynx (P) are normal. Because of this manometric study, achalasia can be excluded from the differential diagnosis.

adenocarcinoma was discovered and removed by esophagogastrectomy. This gave immediate relief of his symptoms and he lived a normal life for 2 years before dying from metastatic adenocarcinoma. Gastric carcinoma must be carefully excluded in patients with achalasia as it can mimic both the radiologic and manometric features of the disease (36–38).

Other rarer causes of dysphagia may pose difficult problems (Fig. 13.14).

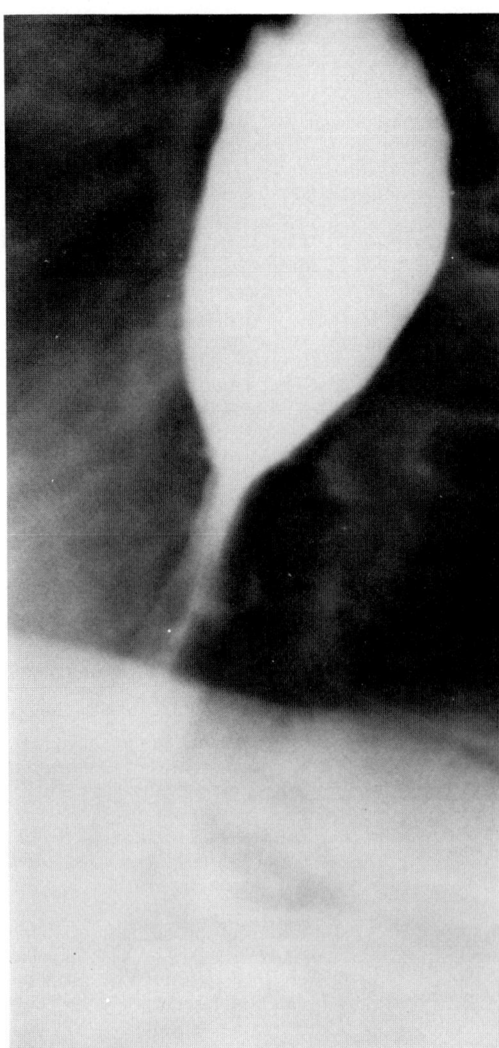

Figure 13.13
Mr. D., age 70, was considered initially to have achalasia. The radiologic appearance was of a tapered lower esophagus with dilatation of the distal esophagus. Manometrically it was shown that he had well-formed peristaltic motor function in the body of his esophagus. Direct biopsy at operation confirmed the presence of adenocarcinoma.

route. Radiologic studies showed a tapered gastroesophageal junction with a very tight stricture (Fig. 13.13). At endoscopy, the stricture was confirmed, but multiple biopsies were all negative for carcinoma. Manometry showed well-formed peristaltic motor waves, incompatible with the diagnosis of achalasia. Achalasia having been excluded by manometric study, the differential diagnosis was peptic stricture or carcinoma. Clinically it was felt that carcinoma was more likely. An exploratory thoracotomy was performed. At operation a gastric

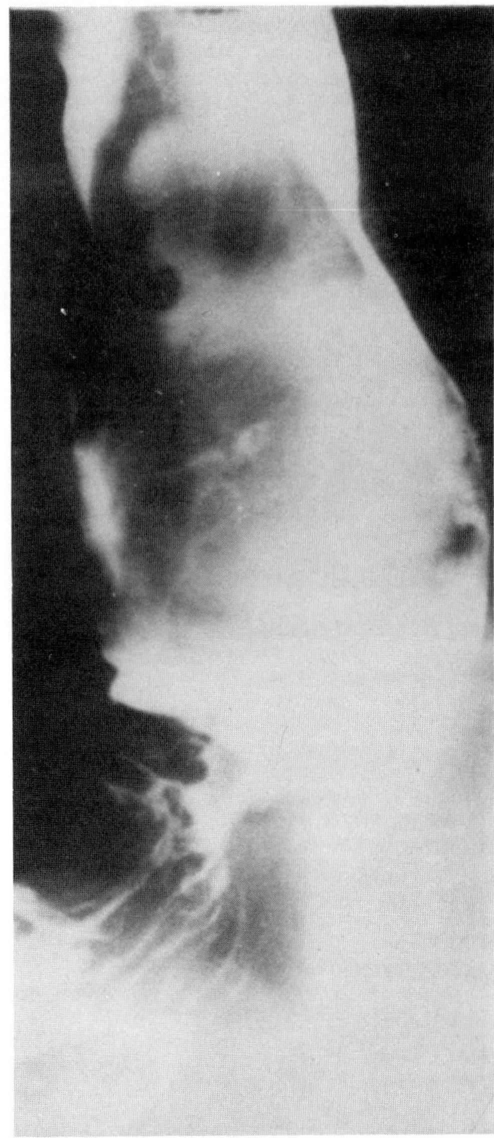

Figure 13.14
Mr. S. (Case 5), age 53, had a distended retention esophagus. At operation he was found to have a very large pharyngeal polyp which had prolapsed into the esophagus and was suspended on a long vascular pedicle.

Case 5. Mr. S., age 53, presented elsewhere with dysphagia and, after radiologic studies, a diagnosis of achalasia was made and he was subjected to a Heller myotomy. When first seen, he had very disordered esophageal function and poor emptying. At endoscopy we did not discover a pedunculated polyp, because the esophagoscope passed along the side of the polyp without displaying its margins. Manometrically there was peristalis in the proximal esophagus, but because of the earlier myotomy there was no effective motor activity in the lower esophagus. On this evidence we could exclude achalasia, but a positive tissue diagnosis was made only at thoracotomy, when the polyp was recognized and removed. His esophageal myotomy was closed and he had excellent return of esophageal motor function and total relief of his symptoms.

These five cases illustrate a variety of differential diagnostic problems. In most patients, however, an accurate diagnosis can be made and appropriate therapy instituted if all steps in the investigation are completed carefully. Anything less than full investigation (39) may lead to a major therapeutic disaster.

References

1. Ellis, F. H., Jr., and Olsen, A. M.: *Achalasia of the Esophagus.* W. B. Saunders Co., Phildelphia, 1969.
2. Plummer, H. S.: Cardiospasm, with a report of forty cases. J.A.M.A., *51:* 549, 1908.
3. Ellis, F. G.: The natural history of achalasia of the cardia (abridged). Proc. R. Soc. Med., *53:* 663, 1960.
4. Just-Viera, J. O., Morris, J. D., and Haight, C.: Achalasia and esophageal carcinoma. Ann. Thorac. Surg., *3:* 526, 1967.
5. Henderson, R. D., Barichello, A. M., Pearson, F. G., Mugashe, F., and Szczepanski, M.: Diagnosis of achalasia. Can. J. Surg., *15:* 190, 1972.
6. Westley, C. R., Herbst, J. J., Goldman, S., and Wiser, W. C.: Infantile achalasia. J. Pediatr., *87:* 243, 1975.
7. Willich, E.: Achalasia of the cardia in children. Manometric, cinematographic and pharmacoradiographic studies. Pediatr. Radiol., *1:* 229, 1973.
8. Olsen, A. M., Holman, C. B., and Andersen, H. A.: Diagnosis of cardiospasm. Dis. Chest, *23:* 477, 1953.
9. Menziew-Gow, N., Gummer, J. W., and Edwards, D. A.: Results of Heller's operation for achalasia of the cardia. Br. J. Surg., *65:* 483, 1978.
10. Plummer, H. S., and Vinson, P. P.: Cardiospasm; report of 301 cases. Med. Clin. North Am., *5:* 355, 1921.
11. Andersen, H. A., Holman, C. B., and Olsen, A. M.: Pulmonary complications of cardiospasm. J. A. M. A., *151:* 608, 1953.
12. Westley, C. R., Herbst, J. J., Goldman, S., and Wiser, W. C.: Infantile achalasia; inherited as an autosomal recessive disorder. J. Pediatr., *87:* 243, 1975.
13. Pierce, W. S., MacVaugh, H., III, and Johnson, J.: Carcinoma of the esophagus arising in patients with achalasia of the cardia. J. Thorac. Cardiovasc. Surg., *59:* 335, 1970.
14. Ellis, F. G.: The causes of death in achalasia of the cardia. Ann. R. Coll. Surg. Engl., *53:* 663, 1960.
15. Belsey, H. R.: Personal communication, 1975.
16. Gautam, H. P.: Oesophageal carcinoma following achalasia of cardia. Br. J. Dis. Chest. *60:* 208, 1966.
17. Templeton, F. E.: Movements of esophagus in presence of cardiospasm and other esophageal diseases; roentgenologic study of muscular action. Gastroenterology, *10:* 96, 1948.
18. Sanderson, D. R., Ellis, F. H., Jr., Schlegel, J. F., and Olsen, A. M.: Syndrome of vigorous achalasia; clinical and physiologic observations. Dis. Chest, *52:* 508, 1967.
19. Edwards, D. A. W.: Drinking time in dysphagia. Rend. Roman Gastro-enterol., *3:* 142, 1971.
20. Holman, C. B.: Roentgenologic observations concerning pulmonary complications of achalasia. J. Med. Assoc. Ga., *54:* 391, 1965.
21. Butin, J. W., Olsen, A. M., Moersch, H. J., and Code, C. F.: Study of esophageal pressures in normal persons and patients with cardiospasm. Gastroenterology, *23:* 278, 1953.
22. Ingelfinger, F. J., Kramer, P., and Sanchez, G. C.: Gastroesphageal vestibule, its normal function and its role in cardispasm and gastroesophageal reflux. Am. J. Med. Sci., *228:* 417, 1954.
23. Cohen, S., and Lipshutz, W.: Lower esophageal sphincter dysfunction in achalasia. Gastroenterology, *61:* 814, 1971.
24. Vantrappen, G., Van Goidsenhoven, G. E., Verbeke, S., VanDenBerghe, G., and Vandenbroucie, J.: Manometric studies in achalasia of the cardia, before and after pneumatic dilations. Gastroenterology, *45:* 317, 1963.
25. Vantrappen, G., Janssens, J., Hellemans, J., and Coremans, G.: Achalasia, diffuse esophageal spasm, and related motility disorders. Gastroenterology, *76:* 450, 1979.
26. Flood, C. A.: Relaxation of the cardia in achalasia. Gastrointest. Endosc., *18:* 114, 1972.
27. Mellow, M. H.: Return of esophageal peristalsis in idiopathic achalasia. Gastroenterology, *70:* 1148, 1976.
28. Sanderson, D. R., Ellis, F. H., Jr., and Schlegel, J. F.: Syndrome of vigorous achalasia; clinical and physiologic observations. Dis. Chest., *52:* 508, 1967.
29. Olsen, A. M., and Creamer, B.: Studies of oesophageal motility, with special reference to the differential diagnosis of diffuse spasm and achalasia (cardiospasm). Thorax, *12:* 279, 1957.
30. Henderson, R. D., Ho, C. S., and Davidson, J. W.: Primary disordered motor activity of the esophagus (diffuse spasm). Ann. Thorac. Surg., *18:* 327, 1974.
31. Kramer, P., Harris, L. D., and Donaldson, R. M., Jr.: Transition from symptomatic diffuse spasm to cardiospasm. Gut, *8:* 115, 1967.
32. Kramer, P., and Ingelfinger, F. J.: Esophageal sensitivity to Mecholyl in cardiospasm. Gastroenterology, *19:* 242, 1951.
33. Hightower, N. C., Jr., Olsen, A. M., and Moersch, H. J.: Comparison of effects of acetyl-beta-methyl-choline chloride (Mecholyl) on esophageal intraluminal pressure in normal persons and patients with cardiospasms. Gastroenterology, *26:* 592, 1954.
34. Beck, I. T., Hernandez, N. A., and Solymar, J.: Dyschalasia; a variant or early phase of achalasia? Can. Med. Assoc. J., *95:* 941, 1966.

35. Henderson, R. D., and Pearson, F. G.: Surgical management of esophageal scleroderma. J. Thorac. Cardiovasc. Surg., *66:* 686, 1973.
36. Tucker, H. J., Snape, W. J., Jr., and Cohen, S.: Achalasia secondary to carcinoma; manometric and clinical features. Ann. Intern Med., *89:* 315, 1978.
37. Lawson, T. L., and Dodds, W. J.: Infiltrating carcinoma simulating achalasia. Gastrointest. Radiol., *1:* 245, 1976.
38. McCallum, R. W.: Esophageal achalasia secondary to gastric carcinoma. Report of a case and a review of the literature. Am. J. Gastroenterol., *71:* 24, 1979.
39. Margulis, A. R., and Koehler, R. E.: Radiologic diagnosis of disordered esophageal motility; a unified physiologic approach. Radiol. Clin. North Am., *14:* 429, 1976.

CHAPTER 14

Achalasia: Treatment

Two approaches to the treatment of achalasia are effective. Both have been reported widely and both have their advocates. The early success of dilatation at the beginning of the 20th century relegated operative procedures to the management of dilatation failures. In the past few decades a more balanced approach was adopted, as with increased experience the results of surgical management have improved. For years the Mayo Clinic (1) has pioneered in the therapy of achalasia, and in so doing has accumulated a vast experience with this disease. This accumulated and shared experience forms the scientific basis upon which the profession has achieved a rational approach to therapy in achalasia.

Dilatation Therapy

Two types of dilatation therapy have been used in the management of achalasia. The mercury-weighted bougie permits the esophagus to be dilated up to #60 Fr—a degree of stretching that produces temporary and incomplete relief, usually of short duration (2). Occasionally in the very sick patient dilatation can be used to improve esophageal drainage until the patient can be offered more effective bag dilatation or myotomy at a later stage. Two of my patients responded well enough to the mercury bougie to permit continued care with this method alone.

Bag dilatation has now replaced the mercury-filled bougie. The inflatable bag makes it possible to introduce the dilator and position it before pressure is applied. Mercury bougies up to #60 Fr produce dilatation only to the normal esophageal diameter, but a bag system produces deliberate overdistention in order to disrupt the esophageal muscle bundles while preserving the overlying mucosa. It is this overdistention which has so greatly improved the results obtained from dilatation.

Russell (3) first described bag dilatation in 1898 after he used a water system to distend the positioned bag and dilate the esophagus. He described 7 patients; 4 had an excellent result, 1 had a good result and 2 had no improvement. These results compare favorably with those achieved by modern dilatation therapy. His success was remarkable when one considers that he had no radiologic control when he positioned the dilatation bag. We can concede that Russell made a major advance even while questioning the accuracy of his clinical diagnosis, working as he did without the assistance of radiologic, manometric and endoscopic techniques.

In 1908 Plummer (4) described his hydrostatic bag. His water pressure system has been used now for almost 70 years and continues to be a safe and effective method of dilatation in patients with achalasia. An adaptation of this principle, the Browne-McHardy (5) bag (Fig. 14.1), allows the bag to be distended by air pressure and this device is the most commonly used of the air distention bags. In both of these systems, dilatation is carried out under fluoroscopic control—that is, the bag is placed at the gastroesophageal junction before distention. The Negus bag (6), which also employs distention but is positioned under direct visual control using an esophagoscope, has gained its widest acceptance in Great Britain. The bag is dilated by instilling 30 to 40 ml of water. The maneuver, which is repeated 3 or 4 times at different levels to ensure that the gastroesophageal junction has been adequately dilated, gives highly satisfactory results.

Case 1. Mrs. F., age 78, had been treated by bag dilatation in Italy 20 years before she emi-

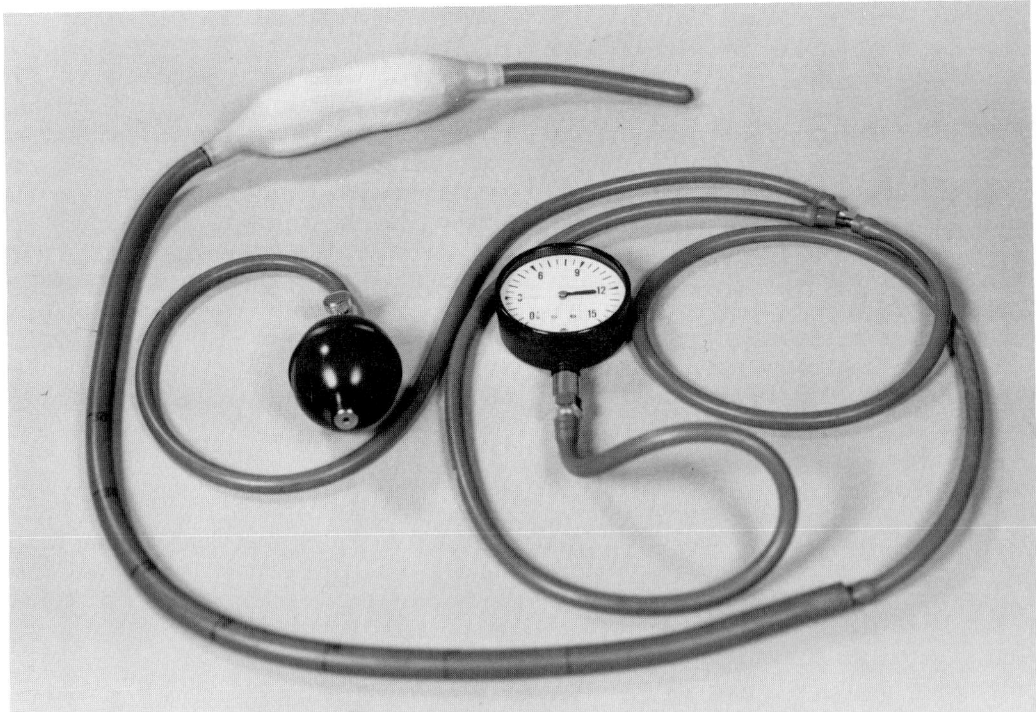

Figure 14.1. Browne-McHardy Bag
The Browne-McHardy dilator uses air pressure in a restricted cuff to apply controlled stress to the gastroesophageal junction. The component parts are a dilator bag with restraining mesh to avoid overdistention, an air pump and a gauge. The bag is inserted under topical anesthesia and placed across the gastroesophageal junction using fluoroscopic control.

grated to Canada. When I first saw her, she had major motor obstruction with regurgitation and had lost 50 pounds. Her general condition was so poor that she could not have been considered for surgical myotomy. Evidence obtained on radiologic, manometric and endoscopic study showed an advanced Stage III achalasia. Following endoscopy we passed a #60 Fr Malloney bougie in an attempt to gain temporary relief and improve nutrition. After dilatation, she was able to swallow mashed and puréed foods; she gained 10 pounds and stopped regurgitating her feedings. Two years have passed since her dilatation, and because of her age and poor condition we have accepted as adequate this degree of improvement.

In most patients this form of dilatation is no longer acceptable treatment, but, as Mrs. F. illustrates, it does play a limited role in the elderly or debilitated patient.

Case 2. Mrs. L., age 52, had had profound dysphagia and regurgitation as her dominant symptoms for 10 years. Following evaluation she was diagnosed radiologically as having achalasia. Her physician decided to manage her at that time by training her to pass a #60 Fr mercury bougie. She gained some improvement initially; however, to maintain normal nutrition it was necessary for her to pass the bougie 5 to 6 times per week. Even with this vigorous form of bougienage her dysphagia has been progressively worsening. Having reviewed this situation it was decided to proceed to Heller myotomy. She is now progressing well and eating normally without bougienage.

The original method of management was not optimal; however, it illustrates the value of this approach when more definitive procedures are contraindicated.

Technique of Dilatation

Great care should be taken in preparing the patient before using the hydrostatic bag. If the esophagus contains retained food, it should be lavaged daily for 3 or 4 days until clear. Feeding of puréed food followed by clear liquids for 24 hours will further cleanse the esophagus. Before the dilator is inserted, mercury-weighted dilators can be passed gently to begin the process. If only the weight of the bougie is used and it is passed under local anesthesia, the risk of perforation is negligible. However, any attempt at forceful dilatation carries a major risk of perforation. If the mercury-weighted bougies should fail, an olive-tipped bougie can be passed safely through the gastroesophageal junction on a weighted thread that has been swallowed over the preceding 24 hours. Once it has passed into the small bowel, the thread is held firmly and is used to guide the dilator.

The hydrostatic dilator must be put in place across the gastroesophageal junction under fluoroscopic control, and pressure is increased gradually to stretch and disrupt the gastroesophageal junction. This procedure is done using topical anesthesia in order that the patient's pain will provide a guide to effective dilatation. Pain appears at the time of maximal stretch, but should subside rapidly. These patients are observed carefully for 48 hours and during this time clear fluids are gradually introduced again.

The most common complication of dilatation is perforation. At the Mayo Clinic, Sanderson and colleagues (7) reported a 3 per cent incidence of perforation in 456 patients during dilatation and that 24 per cent of these required thoracotomy. Although this complication is reported to be rare, it is probably more frequent when dilatation is performed by less experienced people. The other common complications are hemorrhage and aspiration. Aspiration is much less likely if dilatation is preceded by careful lavage of the esophagus. Other reported complications include hemorrhage and esophageal obstruction (8, 9) from the development of an intramural haematoma. Because of these difficulties radiologic examination (10) of the esophagus is a sensible precaution following dilatation and certainly should be performed at an early stage if symptoms suggest perforation.

In the 456 patients treated at the Mayo Clinic, the results of dilatation therapy as judged on a 4-year follow-up were satisfactory in 60 per cent after one dilatation and in 80 per cent after two dilatations. Experience suggests that if two dilatations have failed little is gained by further dilatation.

Higher success rates have been reported in smaller series. Crump and colleagues (11) treated 72 patients by the metal Starck dilator or an air-bag dilator. Patients received nightly lavage for several weeks before dilatation and were maintained on puréed foods and antacids. The dilator was placed over a flexible, tipped piano wire and slipped into the stomach under fluoroscopic control. The dilator was then opened, withdrawn into the gastroesophageal junction, then closed and removed. After an average follow-up of 3.8 years, 82 per cent of these patients had achieved a satisfactory result after one dilatation.

Dilatation gave good results in achalasia, particularly in the early years of this century when surgical correction carried a much higher risk. This success delayed the development of surgical approaches to this disease, and only in recent years has operative correction become popular.

Surgery in Achalasia

Early Surgical Approaches

The earliest surgical approach involved dilatation of the gastroesophageal junction via

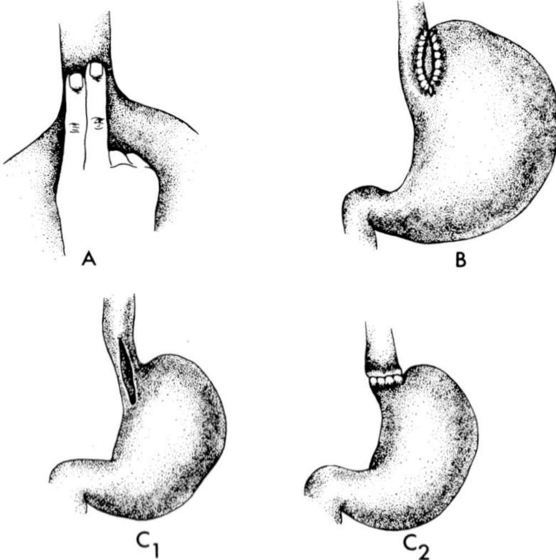

Figure 14.2. Older Surgical Approaches to Achalasia
Various procedures have been used in surgical treatment of achalasia. Direct finger dilatation (A) is no more effective than the various bag methods. The various types of cardioplasty (B, C_1 and C_2) have been discarded because of a high incidence of complication, particularly reflux, and stricture formation.

a gastrotomy. Although these procedures brought relief, they were no more effective than the hydrostatic bag (Fig. 14.2). Achalasia has also been treated by various forms of cardioplasty, in which the lower esophagus was sewn to the fundus of the stomach. This procedure relieves dysphagia instantly, but reflux is common and secondary peptic esophagitis and stricture often follow. Follow-up studies of these patients showed a high failure rate (12, 13).

Various esophageal resections and bowel replacement procedures have been used, but they may be followed by reflux and, in addition, are major operations which carry a much higher risk of morbidity and mortality than the popular Heller myotomy (14, 15). Thal has recommended his operation in patients with achalasia (16). This procedure produces instant relief of dysphagia, but it also carries the risk of reflux and reflux complications. The addition of Nissen fundoplication to the Thal operation may give more effective control of reflux, but at present the follow-up is too short to permit assessment.

Variations of the Thal procedure have been described (17, 18) in which the gastroesophageal junction is split and a prepared flap of stomach is sewn into the junction giving an actual mechanical widening of the junction. This procedure is described as being safe, more effective than Heller myotomy and gives more effective drainage of the esophagus. Follow-up examination shows a return to normal of esophageal emptying, using a timed swallow of barium. Reflux is not considered a problem. While this method is clearly described with good follow-up, it must still be considered experimental and lacking the extensive reporting necessary to establish it as an alternate form of surgical therapy.

Heller Myotomy

The surgeon who performs a Heller myotomy (19, 20) observes certain precautions:

1. He avoids aspiration.
2. He avoids laceration of the mucosa.
3. He provides an adequate length of myotomy.
4. He seeks to avoid reflux as a later complication.

With careful observation of these points, this procedure can be performed with a low mortality and morbidity and with excellent results.

Aspiration is avoided by careful lavage of the esophagus in days preceding. Lavage is carried out again on the morning of operation, using a large-bore stomach tube. Anesthesia is induced with the patient's head elevated and, if necessary, he can be intubated under local anesthesia.

When a general anesthetic is used, the technique of "crash induction" is valuable. The patient is rapidly induced, the trachea compressed by an assistant, the endotracheal tube with inflation syringe attached is rapidly introduced and the bag immediately inflated. In skilled hands the risk of aspiration is minimal.

Esophagoscopy can be performed following intubation to further ensure complete esophageal emptying and lessen the risk of immediate postoperative aspiration. These precautions are mandatory because aspiration poses a major threat to life.

The Heller myotomy can be done using either a transthoracic or transabdominal approach. The transthoracic approach allows careful palpation and inspection of the esophagus and helps to confirm the diagnosis (Fig. 14.3). The typical achalasia esophagus is dilated; however, the gastroesophageal junction remains normal in caliber. In the body the muscle is usually thickened and may be mildly spastic on palpation. In the dilated Stage II and Stage III esophagus the lumen is readily palpable. With experience the achalasia esophagus can be clearly distinguished from the thickened and motor spastic esophagus of diffuse spasm or from the woody thickening of peptic esophagitis. Recognition of the pathology is an important final step in diagnosis.

The esophagus can be mobilized, as for a transthoracic hiatal repair, and the gastric fundus delivered into the chest. An alternate approach, described by Ellis and colleagues, carefully preserves the position of the gastroesophageal junction and by so doing hopes to avoid reflux (21–23). If the technique of full mobilization of the gastroesophageal junction is used, subsequent hernia repair is mandatory (24, 25).

Following full mobilization, a #46 Fr bougie is passed through the mouth and guided into the stomach. When the organ is thus supported, the myotomy can be done safely using blunt tipped Allison scissors with little risk to the underlying mucosa. The my-

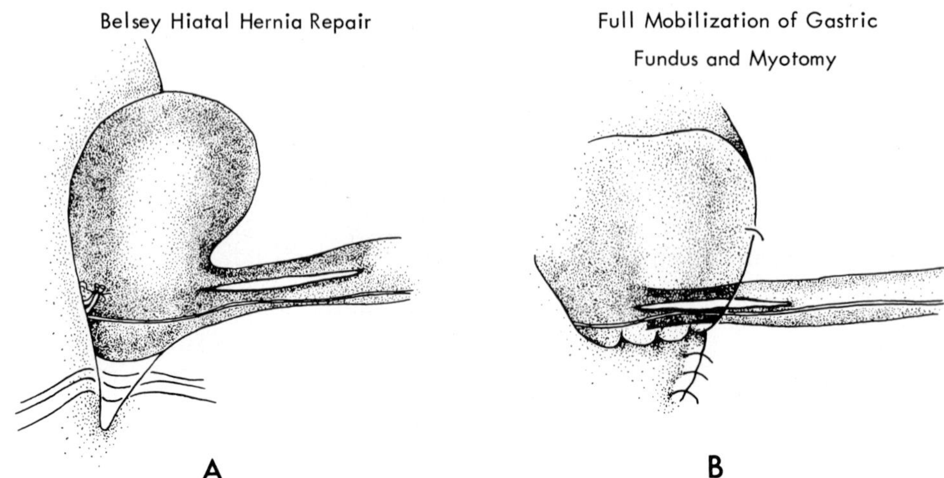

Figure 14.3. Stages of Heller Myotomy
Using a transthoracic approach to Heller myotomy, the surgeon mobilizes the fundus into the chest
and removes the gastric fat pad. A 10-cm myotomy is carried from the stomach to the body of the
esophagus. Reflux is controlled by a modified Belsey hiatal hernia repair (B).

otomy is extended from 1 cm into the stomach
to 2 to 3 cm above the constricted lower
esophagus. The landmarks are easy to recognize. The proximal stomach has short,
transverse, extramucosal veins, which are
quite different from those in the esophageal
mucosa. Proximal extension carries the myotomy for approximately 10 cm and it terminates in the thickened lower esophagus
above the constricted gastroesophageal junction.

A Belsey or Nissen fundoplication may be
added, as previously described, to bring a 3-
to 4-cm segment of esophagus below the diaphragm. This is accompanied by a loose
crural repair.

My present preference is to use a modified
Nissen fundoplication, although I have used
a Belsey in the past with satisfactory results.
The Nissen is sewn in two layers to one edge
of the fundoplication. This allows fixation of
the fundus for a distance of 3 cm above the
esophagogastric junction. Fundus is now
rolled around the lower esophagus and approximated for a distance not exceeding 1 cm
of total fundoplication using fundic sutures
without esophageal incorporation. In this
manner fundus of stomach is fixed to esophagus using sutures which are separate from
those used in the fundoplication. The wrap is
loose and very short. Dysphagia from a Nissen fundoplication is more dependent on total
length of wrap, and the experienced operator
should easily be able to avoid tightness.

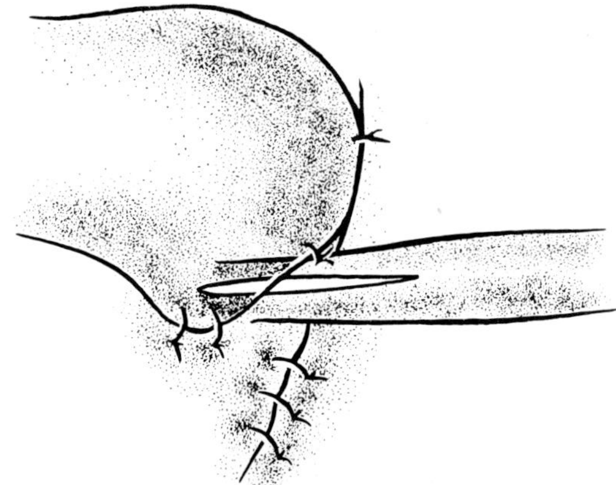

**Figure 14.4. Achalasia—Myotomy with Short
Nissen Fundoplication**
In achalasia reflux control can be achieved by
a short Nissen fundoplication. The anterior surface of the esophagus is sutured to gastric
fundus for a distance of 3½ cm; however, the
completed fundoplication is reduced to ½ to 1
cm in length. Using the short fundoplication
dysphagia is not a problem postoperatively.

Crural sutures are placed and tied following
fundoplication (Fig. 14.4).

The operator and the anesthetist must
make avoidance of aspiration a cardinal principle in this type of surgery and devote all
possible attention to this goal. The technique
of myotomy is a matter of individual choice.
The method described here, that using Allison scissors, is safe and is easily taught to the
resident staff. However, the length of my-

otomy and also its completeness are critical. When myotomy is correctly performed, the mucosa pouches out and the operator can detect no recognizable residual muscle bundles. The muscle should be dissected laterally to prevent scar from closing the myotomy during healing. Hill (26) advocates the use of intraoperative manometry as a method of confirming the completeness of his myotomy; however, in experienced hands the completed myotomy is obvious and this seems an unnecessary addition.

Surgeons agree that late reflux must be avoided but disagree on the method which best achieves success. Two approaches are possible and each has strong advocates. If it is decided to myotomize without the use of a concomitant hiatal hernia repair then the surgeon must take great care not to destroy the normal anatomy while exposing and myotomizing the gastroesophageal junction. Should the choice be to use a hernia repair, then full mobilization is necessary for repair and, of course, this also facilitates the myotomy.

Using myotomy without hernia repair, the reported incidence of reflux is significant. Early occurrence of a hiatal hernia and reflux are reported and reflux accounts for (27–29) a late incidence of heartburn and dysphagia of 16 to 50 per cent. In studies comparing the results of Heller myotomy with and without concomitant hernia repair, the incidence of reflux was reported as 18.5 per cent in the absence of hernia repair and 0 per cent with repair (30).

In my own practice I have always incorporated a Belsey or modified short fundoplication Nissen repair with the myotomy, and reflux has not been a problem in late follow-up (Fig. 14.4).

To some extent the achalasia esophagus is protected from reflux. The esophagus has increased length, so that an anatomic hernia is uncommon. In addition, with Stage III achalasia some mucus retention is common even after myotomy, and this will reduce the damaging effect of reflux. Finally with a vagal nerve degenerative process gastric acidity is often reduced so that the irritant effect of the refluxed bolus is less marked. However, patients with achalasia have not, in my experience, developed this increased incidence of reflux after myotomy. This difference in response has not been explained, although in achalasia the esophagus becomes distended and elongated and the hernia repair may draw a longer length of esophagus below the diaphragm, adding this length as a further barrier to reflux. In addition, gastric acidity is often reduced and the refluxed bolus, if it reaches the esophagus, is often pooled in a reservoir of retained esophageal secretions, which often, being alkaline, may act to neutralize the acidic reflux.

Choice of Treatment—Dilatation vs. Myotomy

The choice of therapy remains open, but the Heller myotomy is gaining in popularity. Myotomy gives a high incidence of satisfactory results—95 per cent (22)—and has a low mortality—less than 1 per cent. Although the incidence of perforation from bougienage is more than 3 per cent (7, 31), the true incidence of major complications favors myotomy. The Heller myotomy is technically easy, and the surgeon is more likely to have the necessary experience to handle the operative procedure and any complication which may arise. In the hands of an expert, dilatation therapy is excellent, but the occasional practitioner is hardly likely to approach the success rate described by the Mayo Clinic, namely 60 per cent satisfactory results on the first dilatation and an incidence of perforation of 3 per cent.

Operative treatment is now recommended in the patient who has achalasia and an associated hiatal hernia. Reflux is much more common if the sphincter is destroyed by dilatation in these patients. Surgery is also recommended in children since dilatation carries a high failure rate (32, 33). Furthermore, rapid and effective correction is mandatory because a reduced dietary intake will rapidly impair growth. Dilatation gives poorer results in "vigorous" achalasia than in the other forms and hence surgery is the primary treatment in this variant. Dilatation is less effective in those with advanced disease and a dilated Stage III esophagus, as accidental perforation is more likely to precipitate serious illness. Thus, excluding these exceptions, operative treatment should be recommended in most healthy adults, unless the patient wishes a trial of dilatation therapy and is in an appropriate category. If dilatation is tried and is not successful after two attempts, an operation should be done forthwith because further dilatation is unlikely to succeed (34–36).

Failures of Operative Therapy

A small group of patients do not respond to myotomy and they should be evaluated carefully to determine the cause of failure; e.g., reassessment must confirm the preoperative diagnosis of achalasia. In most of these patients treatment failure is related to an incorrect diagnosis, and subsequent measures are aimed at recognition and effective therapy of the primary disease. The most common error in differential diagnosis is to do a myotomy in patients with gastroesophageal reflux or in those suffering from linitus plastica.

Those who do have achalasia, yet do not respond to myotomy, present a difficult problem. If myotomy has not given even temporary relief, the myotomy is probably incomplete or was incorrectly placed (37). Under these circumstances manometric study will demonstrate that gastroesophageal junction is intact.

Patients who gain effective relief but later complain of dysphagia usually have developed reflux and peptic stricture. These patients may have the additional symptoms of heartburn and may have signs of reflux into the throat. Treatment is aimed at correction of reflux.

The final group, those with malignancy (38–40), are rare but important. Usually esophageal cancer is recognized late because the esophagus is dilated. Thus, only the most meticulous long-term follow-up will detect the malignancy early and permit complete excision.

In summary, achalasia is a unique esophageal disorder which can be effectively treated with long-lasting satisfactory results. Most of the problems encountered in these patients reflect inadequate investigation and management. If the physician makes a complete evaluation and reaches the correct diagnosis, the patient can be assured relief after effective dilatation or by myotomy. Responsibility for these patients does not end with the relief of dysphagia. The possibility of malignant change makes essential careful follow-up for the remainder of the patient's life.

References

1. Ellis, F. H., Jr., and Olsen, A. M.: *Achalasia of the Esophagus.* W.B. Saunders Co., Philadelphia, 1969.
2. Vinson, P. P.: Diagnosis and treatment of cardiospasm. South. Med. J., *40:* 387, 1947.
3. Russell, J. C.: Diagnosis and treatment of spasmodic stricture of the oesophagus. Br. Med. J., *1:* 1450, 1898.
4. Plummer, H. S.: Cardiospasm, with a report of forty cases. J.A.M.A., *51:* 549, 1908.
5. Browne, D. C., and McHardy, G.: New instrument for use in esophagospasm. J.A.M.A., *113:* 1963, 1939.
6. Wooler, H.: Cardiospasm. Gastroenterologia, *78:* 342, 1952.
7. Sanderson, D. R., Ellis, F. H., Jr., and Olsen, A. M.: Achalasia of the esophagus; results of therapy by dilation, 1950–1967. Chest, *58:* 116, 1970.
8. Heceta, W. G., Wruble, L. D., and Pate, J. W.: Esophageal obstruction due to intramuscular hematoma following pneumatic dilatation. Chest, *69:* 115, 1976.
9. Heimlich, H. J., O'Connor, T. W., and Flores, D. C.: Case for pneumatic dilatation in achalasia. Ann. Otol. Rhinol. Laryngol., *87:* 519, 1978.
10. Stewart, E. T., Miller, W. N., Hogan, W. J., and Dodds, W. J.: Desirability of roentgen esophageal examination immediately after pneumatic dilatation for achalasia. Radiology, *130:* 589, 1979.
11. Crump, A. C., Flood, C. A., and Hennig, G. C.: Results of medical treatment of idiopathic cardiospasm. Gastroenterology, *20:* 30, 1952.
12. Barrett, N. R., and Franklin, R. H.: Concerning the unfavourable late results of certain operations performed in treatment of cardiospasm. Br. J. Surg., *37:* 194, 1949.
13. Maingot, R.: Surgical treatment of cardiospasm. Postgrad. Med. J., *5:* 351, 1949.
14. Wangensteen, O. H.: Physiologic operation for mega-esophagus (dystonia, cardiospasm, achalasia). Ann. Surg., *134:* 301, 1951.
15. Merendino, K. A., and Dillard, D. H.: Concept of sphincter substitution by interposed jejunal segment for anatomic and physiologic abnormalities at esophagogastric junction, with special reference to reflux esophagitis, cardiospasm and esophageal varices. Ann. Surg., *142:* 486, 1955.
16. Thal, A. P., and Kurtzman, R.: A new method for reconstruction of the esophagogastric junction. Surg. Gynecol. Obstet., *120:* 1225, 1965.
17. Hirashima, T., Sato, J., Hara, T., Nakamura, H., Kawamura, I., Takeuchi, H., Muto, M., and Ohkawa, H.: Results of esophagocardioplasty with gastric patch in the treatment of esophageal achalasia. Ann. Surg., *188:* 38, 1978.
18. Seta, K., and Hatafuku, T.: Definitive treatment of advanced achalasia with fundic patch method. Bull. Soc. Int. Chir., *33:* 456, 1974.
19. Heller, E.: Extramuköse Cardiaplastik beim chronischen Cardiospasmus mit Dilatation des Oesophagus. Med. Chir. (Jena), *27:* 141, 1913.
20. Zaaijer, J. H.: Cardiospasm in aged. Ann. Surg., *77:* 615, 1923.
21. Sawyers, J. L., and Foster, J. H.: Surgical considerations in the management of achalasia of the esophagus. Ann. Surg., *165:* 780, 1967.
22. Ellis, F. H., Jr., Kiser, J. C., Schlegel, J. F., Earlam, R. J., McVey, J. L., and Olsen, A. M.: Esophagomyotomy for esophageal achalasia; experimental, clinical and manometric aspects. Ann. Surg., *166:* 640, 1967.
23. Silber, W.: Achalasia. Lancet, *2:* 1287, 1965.

24. Jekler, J., and Lhotka, J.: Modified Heller procedure to prevent postoperative reflux esophagitis in patients with achalasia. Am. J. Surg., *113:* 251, 1967.

25. Nemir, P., Jr., Fallahnejad, M., Bose, B., Jacobowitz, D., Frobese, A. S., and Hawthorne, H. R.: A study of the causes of failure of esophagocardiomyotomy for achalasia. Am. J. Surg., *121:* 143, 1971.

26. Hill, L. D.: Intraoperative measurement of lower esophageal sphincter pressure. J. Thorac. Cardiovasc. Surg., *75:* 378, 1978.

27. Henderson, R. D., Ho, C. S., and Davidson, J. W.: Primary disordered motor activity of the esophagus (diffuse spasm). Ann. Thorac. Surg., *18:* 327, 1974.

28. Wingfield, H. V., and Karwowski, A.: The treatment of achalasia by cardiomyotomy. Br. J. Surg., *59:* 281, 1972.

29. Douglas, K., and Nicholson, F.: The late results of Heller's operation for cardiospasm. Br. J. Surg., *47:* 250, 1959.

30. Black, J., Vorbach, A. N., and Collis, J. L.: Results of Heller's operation for achalasia of the oesophagus. The importance of hiatal repair. Br. J. Surg., *63:* 949, 1976.

31. Clagett, O. T.: Achalasia; dilatation or myotomy? J. Thorac. Cardiovasc. Surg., *53:* 757, 1967.

32. Payne, W. S., Ellis, F. H., Jr., and Olsen, A. M.: Treatment of cardiospasm (achalasia of the esophagus) in children. Surgery, *50:* 731, 1961.

33. Tachovsky, T. J., Lynn, H. B., and Ellis, F. H.: The surgical approach to esophageal achalasia in children. J. Pediatr. Surg., *3:* 226, 1968.

34. Fletcher, P. R.: Acute hiatal hernia with oesophageal perforation following Heller's operation. Br. J. Surg., *65:* 486, 1978.

35. Menzies-Gow, N., Gummer, J. W., and Edwards, D. A.: Results of Heller's operation for achalasia of the cardia. Br. J. Surg., *65:* 483, 1978.

36. Csendes, A., Larrain, A., Strauszer, R. E., and Ayala, M.: Long term clinical, radiological and manometric follow-up of patients with achalasia of the esophagus treated with esophagomyotomy. Digestion, *13:* 27, 1975.

37. Ellis, F. H., Jr., and Gibb, S. P.: Reoperation after esophagomyotomy for achalasia of the esophagus. Am. J. Surg., *129:* 407, 1975.

38. McCallum, R. W.: Esophageal achalasia secondary to gastric carcinoma. Report of a case and a review of the literature. Am. J. Gastroenterol., *71:* 24, 1979.

39. Tucker, H. J., Snape, W. J., Jr., and Cohen, S.: Achalasia secondary to carcinoma; manometric and clinical features. Ann. Intern. Med., *89:* 315, 1978.

40. Lawson, T. L., and Dodds, W. J.: Infiltrating carcinoma simulating achalasia. Gastrointest. Radiol., *1:* 245, 1976.

CHAPTER 15

Diffuse Spasm of the Esophagus

Diffuse spasm of the esophagus (DES) is a condition in which the lower two-thirds of the esophagus loses its normal peristaltic motor coordination and responds to deglutition by segmental spasm. It must be distinguished from other primary esophageal motor disorders and from the secondary disordered motor activity associated with hiatal hernia. Osgood (1) recognized DES in 1889, and Moersch and Camp (2) at the Mayo Clinic gave the first clinical description in 1934; however, their descriptions were not sufficiently specific to permit definite diagnosis and their investigations did not separate DES from achalasia. Indeed, DES was not clearly separated from similar dysfunctions until esophageal manometric studies (3, 4) revived interest in this disorder and led to the development of more specific diagnostic criteria.

Many terms have been used to describe this disorder, e.g., primary disordered motor activity, pseudodiverticulosis, functional diverticula, ripple esophagus, and curling or corkscrew esophagus. These terms are equally appropriate in describing the radiologic appearances of marked secondary disordered motor activity in hiatal hernia or in presbyesophagus (5, 6).

Diffuse spasm (6) is the term most commonly used in the literature and for this reason will be used in the present text. Diffuse spasm must be clearly separated from other primary disorders such as achalasia and scleroderma and must also be separated from secondary disordered motor activity related to hiatal hernias, caustic burns or obstruction. Pain and dysphagia are the dominant symptoms in DES. In addition, several radiologic and manometric features are of diagnostic value, and at operation the pathologic features are highly specific.

The following outline of this disease is based on wide personal exprience. The patients described here exhibited all the characteristic features, including the pathologic changes at operation.

Etiology

The cause of DES is unknown. The similarity between its symptoms and those of achalasia and the difficulty of differentiating the two suggest that they may be related or may be variants of the same fundamental disease process. In two patients, followed up for several years, the manometric findings evolved from one of diffuse spasm to one of achalasia (7, 8). Bennett and colleagues (9) described a patient in whom DES resolved completely following dilatation and esophageal motor function returned to normal.

In this particular case one must question the validity of the original diagnosis. In the patients described as evolving from diffuse spasm to achalasia this is a manometric change and the differentiation of diffuse spasm and achalasia is often difficult. More extensive studies would be necessary before one could say that the two diseases can blend together.

In patients with DES, tissue studies, including electron microscopy (10), show only mild changes in the esophageal muscle cells. The vagal nerve fibers show Wallerian degeneration. (The histologic changes found in the nerves are more extensive than those found in achalasia, suggesting that the disorders are distinct entities.) Ganglion cells are normal in DES, in contrast to ganglion cell depletion usually encountered in achalasia (11). Biochemical investigation has shown that the esophagus responds vigorously to pentagastrin and other cholinergic stimuli suggesting a denervation response (12, 13). This finding is in keeping with the described histology. In short, no specific cause has been assigned, but the disorder seems to be related to some form of vagal degeneration.

Symptoms

There is no particular sex ratio, and DES may appear at any age from the late teens to old age. In 21 cases Henderson and his colleagues (14) reported that the most common symptoms were pain, dysphagia, regurgitation and weight loss. The reported frequency of symptoms varies somewhat, and some authors stress the higher incidence of pain alone, whereas others stress dysphagia (Table 15.1) (15, 16). Having gained further surgical experience with 51 cases of diffuse spasm the dominant symptoms remain pain and dysphagia; however, reflux and related symptoms also occur (Table 15.2) and merit more detailed documentation.

Table 15.1
Symptoms in Diffuse Spasm*

Symptoms	Series (No. of Patients)		
	Henderson et al. (14) (21)	Ellis et al. (16) (31)	Gillies et al. (15) (21)
Pain alone	1	11	0
Pain and dysphagia	20	16	13
Dysphagia alone	0	4	8

* These three series show much variation in symptomatology. In the series by Henderson et al. and by Gillies et al., both pain and dysphagia predominate, whereas in that by Ellis et al. pain alone is a common symptom.

The widely different clinical presentations in the two cases which follow illustrate the difficulties of differential diagnosis:

Case 1. Mrs. W., age 52, presented with dominant dysphagia of many years' duration. She had pain on swallowing, which was felt in the retrosternal area and in the back. Her dysphagia was very severe and occurred with all meals, and she frequently regurgitated.

This woman had been the subject of extensive investigation over a period of 22 years. She had submitted to many radiologic and endoscopic studies, but all had been considered normal. She was referred to me only after she had attempted suicide.

The symptom of painful dysphagia must be considered evidence of esophageal disease until proved otherwise. On radiologic examination the esophageal caliber was normal, but the esophageal wall was thickened and the organ showed a pattern consistent with motor spasm. On manometry the gastroesophageal junction was normal and relaxed well, but there was a marked degree of high amplitude disordered motor activity. Endoscopy was normal.

This evidence supported a diagnosis of DES and the subsequent extended myotomy effectively controlled her symptoms. This woman's long and uncomfortable experience illustrates the severe dysphagia which may develop in some of these patients.

Case 2. Mr. S., age 52, presented with a much different history than Mrs. W. For 3 years he had had recurrent episodes of retrosternal, epigastric and back pain. Occasionally the pain was associated with eating, but was more often related to

Table 15.2
Symptoms of Diffuse Spasm in 51 Patients*

Esophageal pain	100.0%	Reflux	41.2%
Epigastric	72.0%	Aspiration	9.8%
Retrosternal	98.0%	Respiratory symptoms	5.9%
Back	25.5%		
Arms	17.6%		
Eructation	35.3%	Nausea	41.5%
Hiccoughs	5.9%	Vomiting	23.5%
Waterbrash	33.3%		
Dysphagia	96.1%		
Cricopharyngeal	37.3%	Gastroesophageal	88.2%
Liquids	27.5%	Liquids	76.5%
Solids	33.3%	Solids	86.3%
Aspiration	21.6%	Regurgitation	52.9%

* Pain and dysphagia are the most common symptoms in diffuse spasm. Reflux is commonly present and associated symptoms are often present including eructation, nausea and vomiting.

walking and lifting. Initially he was believed to suffer from coronary artery disease, but extensive investigation, including an exercise cardiogram, failed to show any evidence of cardiac abnormality. Radiologic examination revealed a 6-cm hiatal hernia On manometry his gastroesophageal junction was normal, but the body of the esophagus showed a high percentage of abnormal contractions of high amplitude and prolonged duration.

At thoracotomy, because his esophagus was thick-walled and spastic, we carried out an extended myotomy and gastroplasty. After operation he had excellent symptomatic relief which has continued.

Case 3. Mrs. C., age 25, was an emotional young woman with a very limited command of English. She presented to an ENT surgeon with recurrent episodes of very severe laryngospasm. Following emergency admission she required tracheostomy because of rapidly deteriorating respiratory function and anoxia. At this time bilateral vocal cord paralysis was considered probable. As the laryngospasm subsided vocal cord function was noted to be normal and she was extubated.

Reviewing her history the triggering mechanism for laryngospasm was noted to be cricopharyngeal dysphagia and food aspiration. More detailed history was obtained of severe gastroesophageal junctional dysphagia, regurgitation, reflux and night aspiration.

Esophageal radiology was normal without a hernia and without radiologic reflux. Endoscopy demonstrated a patulous gastroesophageal junction with free reflux and a small hiatal hernia. Manometry was the most important investigation. The high pressure zone of normal tone with good relaxation; however, in the body of the esophagus there was 86 per cent DMA of a low amplitude type. These findings were compatible with diffuse spasm.

At operation the esophageal wall was thickened and motor spastic confirming the presence of diffuse spasm. She was treated by extended esophageal myotomy and short standard Nissen fundoplication. Her postoperative course has been excellent. She has returned to a normal diet and has had no further episodes of laryngospasm.

All of these patients have DES and presented difficult diagnostic problems. In all the response to extended myotomy has been excellent. The histories were very different: one presented with dominant dysphagia, the one with the complaint of chest pain, and the last presented with laryngospasm as a complication of aspiration. this variety of clinical presentations challenges the physician to study esophageal disease, to school himself in its various manifestations and to listen to the patient's story with care.

The pain distribution is not characteristic; it may be epigastric or retrosternal and often it is referred to the back and to the base of the neck. Like achalasia, the pain may come on spontaneously and is more frequent when the patient is tired and anxious. Unlike achalasia, the pain often is triggered by swallowing. Some patients in whom painful dysphagia is dominant find eating such an unpleasant experience that they may suffer weight loss.

The dysphagia involves both liquids and solids, and tends to be more marked with solids. Specific foods may give rise to more marked symptoms, e.g. tough solids, carbonated beverages and very hot or very cold liquids.

Nine of the 21 patients with DES described pharyngoesophageal dysphagia and 7 of these coughed and choked with swallowing—an indication of obstruction at the pharyngoesophageal level and spillage of food onto the vocal cords. Fifteen of the 21 complained of regurgitation, which usually occurred soon after swallowing. The regurgitated material tastes like food and is accompanied by large quantities of thick bubbly mucus. The frequency of regurgitation varied, but in some patients constituted a major social embarrassment, keeping them from eating in public. Regurgitation almost always occurs soon after eating, while the patient is awake, and hence aspiration is not usually a problem.

As is characteristic of all motor disorders, the dysphagia is usually provoked by both liquids and solids. If it is severe the patient cannot take adequate nourishment and weight loss becomes a significant problem. Twelve of the 21 patients described by Henderson and colleagues (14) had weight loss; in 3 it was in excess of 30 pounds. This weight loss is in marked contrast to that in hiatal hernias or in nonmalignant strictures, where adequate nourishment can be obtained from liquids. Such severe weight loss, in the absence of stricture, is seen only in Stage III achalasia, DES and in the occasional patient with severe motor disorders of the pharyngoesophageal junction.

Case 4. Miss F., age 26, presented with retrosternal pain and dysphagia. Both symptoms were severe and both had rapidly worsened over a period of 6 months. The pain came on spontaneously and was associated with dysphagia.

The dysphagia was present at almost all meals and was associated with frequent regurgitation. She could take neither liquids nor solids, and eating became so painful that she reduced her intake to a minimum. During this 6-month period she had a progressive and rapid weight loss of 50 pounds.

Manometry and radiologic examination confirmed the presence of DES and subsequently surgical myotomy gave effective relief of her symptoms. Since operation she has gained 20 pounds and is now controlling her diet to avoid excessive weight gain.

Radiology

The radiologic changes in DES are difficult to detect unless the radiologist has this diagnosis in mind and looks specifically for motor spasm and esophageal wall thickening (17–20). In one study, 8 of 9 patients with symptomatic DES could not be shown to have motor spasm on routine esophagogram (21). Of our 21 patients (14), 7 were diagnosed as having hiatal hernias, 4 as having achalasia, 5 as normal and 5 were noted to have disordered motor activity compatible with DES. In retrospective review of 11 radiologic studies of good quality, we considered that the films permitted a radiologic diagnosis of DES in 8 patients (72.7 per cent).

With increasing experience our radiologic diagnosis has not been improved. Presently having operated on 51 patients with diffuse spasm the radiologic diagnosis was correct in only 43.1 per cent, hiatal hernia alone was diagnosed in 25.5 per cent, achalasia in 13.7 percent and the studies were normal in 17.7 per cent (Table 15.3).

The major radiographic features are marked motor spasm in the lower two-thirds of the organ and an increase in esophageal wall thickness to 5 mm or more (19, 20, 22) (Fig. 15.1). Seven of our 21 patients had an associated hiatal hernia. Wall thickness can be demonstrated only if the radiologic penetration is correct and if the patient is rotated to separate the esophagus from the vertebral column. The medial wall of the esophagus is ideal for such assessment because it is adjacent to the pleura of the right lung (Fig. 15.2).

Mid- and epiphrenic diverticula may be recognized radiologically. Both of these may

Table 15.3
Radiologic Diagnosis of Diffuse Spasm—51 Patients*

Correct diagnosis (43.1%)		
Diffuse spasm	13	(25.5%)
Diffuse spasm and hiatal hernia	7	(13.7%)
Diverticulum and diffuse spasm	2	(3.9%)
Incorrect Diagnosis (56.9%)		
Hiatal hernia	13	(25.5%)
Achalasia	7	(13.7%)
Normal	9	(17.7%)

* Radiology is inaccurate in this disease even when films were reviewed retrospectively. It is this lack of specific radiologic features which leads to the relatively high incidence of misdiagnosis and incorrect surgical treatment.

be associated with diffuse spasm of the esophagus; however, this aspect of the disease will be discussed in Chapter 20.

In our study we noted an additional radiologic feature (14). Three of these 21 patients had proximal esophageal dilatation and a "retention" esophagus. Two presented with a radiologic density in the right upper posterior mediastinum and a fluid level at the base of the neck (Fig. 15.3). A barium esophagogram demonstrated esophageal retention and confirmed that the mediastinal enlargement was due to esophageal dilatation. In these patients, unlike those with achalasia, the distal esophagus is narrow and tortuous from persistent motor spasm.

Early experience with esophageal scintigraphy suggests that it may be of some value in quantitating esophageal emptying times.

Manometric Features

Manometric studies are of great diagnostic value in DES (3, 6, 23–29). In conjunction with history and radiology, they permitted a specific diagnosis of DES in 17 of our 21 patients. The gastroesophageal junction shows normal tone (average 21.1 cm of water) and normal or slightly reduced relaxation in response to deglutition (Fig. 15.4). The lower two-thirds of the esophagus has spastic motor waves of prolonged duration and high amplitude. Manometrically the upper third of the esophagus, the cricopharynx and phar-

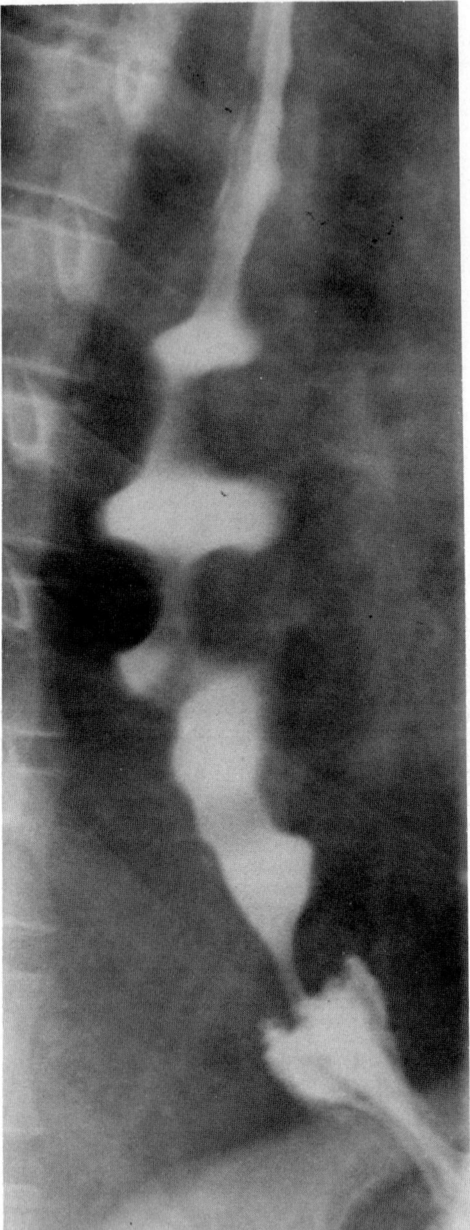

total disordered motor activity in the lower two-thirds of the esophagus and the remaining 9 patients had more than 85 per cent disordered motor activity. The amplitude of motor contraction, which also varied, averaged between 50 and 129 cm of water in 6 patients, between 15 and 49 cm in 13 and below 14 cm in 2. We considered all of these studies compatible with the diagnosis of DES. The amplitude of motor contraction could not be correlated with the thickness of the esophageal wall. One of the two patients with a low amplitude motor wave (average less than 14 cm of water) had an esophageal wall that was 1.4 cm thick (normal, 1 to 3 mm).

Of four patients who had an incorrect diagnosis before operation, two had hiatal hernias and two, although considered to have DES, could not be conclusively diagnosed. In these patients we could now show satisfactory relaxation of the gastroesophageal junction or peristalsis in the proximal third of the

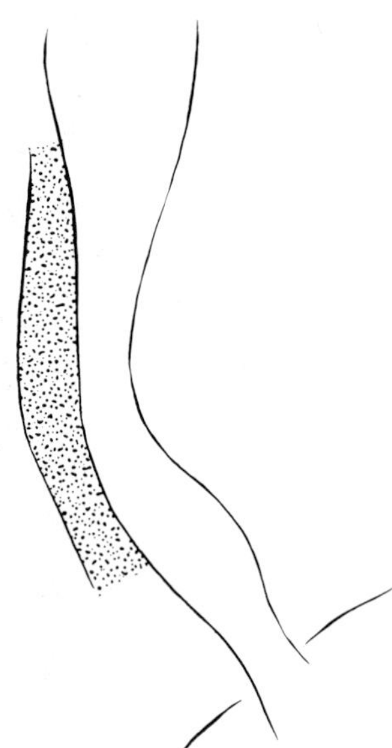

Figure 15.1
Radiologic features are characteristic of DES. A small hiatal hernia is present. In the distal esophagus, severe disordered motor activity is present.

ynx are normal. The motor waves in the lower esophagus are the most typical because they are often of very high amplitude, unlike the spastic waves seen in hiatal hernia.

Some variation of the motor pattern is acceptable. In our study 12 of 21 patients had

Figure 15.2. Diffuse Spasm and Esophageal Wall Thickening
Distal esophagus in this study shows motor spasm. Films were taken with the esophagus projected off the thoracic spine to allow visualization and measurement of the thickened esophageal wall. In this particular study the esophageal wall thickness was 9 mm, and this was confirmed at operation. Reproduction of an x-ray does not clearly show the wall change, and for this reason an exact diagrammatic representation is used.

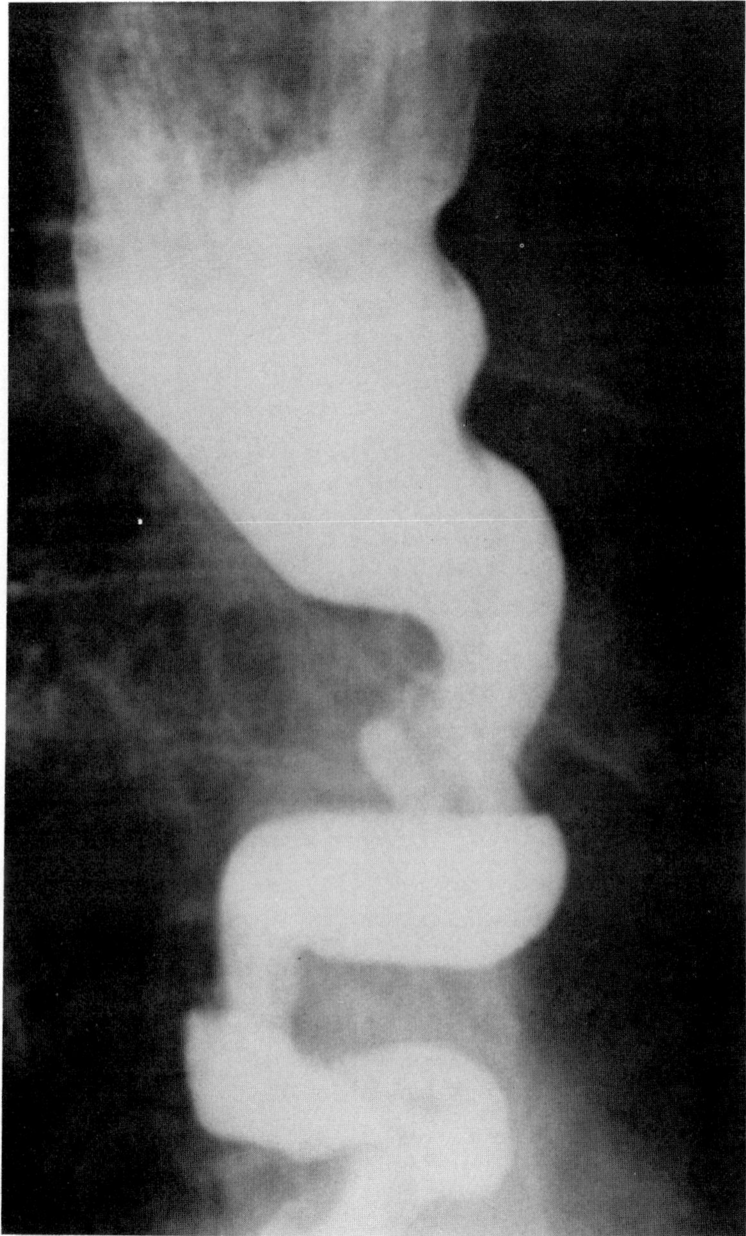

Figure 15.3. Advanced Diffuse Spasm with Esophageal Retention
Barium swallow in a patient with a 20-year history of dysphagia, including a clear history of night aspiration, due to spillage of esophageal content into the pharynx. The distal esophagus is spastic and the esophageal wall is thickened. The proximal esophagus is dilated and is retaining food. This particular radiologic feature—a retention esophagus—must be differentiated from achalasia.

esophagus; the apparent absence of peristalsis may have been due to fluid retention in the esophagus, which so transmits pressure change that it makes motor waves appear simultaneous.

Case 5. Mr. J., age 67, had had dysphagia for 20 years and also had occasional epigastric and retrosternal distress. Initially he was considered to have a bronchogenic carcinoma because of radiologic enlargement of his mediastinum (Fig. 15.3).

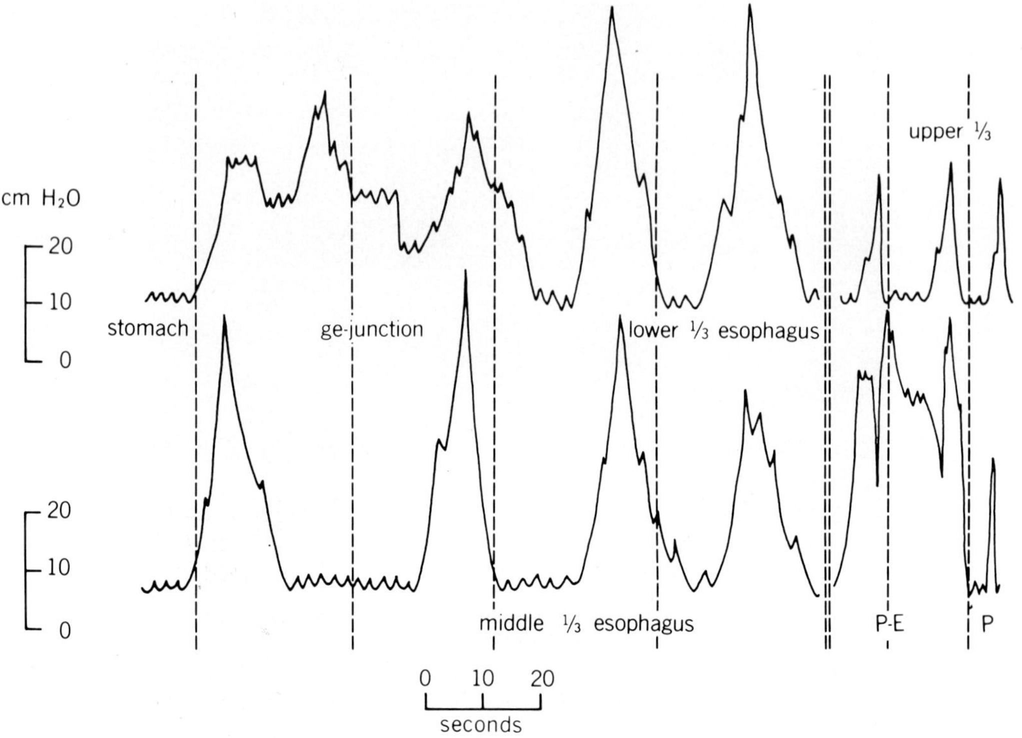

Figure 15.4. Diffuse Spasm
In diffuse spasm, the gastroesophageal (ge) junction is normal and relaxes and contracts in response to deglutition. In the distal esophagus, disordered motor activity is marked and usually of high amplitude and prolonged duration. In the proximal esophagus, cricopharynx (P-E) and pharynx (P) the motor activity is normal. Simultaneous recordings are done 5 cm apart, the lower recording being 5 cm proximal. The single dotted line marks a 1-cm proximal move of the recording catheter and the double dotted line is used to separate tracings in the lower esophagus from tracings in the upper esophagus.

Manometric studies were attempted on two occasions before operation, but the catheter could not be passed into his stomach and hence the gastroesophageal junction could not be studied. Fluid retention distorted his upper esophageal motor pattern and may have dampened out the peristalsis.

At operation his esophagus was thick-walled and spastic. Since the extended myotomy carried out at that time, he has remained well and has had complete remission of symptoms for 5 years. Manometric studies after operation showed that he had normal peristalsis in the upper third of his esophagus.

Analysis of Motor Change in Diffuse Spasm

The same method of manometric classification (29) can be used for diffuse spasm as was used in achalasia. The symbols P can be used for the presence of peristalsis, p for absent peristalsis, R for relaxation, r for absent relaxation, V for vigorous motor activity with 20 per cent or more of motor waves over 50 cm of water and v for low amplitude motor activity. Using this symbol classic diffuse spasm would be represented as PRV in which the high pressure zone (HPZ) relaxed in response to deglutition some peristalsis is present and the motor activity is vigorous.

In 51 patients the following manometric data were obtained:

PRV (47.5 per cent)—classic change of diffuse spasm

pRV (1.9 per cent)—no peristalsis: high amplitude

pRv (9.7 per cent)—no peristalsis: low amplitude

PRv (41.1 per cent)—low amplitude disordered motor activity (DMA)

The classic motor pattern of diffuse spasm is the high amplitude vigorous motor activity in the body of the esophagus. In my experience low amplitude DMA is almost as frequent and indeed can be associated with just as severe symptoms. Most patients have peristalsis and relaxation is present at the gastroesophageal junction. In this study group all patients had relaxation (rare with achalasia), and all but 6 patients had esophageal peristalsis. In the 6 patients without peristalsis mucus and fluid retention is probably interfering with our ability to record peristalsis in the upper esophagus. Four of those patients had postoperative manometry, and all had peristalsis demonstrated in the follow-up study (Fig. 15.5). The finding of peristalsis in follow-up studies almost excludes achalasia from the differential diagnosis.

Manometric Comparison: Achalasia and Diffuse Spasm

The HPZ tone is high normal in both achalasia and diffuse spasm (Table 15.4). Esophageal basal pressure is significantly higher with achalasia. Peristalsis almost never occurs with achalasia and is present in most patients with diffuse spasm. This is the single most important point of manometric differentiation. I have seen only one patient with classic achalasia who had possible peristaltic waves in the proximal esophagus. Relaxation can occur with both achalasia and diffuse spasm; however, with achalasia relaxation is of short duration and is weak. With diffuse

Table 15.4
Manometric Comparison of Achalasia and Diffuse Spasm*

	Achalasia	Diffuse Spasm
No. patients	40	51
HPZ tone	15.6 cm H_2O	16.7 cm H_2O
Esophageal basal pressure	16.8 cm H_2O	7.5 cm H_2O
Average tone of motor waves	14.5 cm H_2O	34.6 cm H_2O
	prv 86.3%	PRV 47.5%
	pRv 6.8%	pRV 1.9%
	prV 4.6%	pRv 9.7%
	Prv 2.3%	PRv 41.1%

* Comparison is made between achalasia and diffuse spasm. Although a clear distinction can usually be made, the occasional patient will have features of both disorders.

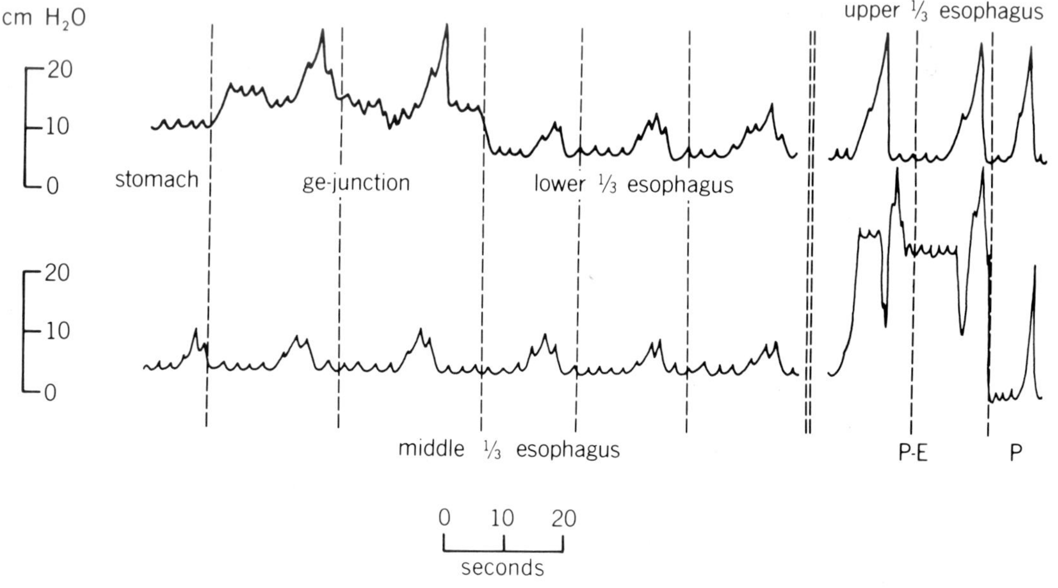

Figure 15.5. Diffuse Spasm—Motor Function after Myotomy
Following myotomy the pressure in the gastroesophageal (ge) junction is reduced. Relaxation may still be recognizable. The distal esophagus shows low amplitude disordered motor activity. In the proximal esophagus there are peristaltic motor waves. Motor function in the cricopharynx (P-E) and pharynx (P) is normal.

spasm relaxation is almost always present and well formed.

In the majority of patients a clear distinction can be made between the manometric patterns of achalasia and diffuse spasm.

Mecholyl Test

Mecholyl has been used as a diagnostic test for achalasia; 6 to 10 mg given subcutaneously produces increased motor spasm and a rise in the baseline esophageal pressure (24). Some patients with achalasia do not respond to Mecholyl, but these usually have Stage III achalasia and a dilated and flaccid esophagus. A standard Mecholyl test, although of some diagnostic value in achalasia, can also be positive in symptomatic DES (30); therefore, this test has limited value in separating these diseases. With the graded Mecholyl test described by Pope (31), the esophagus in achalasia is more sensitive than in DES. This test (31) uses a distended balloon in the body of the esophagus and constantly monitors pressure changes. Most patients with DES develop increased esophageal pressure when given 5 to 7.5 mg of Mecholyl, but a smaller dose usually increases esophageal pressure in patients with achalasia.

Endoscopy

There are no specific endoscopic findings of DES, but endoscopy is valuable in differential diagnosis and in the assessment of associated disease. Using a flexible fiberoptic esophagoscope under local anesthesia, the operator may see marked motor spasm, but he cannot quantitate the spasm; hence this procedure lacks diagnostic accuracy. As in all esophageal disease, the surgeon must exclude related disorders and, in particular, carcinoma of the gastric cardia, which can produce radiologic and manometric changes compatible with DES. Gastroesophageal reflux, although frequently present does not exclude the presence of diffuse spasm.

Differential Diagnosis

The major items in differential diagnosis are achalasia and various forms of secondary disordered motor activity, chiefly that associated with hiatal hernia. Occasionally noesophageal disease is important in differen-

tial diagnosis, particularly when the pain of DES mimics that of myocardial ischemia.

Case 6. Mr. M., age 50, had had three admissions to hospital for suspected myocardial infarction, but no electrocardiographic changes were recognized. On each occasion he presented with major retrosternal chest pain and radiation of pain to the left upper arm. Coronary angiography performed during his third admission showed normal coronary arteries. A small hiatal hernia was present radiologically. Manometric studies showed high amplitude disordered motor activity compatible with DES. An acid perfusion study clearly reproduced his chest pain. He did not respond to conservative management and was treated by extended myotomy. At operation his esophageal wall was 1 cm thick and typically spastic. Two years after operation he remains free of symptoms.

In making a diagnosis history, radiology, manometry and endoscopy are important. To avoid error all of these investigations should be completed and the evaluation tempered with experience. For optimal diagnostic accuracy the interpretation of the data should be in the hands of one investigator as any one investigative parameter taken by itself may be very misleading.

Case 7: Mr. B., age 48, had duodenal ulcer symptoms treated 3 years previously by Billroth I gastrectomy. He presented with intractable heartburn, precipitated by all meals and aggravated by postural change. He described reflux of gastric content but no history of aspiration. Eructation was excessive and he had periodic nausea and vomiting. Gastroesophageal junctional dysphagia was a concomitant symptom, occurring to both liquids and solids and associated with periodic regurgitation of food tasting material.

Radiology showed poor gastric emptying and massive reflux. Solid food obstruction was demonstrable and required liquids to wash the solids into the stomach.

Manometric evaluation showed a low tone gastroesophageal junction without relaxation. The body of the esophagus was totally disordered with motor waves of very low amplitude and a mirror image pattern characteristic of achalasia (prv).

This one finding, manometry, indicated a diagnosis of achalasia; however, symptoms and radiology indicated that reflux was the dominant problem. Endoscopy showed marked chronic epithelial change with a patulous gastroesophageal junction and gastric retention of bile stained food products.

One feature of the investigation was misleading; however, had this been taken in isolation and the patient treated by Heller myotomy the resultant reflux would have been disastrous. Repeat manometry on this occasion demonstrated peristalsis, and the motor changes were then considered compatible with the marked secondary DMA of severe reflux. Surgical correction of reflux and revision of his gastrectomy have successfully corrected his symptoms.

Comparison of the symptoms of achalasia (32), diffuse spasm and reflux are helpful in illustrating their differences (Table 15.5). It can be seen from this analysis that the symptoms of achalasia are quite different with a presentation which is dominantly dysphagia. Pain, although present in 85.4 per cent, is not usually severe and is more a general food-related discomfort. Spontaneous pain, although helpful, is rare (12.2 per cent) and also occurs with diffuse spasm (23.5 per cent). Aspiration, when it occurs, is frequently associated with significant secondary respiratory infection as the aspirated esophageal content is often infected. Patients with achalasia may describe eructation; however, the gas return is esophageal in origin. When vomiting is described by the patient it probably represents spontaneous regurgitation and is not usually associated with nausea.

The symptoms of diffuse spasm and reflux are more difficult to separate; however, with diffuse spasm, pain and dysphagia are usually the dominant symptoms and this may help in deciding what further studies are necessary.

Radiology is very helpful (Table 15.6); however, a specific diagnosis cannot always be made. In the present series almost all patients with achalasia were correctly diagnosed (96.7 per cent); however, 13.7 per cent of patients with diffuse spasm were diagnosed as having achalasia so that the incidence of a false positive diagnosis of achalasia is significant. In my experience patients seen because of failure of Heller myotomy most often never had achalasia and the error in diagnosis was based on radiology. Diffuse spasm is very difficult to accu-

Table 15.6
Radiologic Diagnoses: Achalasia (41), Diffuse Spasm (51) and Reflux (335)*

	Correct Diagnosis	Incorrect Diagnosis
	%	%
Achalasia	97.6	2.4
Diffuse spasm	43.1	56.9
Reflux	80.0	20.0

* The radiologic diagnosis of diffuse spasm can be quite precise; however, the necessary features of spasm and wall thickening were present in less than 50 per cent of the 51 patients studied.

Table 15.5
Symptom Comparison: Achalasia, Diffuse Spasm and Reflux*

	Achalasia (41)		Diffuse Spasm (51)		Reflux (359)	
	No.	%	No.	%	No.	%
Esophageal pain	35	85.5	51	100.0	359	100.0
Precipitation						
Food	30	73.2	47	92.2	351	97.8
Posture	6	14.6	18	35.3	263	73.3
Exercise	1	2.4	12	23.5	53	14.8
Spontaneous	5	12.2	12	23.5	0	0
Reflux	0	0	21	41.2	304	86.7
Night aspiration	15	36.6	5	9.8	147	41.0
Respiration symptoms	8	19.5	3	5.9	42	11.7
Eructation	13	31.7	18	35.3	254	70.8
Hiccoughs	3	7.3	3	5.9	99	27.6
Waterbrash	0	0	17	33.3	85	23.7
Nausea	3	7.3	23	45.1	251	69.9
Vomiting	6	14.6	12	23.5	123	34.3
Dysphagia						
Total	41	100.0	49	96.1	284	79.1
Gastroesophageal	38	82.6	45	88.2	205	57.1
Pharyngoesophageal	7	17.1	19	37.3	152	42.3

* Although symptoms overlap between achalasia and diffuse spasm, the patient with achalasia usually presents with dysphagia as the dominant symptom.

rately diagnose radiologically even when the films are reviewed retrospectively. Without manometry considerable experience and the recognition of its specific intraoperative pathology, the diagnosis of diffuse spasm will be missed. In the series of 51 patients treated surgically for diffuse spasm 10 (19.6 per cent) had had previous esophageal surgery based on an incorrect diagnosis.

Endoscopy is specific in recognizing the secondary changes of reflux; however, reflux may coexist with diffuse spasm so that this cannot be used for differentiation. In the patients with diffuse spasm two had a short, peptic stricture.

Advanced Stage III achalasia is easily recognized and is the most common form of achalasia seen clinically.

Manometric differentiation has already been presented. In most patients an accurate diagnosis can be based on manometry; however, the findings must be used in conjunction with the other clinical parameters.

At the time of surgery careful inspection and palpation of the esophagus should be carried out. This is often neglected; however it is very important to the patient, as if the pathology is not recognized it can have disastrous consequences. The dilated achalasia esophagus with a tapered gastroesophageal junction is clearly recognizable. Reflux esophagitis when severe produces a thickened esophageal wall; however, this is of woody consistency and is not motor spastic. Very occasionally slight motor spasticity is recognizable in the presence of reflux; however, this can be clearly distinguished from the changes of diffuse spasm.

The following patient illustrates the difficulty is differential diagnosis of achalasia and diffuse spasm.

Case 8. Mrs. R., age 44, had a 5-year history of retrosternal and epigastric pain which came on spontaneously but was also aggravated by eating. In addition, she had gastroesophageal junctional

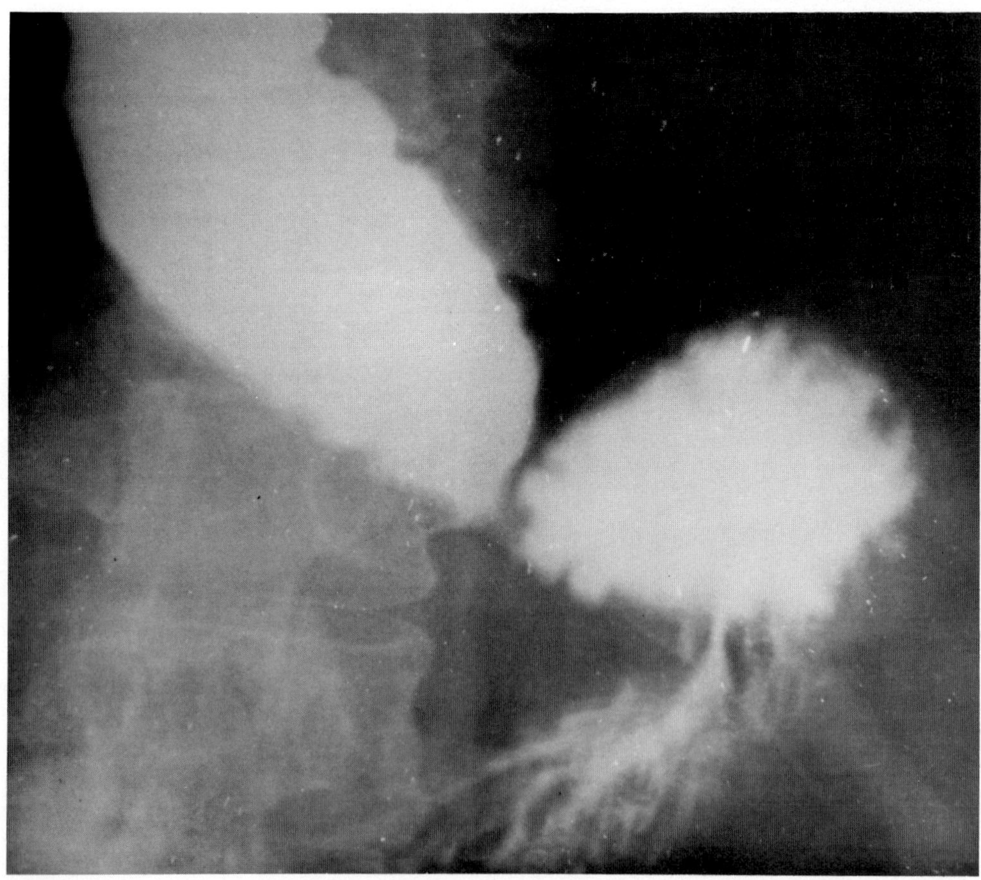

Figure 15.6
Radiologic features consistent with achalasia—diffuse disordered motor activity, esophageal dilation, a "bird beak" deformity of the lower esophagus and no air bubble in the stomach. However, on manometry, Mrs. R. (Case 8) had a typical pattern of diffuse spasm.

dysphagia, which developed during most meals and frequently was associated with regurgitation. Repeated radiologic studies were all considered to show achalasia (Fig. 15.6). Manometry showed a normal gastroesophageal junction and severe, high amplitude disordered motor activity in the lower two-thirds of the esophagus. Peristalsis was present in the upper esophagus. At operation this woman had a thickened and spastic esophagus, and extended myotomy gave her good relief from her symptoms.

Rarely other disorders must be differentiated from diffuse spasm. Occasionally carcinoma can produce high amplitude motor waves (33). However, if radiologic and manometric features are confusing, malignancy must be pursued by endoscopy and biopsy.

Case 9. Mrs. E., age 44, had a 6-month history of painful dysphagia, becoming progressively more severe. The pain was located in the mid-retrosternal area. She had no other significant symptoms. Radiologic study showed only a small hiatal hernia. Manometry showed high amplitude disordered motor waves in the lower esophagus (Fig. 15.7). At this stage of evaluation the motor changes were considered to represent DES; however, endoscopy demonstrated a small and localized circumferential esophageal carcinoma. We concluded that the motor response was related to partial esophageal obstruction. Without endoscopy this patient's symptoms would have been attributed to disordered motor activity and she would not have received definitive therapy for the carcinoma, namely, esophagogastrectomy.

On rare occasions neurologic disease may simulate DES (34). Although DES is so difficult to define that its very existence has been questioned, a group of patients with DES can be separated out by carefully analyzing the history, radiology and manometric evidence (35, 36). The diagnosis must be made before operation because, although the patient has specific pathologic lesions, these will be recognized only at thoracotomy and will be missed entirely if the surgeon uses an abdominal approach. Once a specific diagnosis has been made, a more difficult problem awaits the surgeon: namely, to institute effective therapy.

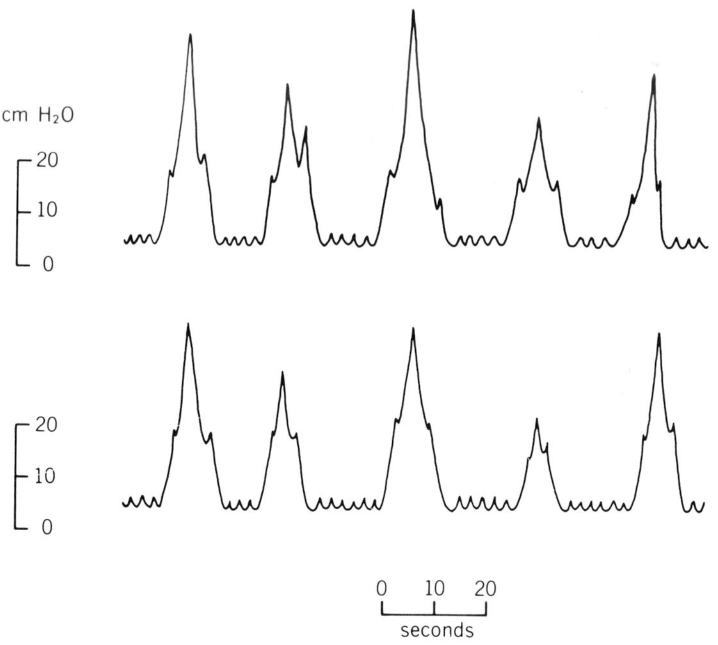

Figure 15.7. Esophageal Carcinoma in Situ
Mrs. E. (Case 9) had a radiologic hiatal hernia but otherwise was considered normal. Manometrically in the body of the esophagus she had high amplitude prolonged duration motor waves compatible with diffuse spasm. On endoscopic examination, we discovered a circumferential carcinoma which was at an early and superficial stage.

References

1. Osgood, H.: A peculiar form of oesophagismus. Boston Med. Surg. J., *120:* 401, 1889.
2. Moersch, H. J., and Camp, J. D.: Diffuse spasm of lower part of esophagus. Ann. Otol. Rhinol. Laryngol., *43:* 1165, 1934.
3. Creamer, B., Donoghue, E., and Code, C. F.: Pattern of esophageal motility in diffuse spasm. Gastroenterology, *34:* 782, 1958.
4. Ingelfinger, F. J.: Esophageal motility. Physiol. Rev., *38:* 533, 1958.
5. Zboralske, F. F., Amberg, J. R., and Soergel, K. H.: Presbyesophagus; cineradiographic manifestations. Radiology, *82:* 463, 1964.
6. Rider, J. A., Moeller, H. C., Puletti, E. J., and Desai, D. C.: Diagnosis and treatment of diffuse esophageal spasm. Arch. Surg., *99:* 435, 1969.
7. Kramer, P., Harris, L. D., and Donaldson, R. M., Jr.: Transition from symptomatic diffuse spasm to cardiospasm. Gut, *8:* 115, 1967.
8. Schroder, S., Achord, J. L., and Rogers, J. V., Jr.: Achalasia preceded by non-cardiospastic diffuse esophageal spasm; a cineradiographic study (Abstract). Gastroenterology, *44:* 849, 1963.
9. Bennett, J. R., Donner, M. W., and Hendrix, T. R.: Diffuse esophageal spasm; return to normality. Johns Hopkins Med. J., *126:* 217, 1970.
10. Cassella, R. R., Ellis, R. H., and Brown, A.: Diffuse spasm of the lower part of the esophagus. J.A.M.A., *191:* 107, 1965.
11. Cassella, R. R., Ellis, F. H., Jr., and Brown, A. L., Jr.: Fine-structure changes in achalasia of esophagus; 1. Vagus nerves. Am. J. Pathol., *46:* 279, 1965.
12. Eckardt, V., and Weingand, H.: Supersensitivity to pentagastrin in diffuse oesophageal spasm. Gut, *15:* 706, 1974.
13. Mellow, M.: Symptomatic diffuse esophageal spasm. Manometric follow-up and response to cholinergic stimulation and cholinesterase inhibition. Gastroenterology, *73:* 237, 1977.
14. Henderson, R. D., Ho, C. S., and Davidson, J. W.: Primary disordered motor activity of the esophagus (diffuse spasm). Ann. Thorac. Surg. *18:* 327, 1974.
15. Gillies, M., Nicks, R., and Skyring, A.: Clinical, manometric and pathological studies in diffuse oesophageal spasm. Br. Med. J., *2:* 527, 1967.
16. Ellis, F. H., Jr., Olsen, A. M., Schlegel, J. F., and Code, C. F.: Surgical treatment of esophageal hypermotility disturbances. J.A.M.A., *188:* 862, 1964.
17. Zboralske, F. F., and Dodds, W. J.: Roentgenographic diagnosis of primary disorders of esophageal motility. Radiol. Clin. North Am., *7:* 147, 1969.
18. McNally, E. F., and Katz, I.: The roentgen diagnosis of diffuse esophageal spasm. A.J.R., *99:* 218, 1967.
19. Johnstone, A. S.: Diffuse spasm and diffuse muscular hypertrophy of the lower esophagus. Br. J. Radiol., *33:* 723, 1960.
20. Zaino, C., and Beneventano, T. C.: *Radiologic Examination of the Orohypopharynx and Esophagus.* Springer-Verlag, New York, Inc., 1977.
21. Roth, H. P., and Fleshler, B.: Diffuse esophageal spasm; clinical, radiological and manometric observations. Ann. Intern. Med., *61:* 914, 1964.
22. Tolin, R. D., Malmud, L. S., Reilley, J., and Fisher, R. S.: Esophageal scintigraphy to quantitate esophageal transit (quantitation of esophageal transit). Gastroenterology, *76:* 1402, 1979.
23. Bradham, R. R., and Sealy, W. C.: Neuromuscular disorders of the esophagus. Ann. Thorac. Surg., *3:* 460, 1967.
24. Kramer, P., and Ingelfinger, F. J.: Esophageal sensitivity to Mecholyl in cardiospasm. Gastroenterology, *19:* 242, 1951.
25. Graham, D. Y.: Hypertensive lower esophageal sphincter; a reappraisal. South Med., J., *71:* Suppl. 1, 31, 1978.
26. Orlando, R. C., and Bozymski, E. M.: Clinical and manometric effects of nitroglycerin in diffuse esophageal spasm. N. Engl. J. Med., *289:* 23, 1973.
27. Swamy, N.: Esophageal spasm; clinical and manometric response to nitroglycerin and long acting nitrites. Gastroenterology, *72:* 23, 1977.
28. Leonardi, H. K., Shea, J. A., Crozier, R. E., and Ellis, F. H.: Diffuse spasm of the esophagus. Clinical, manometric and surgical considerations. J. Thorac. Cardiovasc. Surg., *74:* 736, 1977.
29. Vantrappen, G., Janssens, J., Hellemans, J., and Coremans, G.: Achalasia, diffuse esophageal spasm and related motility disorders. Gastroenterology, *76:* 450, 1979.
30. Kramer, P., Fleshler, B., McNally, E., and Harries, L. D.: Oesophageal sensitivity to Mecholyl in symptomatic diffuse spasm. Gut, *8:* 120, 1967.
31. Sleisinger, M. H., and Fordtran, J. S.: *Gastrointestinal Disease. Pathophysiology, Diagnosis, Management.* W. B. Saunders Co., Philadelphia, 1973.
32. Olsen, A. M., Holman, C. B., and Andersen, H. A.: Diagnosis of cardiospasm. Dis. Chest, *23:* 477, 1953.
33. Kelley, M. L., Jr.: Intraluminal manometry in the evaluation of malignant disease of the esophagus. Cancer, *21:* 1011, 1968.
34. Fischer, R. A., Ellison, G. W., Thayer, W. R., Spiro, H. M., and Glaser, G. H.: Esophageal motility in neuromuscular disorders. Ann. Intern. Med., *63:* 229, 1965.
35. Bennett, J. R., and Hendrix, T. R.: Diffuse esophageal spasm; a disorder with more than one cause. Gastroenterology, *59:* 273, 1970.
36. Demian, S. D. E.: Idiopathic muscular hypertrophy of the esophagus. Postmortem incidental finding in 6 cases and a review of the literature. Chest, *73:* 28, 1978.

CHAPTER 16

Diffuse Spasm: Medical and Surgical Management

Varied approaches have been advocated for the treatment of diffuse spasm (DES) of the esophagus and at present no consensus has been reached concerning the best therapeutic approach. The continued confusion stems from at least two major causes: the relative rarity of the disorder, and the imprecise definitions used by those who write on this subject. Because the disease is rare, only a few investigators have much experience with it, and in most instances the investigator follows one mode of treatment and never accumulates enough patients to randomize his treatment. The confusion is compounded by the failure to apply clear definitions to the disorder, and to separate it from the motor spasm seen in hiatal hernias and in achalasia.

In Chapter 15 the symptoms and findings were described in 21 patients with DES who were treated by operation. This experience has now increased to 51 patients and the operative approach has been modified by increased experience. History alone is not diagnostic. At interview these patients complain of pain and dysphagia, and every patient will have one symptom or the other. Spasm on cineradiography suggests the presence of DES but increased thickness of the esophageal wall at operation is a more specific diagnostic feature. On manometry the gastroesophageal junction should show evidence of relaxation; the lower esophageal tracing should show a profound disorder of motor activity and the upper third of the esophagus should be peristaltic. If these various radiologic, manometric and pathologic findings are present, the disorder can be accurately categorized. Frequently, as noted earlier, the literature is confusing because the criteria are not precise and the reader is often

left in doubt concerning the true identity of the disorder being described.

Medical Management of DES

Few published reports have described drug therapy in the management of DES. Nitrites relax smooth muscle but have been shown to have only limited value in achalasia (1). Short- and long-acting nitrites have been used in the management of DES, but experience is limited. Radiologically and manometrically nitroglycerin decreases disordered motor activity (2, 3), and, if given during manometric studies, will decrease the intensity of motor spasm (4–6). In effect, it produces a medical myotomy and occasional case reports have attributed some value to treatment with short- and long-acting nitrites. Short-acting nitrites can be used to abort the acute attacks of motor spasm and long-acting nitrites to prevent major motor spasms.

My own experience with nitroglycerin and long-acting nitrites does not support these claims. Most patients have a short-term improvement but within 3 months the drugs lose their effectiveness. It is difficult to determine whether the initial improvement is psychogenic or whether there is true relief. As in achalasia, these patients may develop drug tolerance (7). Other drugs, including local anesthetics and combinations of local anesthetics and sedation (8), have not proved effective in controlling the symptoms of DES.

Anticholinergics have been used in patients with hiatal hernia, mostly to reduce gastric acidity, and these drugs may also decrease esophageal motor activity. However, the effects of DES are disappointing. Hyoscine butyl bromide (Buscopan) produces transient relief only, and symptoms rapidly recur in most patients. Cholinergics such as metaclopramide should be avoided as they will overstimulate the esophagus and aggravate the symptoms. Similarly it has been shown that alkalinization of the stomach will increase the tone of the high pressure zone (HPZ). This action was previously considered to be through the gastrin mechanism (9–13); however its exact etiology is now in doubt.

When dietary modifications are employed, a bland diet is prescribed, and the patient is told to avoid any specific food which produces distress. The type of food producing distress varies, but commonly, cold or hot beverages, carbonated drinks and hard solids are major sources of painful dysphagia.

In general, these therapeutic measures are unsuccessful and are used only in patients with mild symptomatology or in those refusing more definitive therapy.

Dilatation Therapy

The two types of dilatation therapy, the mercury-weighted bougie and bag dilator, have been reported to give variable results. All of these series are small and do not provide sufficient evidence to judge the effectiveness of this form of therapy.

Baird (14) reported that simple bouginage with a #40 Fr bougie or with the esophagoscope gives transient relief. This appears to be similar to the relief obtained by bouginage in achalasia (15) and, as such, should not alter the course of the disease significantly.

The various bag forms of forceful dilatation provide more effective bouginage. Using bag dilatation in 9 patients, Rider and colleagues (16, 17) achieved either complete or marked symptomatic relief after 1 to 22 dilatations. This result is satisfactory, but the surgeon must weigh the number of dilatations and the potential hazards of this procedure against our experience in achalasia, where dilatation therapy is discontinued if it is not effective after two dilatations. Using the Negus esophagoscope and bag dilatation in 12 patients, Craddock and associates (18) found that 7 were slightly improved and continued on conservative management, and 5 required surgical myotomy. The 7 who were improved required continued care and some had to be hospitalized for further dilatation therapy.

It is noteworthy that dilatation therapy in achalasia aims to disrupt the outer muscular layers of the gastroesophgeal junction and thus promote esophageal drainage. In DES the gastroesophageal junction is normal, and it is motor spasm in the body of the esophagus that causes obstruction. Logically, dilatation of the gastroesopohageal junction should not relieve the obstructive element in DES.

The results reported in the literature vary greatly and we do not yet have sufficient clinical detail to permit independent assessment of these various dilatation techniques. Hence we must await for further reports concerning these procedures.

I have tried bougienage on many occasions, and the results are either ineffective or give only short-term relief. One patient is an outstanding exception and is worth separate mention.

Case 1. Mr. S., age 75, presented with a 1-year history of food-induced and spontaneous pain associated with severe gastroesophageal junctional dysphagia and a weight loss of 20 pounds. Radiologically he had severe disordered motor activity (DMA) and marked esophageal wall thickening. Manometrically the changes were characteristic of diffuse spasm. At endoscopy a #60 Fr bougie was passed. Following this and for a period of 3 months he had an almost complete remission of symptoms. He has been lost to follow-up so that the long-term value of mercury bougienage can not be assessed; however, this single case is an exception and has responded to an unusual degree.

Pathophysiology of Diffuse Spasm

The pathology of diffuse spasm is best appreciated at thoracotomy since this is rarely a lethal disease. Although death from starvation (19) and perforation (20) have been described most autopsy reports are incidental findings. In one of the rare autopsy reports, 6 patients (21) were reported in 30 months from a series of 1300 autopsies. Two patients had esophageal dilatation proximal to hypertrophic motor obstruction similar to the patients described in Chapter 15. Microscopically all had circular muscle hypertrophy and one had hypertrophy of the longitudinal muscle layer. All had normal ganglion cells in the myenteric plexus. These findings were based on light microscopy. Electron microscopy from biopsy material has been reported as showing slight muscle degeneration and Wallerian degeneration in the vagal nerves (22).

Direct inspection and palpation of the esophagus at operation gives much valuable informtion. Following full mobilization and careful inspection of the esophagus, the degree of muscle hyperplasia will be seen to vary considerably. In a series of 21 reported patients that I studied at operation (23), all showed some degree of muscle thickening. Four patients had a wall thickness of 4 mm (normal, 2 mm) and the remaining 17 had wall thickness of 5 to 15 mm as measured from mucosa to muscle exterior. The circular fibers of the esophagus showed hyperplasia and the longitudinal muscle was normal to gross inspection (Fig. 16.1). Circular muscle fibers were gathered in bundles, and when stimulated immediately after myotomy, the individual bundles contracted in sequence over a distance of 3 to 4 cm from proximal to distal esophagus (Fig. 16.2).

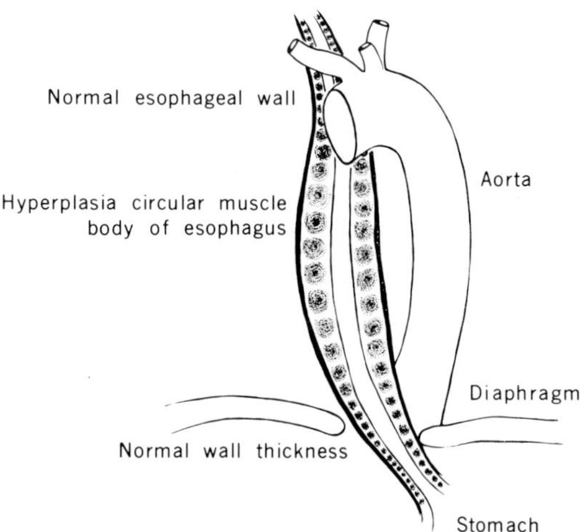

Figure 16.2
In DES, hyperplasia of circular muscle extends from a point close to the aortic arch to the gastroesophageal junction. The proximal esophagus and the gastroesophageal junction are normal.

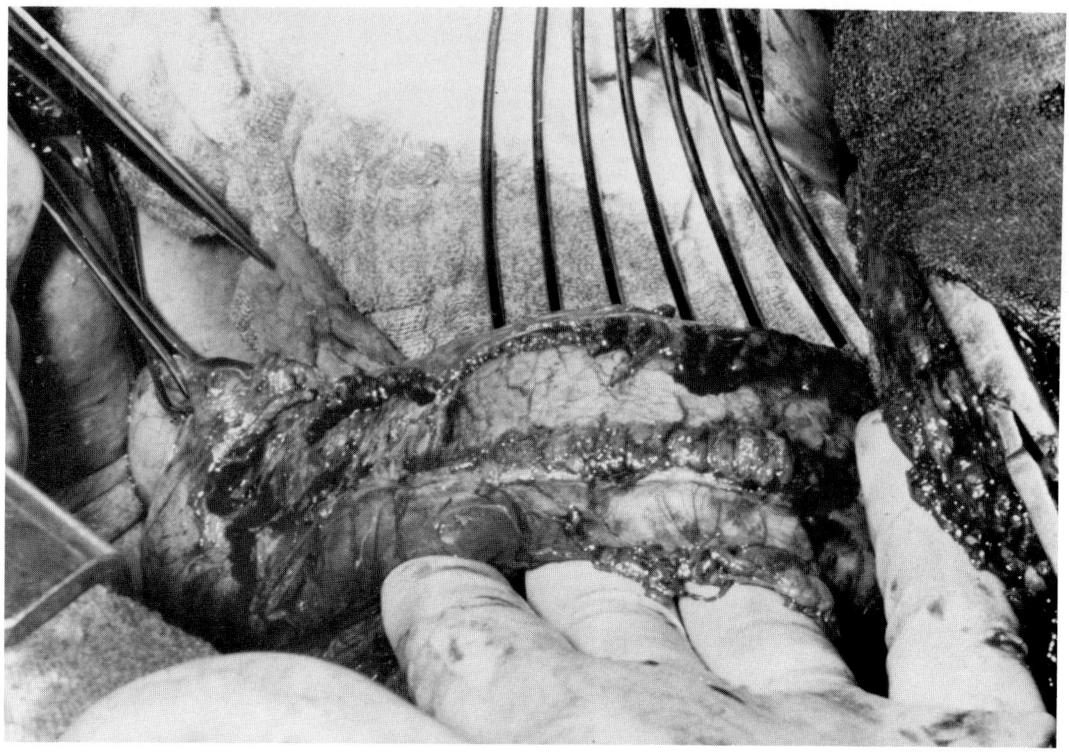

Figure 16.1.   Esophageal Wall in Diffuse Esophageal Spasm
Circular muscle in the body of the esophagus is thickened and hyperplastic. Macroscopically and microcopically the longitudinal muscle layer is normal. In the photograph the esophagus is seen following myotomy, and both the normal longitudinal muscle layers and the hypertrophied circular muscle can be seen.

The gastroesophageal junction appeared normal, but the organ was thickened from the proximal gastroesophageal junction to the aortic arch. At the level of the arch the thickening gradually decreased and the wall became normal again. The exact point at which the muscle wall regained its normal caliber was difficult to determine, but this change took place in the region of the aortic arch (Fig. 16.2).

Palpation of the esophageal wall produces muscle spasm which the surgeon readily recognizes once he becomes familiar with this process. The spasm can be seen and felt as the esophageal consistency changes from flaccid to a firm sausage-like consistency. This phenomenon is referred to as "motor spasticity" and is entirely different from the woody and nonspastic esophageal wall of reflux inflammation. The operative report must describe the pathologic changes in detail, and the detection and recording of these changes should be considered an integral part of the procedure. Although the diagnosis of DES can usually be made before operation, 4 cases in my personal series of 21 were recognized only at operation. In 2 patients considered to have an uncomplicated hiatal hernia the finding was a complete surprise, although in retrospect we had the clinical data necessary for the diagnosis. In the other 2 patients diagnosed at operation, the differential diagnosis had not been settled between DES and achalasia. Follow-up manometric studies in these 4 patients confirmed the presence of proximal esophageal peristalsis; that is, the correct diagnosis was DES and not achalasia. The pathologic findings are important because they confirm the diagnosis and distinguish this process from achalasia, and from the severe secondary disordered motor activity occasionally seen in hiatal hernias. In the patient with hiatal hernia, the surgeon may recognize a slight degree of palpable motor spasm, but it is much less than that found in DES.

Case 2. Mr. J.R., age 48, presented with symptomatic reflux, typical heartburn, severe gastroesophageal junctional dysphagia and food regurgitation once or twice per day. His symptoms, present for 2 years, had become much more severe in the previous 3 months and were unresponsive to vigorous conservative management. Radiologically he had a hiatal hernia but no evidence of spasm or wall thickening (Fig. 16.3). Endoscopically he had a Stage I esophagitis. Manometrically he had a severe disorder of motor activity, but this was believed to be secondary to his hiatal hernia (Fig. 16.4).

At operation the esophageal wall was 1.2 cm thick and exhibited marked motor spasm. An extended myotomy was performed and 3 years later he remains free of symptoms.

This patient had a history compatible with DES. Radiologically had a hiatal hernia with no evidence of motor spasm or wall thickening. The manometric findings did show a high amplitude disordered motor activity, which was more suggestive of DES than of that secondary to hiatal hernia.

Case 3. Mr. S., a patient who is described to provide contrast with Mr. J.R., had a 10-year

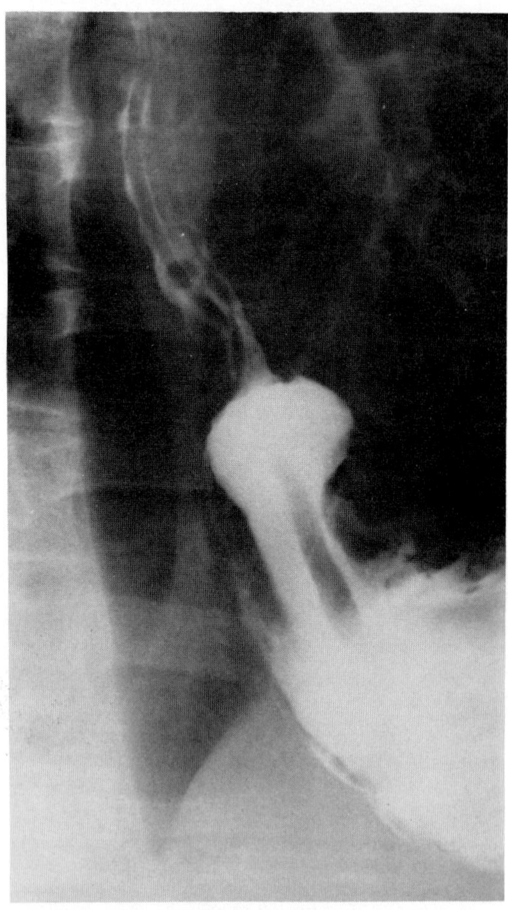

Figure 16.3.   Case 2
Mr. J.R. presented with radiologic features of a hiatal hernia. Motor spasm, although present, was not marked. A diagnosis of DES was made based on manometry and on the findings of muscle hyperplasia and spasticity at operation.

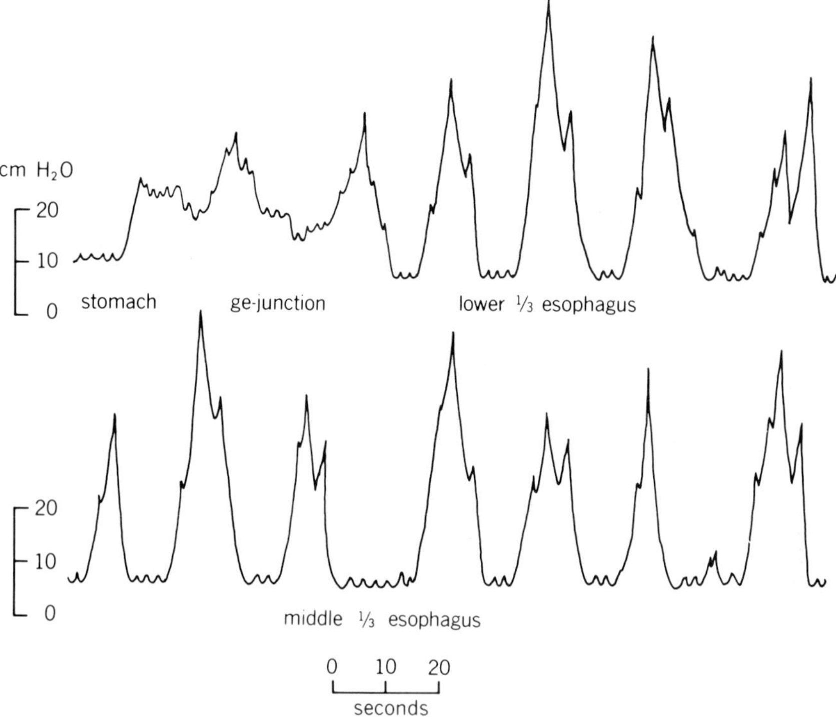

Figure 16.4.   Hiatal Hernia and Diffuse Esophageal Spasm
Manometric findings in Mr. J.R. (Case 2) are typical of DES. His gastroesophageal junction was of normal tone, with good relaxation. Disordered motor activity was very marked and of high amplitude in the lower two-thirds of the esophagus and was normal in the upper third.

history of dysphagia and had been told that he had "cardiospasm." Because of recurrent episodes of severe retrosternal chest pain, he was evaluated by a cardiologist and was hospitalized for a presumed myocardial infarct. However, no evidence of cardiac disease was detected. Radiologically he had a moderate esophageal motor spasm, wall thickening over the distal half of the esophagus, a small hiatal hernia and a peptic stricture. Endoscopically he had a tight stricture, which admitted a #40 bougie. This was dilated to #60 with slight improvement in his dysphagia. Manometrically the tone in his gastroesophageal junction was low and was entirely respiratory-negative. The tracings of the lower two-thirds of his esophagus were completely disordered, and the motor waves, which had an amplitude of 20 to 30 cm of water, were of prolonged duration. Peristalsis was present in the upper esophagus (Fig. 16.5). Acid perfusion studies exactly reproduced his retrosternal pain.

Because of his history, the radiologic spasm and wall thickening, we considered that he was suffering from DES. The disordered motor waves, although of lower amplitude than usually seen in DES, were higher than those usually seen secondary to hiatal hernia. The motor spasm is very

different from that present in Mr. J.R., but despite the lower amplitude of the waves it is completely compatible with DES. At operation his esophagus was 1 cm thick and very spastic. The extended myotomy and gastroplasty done at that time gave him excellent symptomatic relief.

Principles of Surgical Management

In designing an operative approach to diffuse spasm different recommendations have been made and the procedures remain controversial. The arguments used are very similar to those used in achalasia. There is controversy regarding the length of myotomy and also whether or not reflux control procedures should be added following myotomy (23–30).

Length of Esophageal Myotomy

It has been stated that the length of myotomy can be judged by preoperative radiology and manometry (31). Using this approach in most patients myotomy is reported

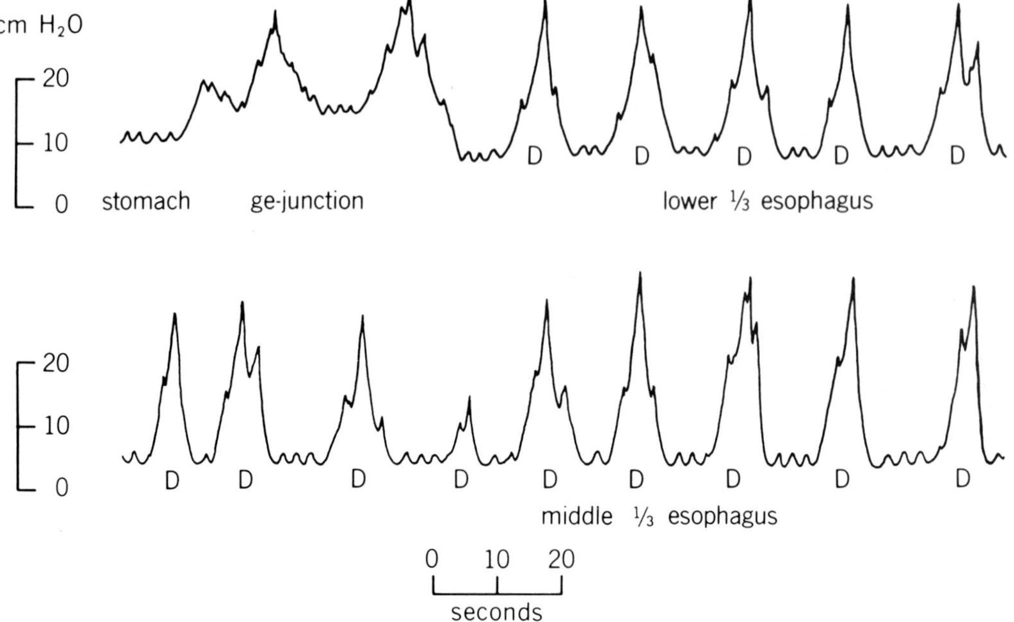

Figure 16.5.   Hiatal Hernia and Stricture with Diffuse Esophageal Spasm
Mr. S. (Case 3) presented withh a small hiatal hernia and peptic stricture. His symptoms were those of chest pain induced by exercise but also related to eating. Manometrically his gastroesophageal (ge) junction was of low tone, but showed slight relaxation. Disordered motor activity was severe and of high amplitude in type. At operation he had the typical circular muscle hyperplasia and spasm of DES.

to be required to the undersurface of the aortic arch only. The fallacy of this approach is the unreliability of the methods used. Radiology in my experience is not always diagnostic of diffuse spasm and even when clearly positive, the extent of the motor spasm will show some variability from one examination to the next and will vary with the type of medium used from liquid barium to solids. Manometry, used in conjunction with fluoroscopy, may accurately localize the level of DMA; however, even under these circumstances localization of the upper limits of spasm must vary by 2 to 3 cm depending upon the response of the upper esophagus to spasm and obstruction in the lower esophagus. In clinical practice I have tried to accurately localize the upper limits of spasm and have been unsuccessful.

We do not presently know the pathophysiology of the muscle spasm; however, most probably diffuse spasm is confined to the smooth muscle component of the esophagus. The point of transition from smooth to striated muscle varies and is a gradual rather than an abrupt transition making its precise localization difficult.

My approach to this controversy has been to extend the myotomy to a level which is certain to be effective. Using this approach in each patient the myotomy has been carried to the apex of the chest, 6 to 10 cm above the aortic arch. This extent of myotomy may be considered excessive; however, the operative technique of extending the myotomy below the aortic arch and to the apex of the chest is simple and safe and has not been associated with any intraoperative or postoperative difficulty. I have seen three patients with residual esophageal pain and dysphagia who were myotomized to the aortic arch level only. In each of these patients relief was obtained by extending the myotomy. Ellis has stated that the myotomy rarely requires this extension and should it be necessary it should be performed through the right chest. He also states that the poor results of this operation (approximately 25 per cent in his hands) are due to persistence or recurrence of pain. This is not my experience and the difference in reported results probably relates to the extent of the myotomy.

Most operations for diffuse spasm included myotomy of the gastroesophageal junction. When the junction is myotomized reflux becomes a problem. Ellis reports reflux in 5 of 30 patients (16.6 per cent) with 2 patients developing a peptic stricture (27). Not all of his patients had radiologic studies, and pH reflux was not documented. Henderson and Pearson (29) report reflux in 8 of 17 patients (47 per cent) following myotomy of the gastroesophageal junction with all patients studied by pH and radiology.

Hiatal hernia is frequently associated with the presence of diffuse spasm. In my present experience with 51 surgically treated patients 39.2 per cent had a hiatal hernia. All of these would certainly require reflux control following myotomy.

Results reported following myotomy in achalasia must be in part similar, and certainly the incidence of reflux in Heller myotomy is significant. The Mayo Clinic reports only a 3.1 per cent of serious reflux complications following Heller myotomy; however, they fail to document the total incidence of reflux and did not use pH reflux testing (32, 33). Others have reported on incidence of reflux following Heller myotomy without hiatal hernia repair which varies from 16 (34) to 50 per cent (35).

The most recent proposal by Leonardi and colleagues (31) to void myotomy of the gastroesophageal junction and instead myotomize only the body of the esophagus would certainly void the controversy of myotomy-induced reflux and deserves careful consideration.

In a series of 11 patients followed 12 to 70 months, extended myotomy was performed for diffuse spasm. The diagnosis was based on history, radiology and manometry and only 6 of the 11 had muscle hypertrophy noted at operation. One had a myotomized HPZ because of hypertonic sphincter (36, 37) and one had a right thoracotomy and total thoracic myotomy because of the extent of manometric spasm. The follow-up is incomplete; however, 9 of 11 are considered to have good or excellent results and only 2 have symptomatic or radiologic reflux (18.1 per cent). This method may well be a significant advance in the management of diffuse spasm;

however, considerably more experience and more detailed follow-up would be necessary. Of particular importance is evaluation of esophageal emptying following myotomy with preservation of the HPZ, as I have seen 3 patients with incomplete esophageal emptying referred to me for evaluation following myotomy with preservation of the HPZ. Two cases illustrate the patient problems which may be encountered.

Case 4. Mrs. K., age 46, was diagnosed as having diffuse spasm by clinical, radiologic and manometric evaluation (38). She had an extended myotomy from stomach to the lower margin of the aortic arch and her esophageal muscle was noted at operation to be thickened and spastic. Following surgery she had persistence of dysphagia and chest pain similar to that present preoperatively.

At this time she was seen for evalution. Radiologically food obstruction was present at the level of the aortic arch. Manometrically DMA was present above the level of her myotomy. No abnormality could be detected endoscopically and a #60 Fr bougie could be passed without resistance.

Through a left thoracotomy her myotomy was extended 10 cm above the aortic arch. Her previous myotomy was inspected and considered to be satisfactory.

The extended myotomy has been effective in giving symptomatic relief and she has now been followed for 6 years.

This patient illustrates the value of extending the myotomy above the aortic arch. She had been operated on by an experienced surgeon and in his judgment at the time of surgery the original myotomy was into healthy muscle.

Case 5. Mr. R., age 38, had a complex past history. Originally he had a transabdominal hernia repair. He did well for 2 years then developed severe dysphagia. At re-evaluation he was considered to have diffuse spasm and an extended myotomy was carried out from the upper margin of the HPZ to the level of the aortic arch. Again he initially did well; however, 1 year following surgery he developed dysphagia which became progressively more severe and required endoscopy on several occasions for removal of impacted food.

He was seen for evaluation at this time. His chief complaint was severe dysphagia. Radiologically his esophagus was dilated to 8 cm in the lower one-third. Manometrically his lower esophagus had low amplitude peristaltic motor waves which did not suggest diffuse spasm. The HPZ was normal. His previous myotomy had produced a motor obstruction at the level of the HPZ and progressive esophageal dilatation was gradually increasing the amount of dysphagia (Fig. 16.6).

Surgically his esophageal muscle was dissected laterally off the mucosa and repaired with interrupted silk sutures. Following surgery his swallowing returned to normal and manometrically he developed a satisfactory return of peristalsis.

I have seen now 3 such patients with esophageal retention and dilatation following myotomy with a preserved HPZ. For this reason I would feel that the operative procedure of myotomy with preservation of the HPZ should be viewed with caution and long-term follow-up should be available before it receives general acceptance.

Reflux Control

The incidence of reflux following extended myotomy with division of the HPZ is reported as 16 to 50 per cent in achalasia and 16 to 47 per cent with diffuse spasm. Despite the controversy that exists as to whether or not hiatal hernia repair is necessary the high incidence of reflux is unacceptable and if reduced by adding repair then this is clearly a good addition to the operative procedure.

Operative Techniques

The operation currently performed at the Womens College Hospital consists of an esophageal myotomy that extends from the proximal stomach to a point 6 to 10 cm above the aortic arch. Esophagogastric competence is maintained by a modified total fundoplication gastroplasty, or more recently by a modified standard Nissen procedure.

The esophagus is approached through a long left thoractomy using the sixth interspace, which gives excellent exposure of the aortic arch and diaphragmatic hiatus. The gastroesophageal junction is fully mobilized and brought into the chest as for hiatal hernia repair. The esophagus is mobilized up to the inferior pulmonary ligament and then, by blunt dissection, is mobilized along its left pleural surface to the aortic arch. To fully expose the left pleural surface of the esophagus between the lung and aorta, I divide one major intercostal artery immediately below the aortic arch. Once this is done a tunnel can be made under the arch and the pleura above

the arch opened for a distance of 10 cm. With experience this maneuver becomes quite easy, and it allows safe myotomy of the esophagus behind the arch at a later stage of the same procedure.

Careful palpation of the esophagus confirms the presence of muscle hyperplasia and spasm. Almost always the muscular thickening can be detected from the upper margin of the gastroesophageal junction to a point just below or just above the aortic arch. Although marked thickening is present in only 70 per cent of the patients I have operated upon, all patients have some degree of thickening and in all patients when the esophagus is palpated it is noted to be motor spastic. Without these findings I would question the accuracy of the diagnosis.

The posterior crural sutures, which are put in place now to be tied later, permit a loose approximation of the crura, but care must be taken to avoid any obstruction to the distal myotomized esophagus.

At this point a #44 Fr Malloney bougie is passed to make the myotomy easier. The myotomy is done using Allison scissors with round tips; these allow free cutting of the muscle with very little risk of cutting into the exposed mucosa. Full myotomy is carried out from a point of 6 to 10 cm above the aortic arch to the level of the proximal transverse gastric veins.

Reflux control is now achieved either by total fundoplication gastroplasty or by modified Nissen fundoplication. Recently we have been using Nissen with excellent results although follow-up is to a maximum of 1½ years only.

From past experience the Belsey wrap is not reliable in reflux control in the presence of a myotomy. If a full Nissen wrap is used motor dysphagia will probably result. Based on past experience and evaluation of patients with dysphagia following Nissen fundoplication I believe that the length of the wrap is more frequently a cause of dysphagia than actual tightness in the wrap mechanism. Tightness in a fundoplication is easily avoided by adequate mobilization; however, once mobilized the temptation to produce too long a wrap is considerable. While this is effective in achieving competence, it also produces obstruction to the forward passage of food. The Nissen wrap totally surrounds dis-

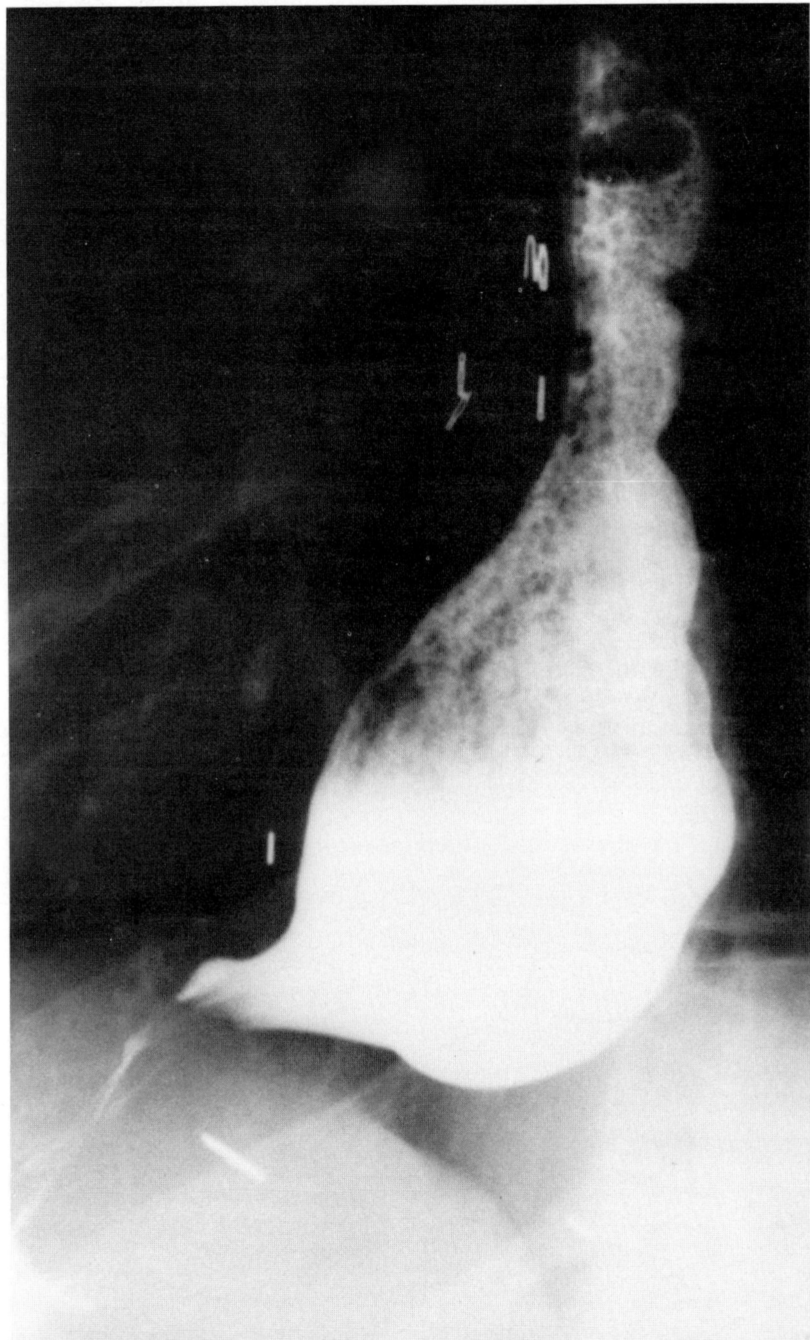

Figure 16.6
Mr. R. (Case 5) had a previous extended myotomy from the lower margin of his aortic arch to immediately above his HPZ. He presented with progressive dysphagia. Radiologically the myotomized esophagus is dilated and retaining food products.

tal esophagus and transmits gastric pressure to the HPZ. As gastric pressure increases the wrap becomes even more competent.

To avoid overcompetence the Nissen wrap is sutured 3 cm up the esophagus with 3 interrupted mattress sutures of 00 silk and the fundus is then wrapped around the HPZ with completion sutures for a distance of only ½ to 1 cm. In this way the total wrap—the point of maximal competence—is kept very short and does not present a barrier to the forward passage of food particles and liquids (Figs. 16.7 and 16.8).

Results with Extended Myotomy

The results achieved with extended myotomy in DES are not as satisfactory as those following myotomy for achalasia. In 1960, Ellis and colleagues (26) reported that 84 per cent of patients showed clinical improvement; in 1964 (27) they reported that 78 per cent were improved and 67 per cent had good or excellent results.

My total experience with extended myotomy for DES is 51 cases with a follow-up of 6 months to 9 years. In this time the extent of myotomy has not varied and has always been continued above the aortic arch. In follow-up evaluation the patient's pain complex has been eliminated and dysphagia at the aortic arch level has not been a problem. As previously noted experience with below arch myotomies in 3 patients with residual pain and dysphagia suggests that this shortened myotomy carries the risk of continued motor spasm (Table 16.1).

Reflux control has been a difficult problem and the Belsey fundoplication with or without gastroplasty has not been a guarantee of reflux control. Eight of 18 patients with a standard Belsey fundoplication of 270° have not had good control and 3 required reoperation. Four of 12 patients with partial fundoplication gastroplasty (Belsey: PFG) have had continued reflux and one required reoperation. Although the PFG was more effective, it was replaced by total fundoplication gastroplasty (TFG) with a modified fundoplication in which the wrap was approximated for a distance of ½ to 1 cm. Using this procedure and with a follow-up of 1 to 4 years no patients have reflux; however, 11.7 per cent have moderate residual dysphagia. In an

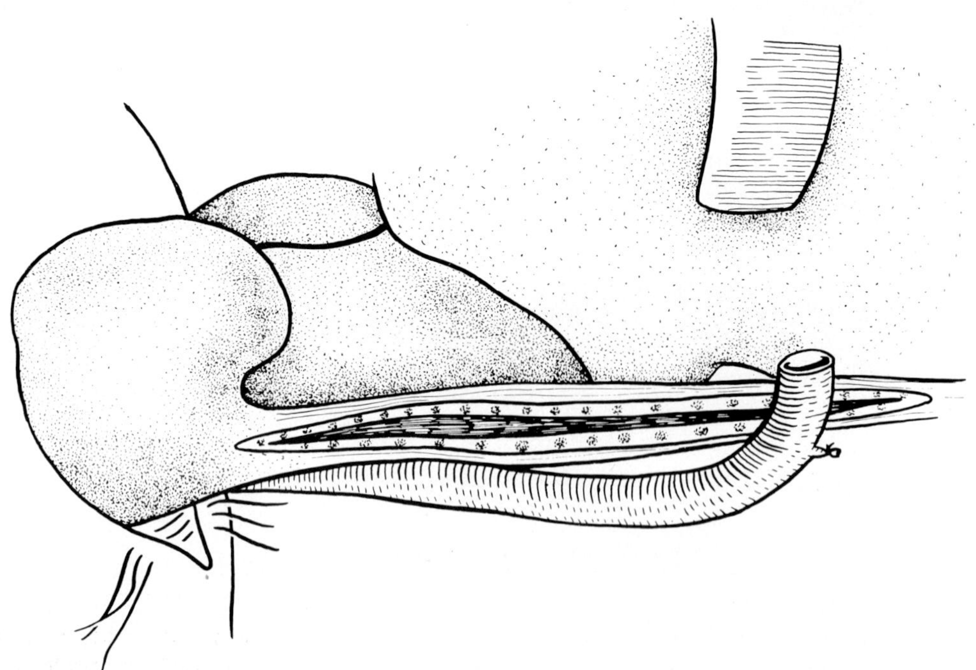

Figure 16.7
The myotomy used in the management of DES is carried from 6 to 10 cm above the aortic arch to the lower margin of the HPZ.

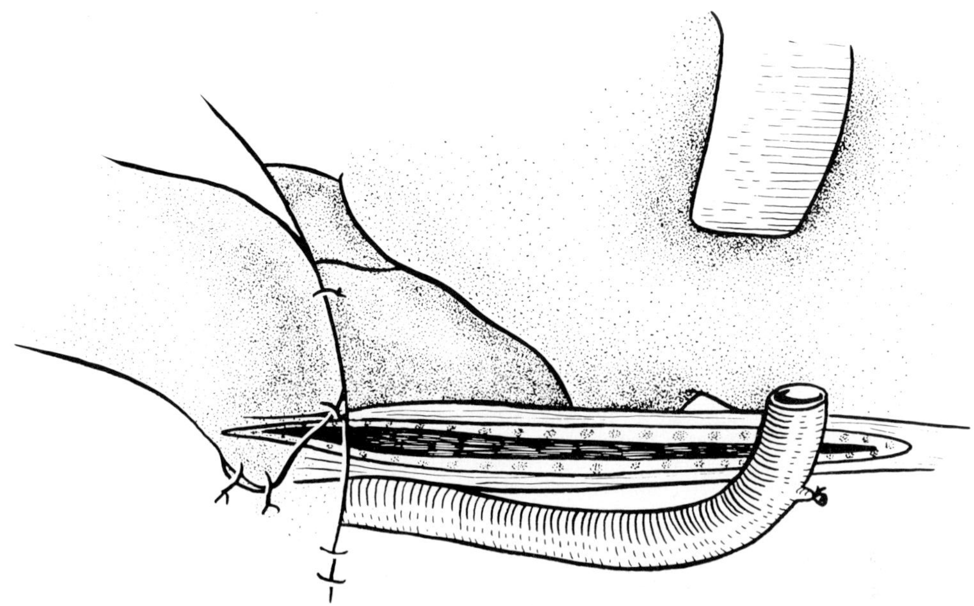

Figure 16.8
After the myotomy is completed, reflux control is achieved by a shortened Nissen fundoplication. The gastric fundus is seen 3½ cm up the anterior aspect of the esophagus with interrupted sutures. Total fundoplication is completed over a distance of only ½ to 1 cm.

Table 16.1
Results of Surgery in Diffuse Spasm—51 Patients with Extended Myotomy*

	Excellent	Good	Poor
Standard Belsey (18)	10	3	5
PFG (12)	8	3	1
Standard Nissen (3)	3	0	0
TFG (18)	17	0	2

* Four groups of patients are reported. In the two groups with Belsey fundoplication (270° wrap) reflux control remains a problem. When a shortened Nissen was used, with or without gastroplasty, effective reflux control was achieved.

effort to eliminate dysphagia in the past 1½ years only a modified Nissen wrap has been added without gastroplasty. In this early follow-up all 3 patients are asymptomatic. There are 6 further patients in short-term follow-up with a short Nissen wrap. None of these patients have reflux or dysphagia.

Certainly the use of a modified Nissen wrap is effective in reflux control. Of the 20 patients treated in this fashion reflux is no longer a problem. In this group excellent results have been achieved in 90 per cent and residual dysphagia is present in 10 per cent.

These results compare favorably with other reported operative approaches to the management of DES and the technique merits further study.

Clearly the surgical management of DES is controversial and the final decision as to the optimal procedure has not been decided. This is a rare disease and time and experience are necessary to evaluate the results of therapy.

Diffuse esophageal spasm remains a diagnostic and therapeutic challenge to those interested in esophageal disease. Although rare, it must be considered in the differential diagnosis of chest pain or dysphagia. Most patients with this disorder remain undiagnosed and some are submitted to inappropriate and sometimes dangerous treatment. Only by continued study and careful evaluation of these patients can we achieve a more complete understanding of this disorder.

References

1. Douthwaite, A. H.: Achalasia of cardia; treatment with nitrites. Lancet 2: 353, 1943.
2. Ingelfinger, F. J.: Esophageal motility. Physiol. Rev., 38: 533, 1958.
3. Sheinmel, A., Priviteri, C. A., and Poppel, M. H.:

Study of effect of certain drugs on curling of esophagus; preliminary report. A.J.R., *62:* 807, 1949.

4. Orlando, R. C., and Bozymski, E. M.: Clinical and manometric effects of nitroglycerin in diffuse esophageal spasm. N. Engl. J. Med., *289:* 23, 1973.

5. Orlando, R. C., and Bozymsiti, E. M.: Clinical and manometric effects of nitroglycerin in diffuse esophageal spasm. J. Engl. J. Med., *289:* 23, 1973.

6. Swamy, N.: Esophageal spasm; clinical and manometric response to nitroglycerin and long acting nitrites. Gastroenterology, *72:* 23, 1977.

7. Dunlop, D.M., Davidson, S., and Alstead, S.: *Textbook of Medical Treatment,* p. 478. E. & S. Livingstone, Ltd., London, 1958.

8. Gillies, M., Nicks, R., and Skyring, A.: Clinical, manometric and pathological studies in diffuse oesophageal spasm. Br. Med. J., *2:* 527, 1967.

9. Dodds, W. J., Dent, J., and Hogan, W. J.: The effect of atropine on esophageal motor function in man. Gastroenterology, *74:* 1028, 1978.

10. Eckardt, V., and Weigand, H.: Supersensitivity to pentagastrin in diffuse oesophageal spasm. Gut, *15:* 706, 1974.

11. Mellow, M.: Symptomatic diffuse esophageal spasm. Manometric follow-up and response to cholinergic stimulation and cholinesterase inhibition. Gastroenterology, *73:* 237, 1977.

12. Eckardt, V. F., and Holtermuller, K. H.: Effects of pentagastrin and gastric alkalinization on lower esophageal sphincter pressure in diffuse esophageal spasm. Digestion, *13:* 1, 1975.

13. DeJesus, R., Peternel, W. W., Orchard, J. L., and Colatrella, A. M.: Diffuse esophageal spasm provoked with prostigmine. (Letter).Gastroenterology, *74:* 332, 1978.

14. Baird, W. L., Jr.: The spastic esophagus. J. Fla. Med. Assoc., *54:* 882, 1967.

15. Vinson, P. P.: Diagnosis and treatment of cardiospasm. South. Med. J., *40:* 387, 1947.

16. Rider, J. A., Moeller, H. C., Puletti, E.J., and Desai, D. C.: Diagnosis and treatment of diffuse esophageal spasm. Arch. Surg., *99:* 435, 1969.

17. Rider, J. A., Moeller, H. C., and Puletti, E. J.: Diffuse esophageal spasm. Am. J. Gastroenterol., *44:* 97, 1965.

18. Craddock, D. R., Logan, A., and Walbaum, P. R.: Diffuse oesophageal spasm. Thorax, *21:* 511, 1966.

19. Hall, A. J.: A case of diffuse fibromyoma of the oesophagus, causing dysphagia and death. Q. J. Med., *9:* 409, 1916.

20. Katz, S. J., Lieberman, A., and Hecktman, H. B.: Spontaneous perforation of the esophagus associated with smooth muscle hypertrophy. Am. J. Surg., *127:* 338, 1974.

21. Demian, S. D., and Vargas-Cortes, F.: Idiopathic muscular hypertrophy of the esophagus. Postmortem incidental finding in six cases and a review of the literature. Chest, *73:* 28, 1978.

22. Cassella, R. R., Ellis, F. H., and Browl, A. L.: Fine-structure changes in achalasia of the esophagus; 1. Vagus nerves. Am. J. Pathol., *46:* 279, 1965.

23. Henderson, R. D., Ho, C. S., and Davidson, J. W.: Primary disordered motor activity of the esophagus (diffuse spasm). Ann. Thorac. Surg., *18:* 327, 1974.

24. Belsey, R.: Functional disease of the esophagus. J. Thorac Cardiovasc. Surg., *52:* 164, 1966.

25. Bradham, R. R., and Sealy, W. C.: Neuromuscular disorders of the esophagus. Ann. Thorac. Surg., *3:* 460, 1967.

26. Ellis, F. H., Jr., Code, C. F., and Olsen, A. M.: Long esophagomyotomy for diffuse spasm of the esophagus and hypertensive gastroesophageal sphincter. Surgery, *48:* 155, 1960.

27. Ellis, F. H., Jr., Olsen, A. M., Schlegel, J. F., and Code, C. F.: Surgical treatment of esophageal hypermotility disturbances. J.A.M.A., *188:* 862, 1964.

28. Henderson, R. D.: Regarding paper on primary disordered motor activity of the esophagus (diffuse spasm) (Letter to Editor). Ann. Thorac. Surg., *19:* 608, 1975.

29. Henderson, R. D., and Pearson, F. G.: Reflux control following extended myotomy in primary disordered motor activity (diffuse spasm) of the esophagus. Ann. Thorac. Surg., *22:* 278, 1976.

30. Lortat-Jacob, J. L.: Myomatoses localisees et diffuse de l'esophage. Arch. Mal. Appl. Dig., *39:* 519, 1950.

31. Leonardi, H. K., Shea, J. A., Crozier, R. E., and Ellis, F. H., Jr.: Diffuse spasm of the esophagus. Clinical, manometric and surgical considerations. J. Thorac. Cardiovasc. Surg., *74:* 736, 1977.

32. Okike, N., Payne, W. S., Neufeld, D. M., Bernatz, P. E., Pairolero, P. C., and Sanderson, D. R.: Esophagomyotomy versus forceful dilatation for achalasia of the esophagus; results in 899 patients. Ann. Thorac. Surg., *28:* 119, 1979.

33. Orringer, M. B.: The treatment of achalasia; controversy resolved (Editorial). Ann. Thorac. Surg., *28:* 100, 1979.

34. Wingfield, H. V., and Karwowski, A.: The treatment of achalasia by cardiomyotomy. Br. J. Surg., *59:* 281, 1972.

35. Douglas, K., and Nicholson, F.: The late results of Hellers operation for cardiospasm. Br. J. Surg., *47:* 250, 1959.

36. Graham, D. Y.: Hypertensive lower esophageal sphincter; a reappraisal. South Med. J., *71:* 31, 1978.

37. DiMarina, A. J., and Cohen, S.: Characteristics of lower esophageal sphincter function in symptomatic diffuse esophageal spasm. Gastroenterology, *66:* 1, 1974.

38. Vantrappen, G., Janssens, J., Hellemans, J., and Coremans, G.: Achalasia, diffuse esophageal spasm and related motility disorders. Gastroenterology, *76:* 450, 1979

Scleroderma

CHAPTER 17

Scleroderma and Related Disorders

Various collagen disorders including scleroderma, Raynaud's disease, disseminated lupus erythematosus and polymyositis may involve the esophagus at some stage during their progress (1). Of these, scleroderma is most frequently associated with esophageal changes and as such illustrates the problems encountered in this group of disorders. The principal motor changes are a reduction in the tone of the gastroesophageal junction and a marked diminution in the amplitude of motor waves in the distal two-thirds of the organ (2–5). The proximal esophagus, pharyngoesophageal junction and pharynx retain normal motor function. In effect the esophagus loses its normal motor power and becomes adynamic, and the symptoms are directly related to loss of motor power and to the secondary effects of gastroesophageal reflux. Although a great deal is now known about the behavior of an adynamic esophagus, we know little about the underlying pathogenic mechanisms.

Esophageal Pathology and its Relation to Motor Function

The pathologic changes in the esophagus in scleroderma have been extensively studied and their extent and distribution correlated with the associated motor changes. In the first reports of this disorder in 1903, Ehrmann (6) described the association between scleroderma and dysphagia.

The most characteristic pathologic features are myogenic atrophy, damage to Auerbach's plexus, deposition of collagen in the connective tissue and a subintimal fibrosis of esophageal arteries. In addition to these primary changes, the patient may develop secondary esophagitis from reflux, and this may obscure the underlying primary pathology (7).

The neurogenic damage is well established (8), and some workers report that the Auerbach's plexuses may be deficient or absent. Unlike those who have achalasia, these patients do not develop hypersensitivity to cholinergic drugs, perhaps because of associated myogenic damage.

The muscle fibers show atrophic changes (9) in the lower two-thirds of the esophagus, but the fibers are preserved in the upper third—the "striated" esophagus. The increased deposition of collagen which may be associated is not as prominent as was originally described. The muscle changes in dermatomyositis may involve the striated esophagus and indeed may be limited to the upper third of the organ. All of these changes, although they help to characterize the esophageal lesion, do not explain the myogenic or neurogenic atrophy and do not establish the etiology.

Autopsy examination of a limited number of patients who had had manometric esophageal studies before death (9, 10) has shown that the extent of muscle atrophy correlates with the degree of loss of motor activity in the esophagus.

Pharmacologic Changes

Cohen and associates (11) have studied the response of the esophagus to various stimuli to determine whether the neurogenic or myogenic changes are primary disorders. Cholinergic stimulation with methacholine, the potentiation of acetylcholine by choline esterase inhibition and stimulation using gastrin I as an acetylcholine-releasing drug, has shown that, in the earlier stages of scleroderma, the esophagus responds to direct stimulation by methacholine. In the very late stages they found no muscle response, probably indicating severe atrophy. When a myogenic response could still be evoked by direct muscle stimulation, there was no response to indirect neurogenic stimulation of the esophageal muscle. This observation suggests that the neurogenic change precedes the myogenic; however, if our methods of testing are more sensitive to neurogenic failure, it is still possible that neurogenic and myogenic changes develop simultaneously.

Vascular Theory

These pathologic and pharmacologic studies define the esophageal injury but do not suggest the cause of the changes. One theory holds that all esophageal changes are secondary to vascular spasm and anoxia. This theory is based upon the higher incidence of Raynaud's phenomenon in patients with an adynamic esophagus than in those with collagen disorders but no esophageal motor changes.

If a relationship exists between Raynaud's phenomenon and the esophageal motor disorders of collagen diseases, they could produce secondary myogenic or neurogenic injury.

In scleroderma, motor deterioration is certainly more common in those patients who exhibit Raynaud's phenomenon (4). However, Raynaud's is common in scleroderma, and the higher frequency of motor disorder does not provide conclusive evidence of their association. In collagen disorders where Raynaud's is less common, the association of this phenomenon and motor change is more striking. In one series of patients with collagen disorders, only 6 per cent has the motor disorder in the absence of Raynaud's, whereas when Raynaud's was present, 63 per cent had motor changes. When Raynaud's phenomenon occurs as an isolated disorder, as many as 56 per cent of patients have associated esophageal motor changes (4).

This striking statistical correlation of Raynaud's phenomenon and esophageal motor change in patients with collagen diseases suggests an etiologic relationship. However, the motor disorder can appear without Raynaud's; hence other factors are likely to be involved.

Symptomatology

The incidence of adynamic esophagus is highest in patients with scleroderma and Raynaud's phenomenon, and much lower in those with systemic lupus erythematosus and other collagen diseases: 86 per cent in scleroderma, 60 per cent in Raynaud's, 30 per cent in lupus erythematosus and 20 per cent in other disorders (4). Aperistalsis and esophageal symptoms are not synonymous. In their series, Stevens and associates (4) found that only 18 of 33 patients with an adynamic esophagus had esophageal symptoms; thus, it seems that by itself the loss of motor power does not produce symptoms (3, 12). Some other factor must be necessary. This factor most probably is associated gastroesophageal incompetence and reflux. A hiatal hernia has been reported in from 30 (13) to 50 per cent (14) of patients with scleroderma. Certainly the heartburn and dysphagia described by scleroderma patients are indistinguishable from those encountered in hiatal hernias (9).

The incidence of symptoms varies, but in one series in which 86.9 per cent of patients had radiologic or manometric abnormalities, only 42 per cent had symptoms (12). My own experience gained from evaluating 26 patients with scleroderma is somewhat skewed because some of the patients were referred for surgical management of reflux and in this group 92 per cent had symptoms. In all of these patients, we had demonstrated an adynamic esophagus manometrically and had made the diagnosis of scleroderma on clinical grounds (15).

When studied radiologically and manometrically, 25 of these 26 patients had reflux,

Table 17.1

Symptoms in 26 Patients with Scleroderma Compared with Those in 200 Patients with Hiatal Hernia

Symptoms	Sclero-derma	Hiatal Hernia
	%	%
Heartburn	84	97
Reflux to throat	60	71.5
Night aspiration	20	24
Peptic stricture*	48	10
Gastroesophageal motor dysphagia	20	50
Pharyngoesophageal motor dysphagia	52	51.5
Total dysphagia	84	76.5

* The striking difference between these two groups is that nearly half of the patients with scleroderma developed peptic stricture.

and 21 of the 25 had a radiologic hiatal hernia. Four of the 26 had no esophageal symptoms and 3 of these had a hiatal hernia with radiologic reflux.

I also compared the esophageal symptoms in these 26 patients with those reported by 200 patients with otherwise uncomplicated gastroesophageal reflux (Table 17.1). The symptoms were comparable, except that 48 per cent of the scleroderma patients had peptic stricture, compared with 10 per cent in the gastroesophageal reflux group. This high incidence of peptic stricture attests to the severity of the reflux in scleroderma. When a refluxed bolus enters the esophagus, particularly when the patient is in a recumbent position, esophageal clearance will be greatly delayed through lack of motor propulsion.

This prolonged exposure to the acid and bile salts probably explains the rapid development of severe esophagitis and peptic stricture.

The similarity of complaints in these two groups emphasizes that the symptoms are those of reflux esophagitis. The patient's complaints are the same as those encountered in hiatal hernia and include typical heartburn aggravated by eating and postural change, and relieved by antacids. They also include reflux to the throat and aspiration, burping, waterbrash, nausea and vomiting.

Dysphagia, when present, is disproportionate in its severity to that seen with an uncomplicated hiatal hernia. The tendency to mechanical obstruction is aggravated by the lack of propulsive motor activity, so that even

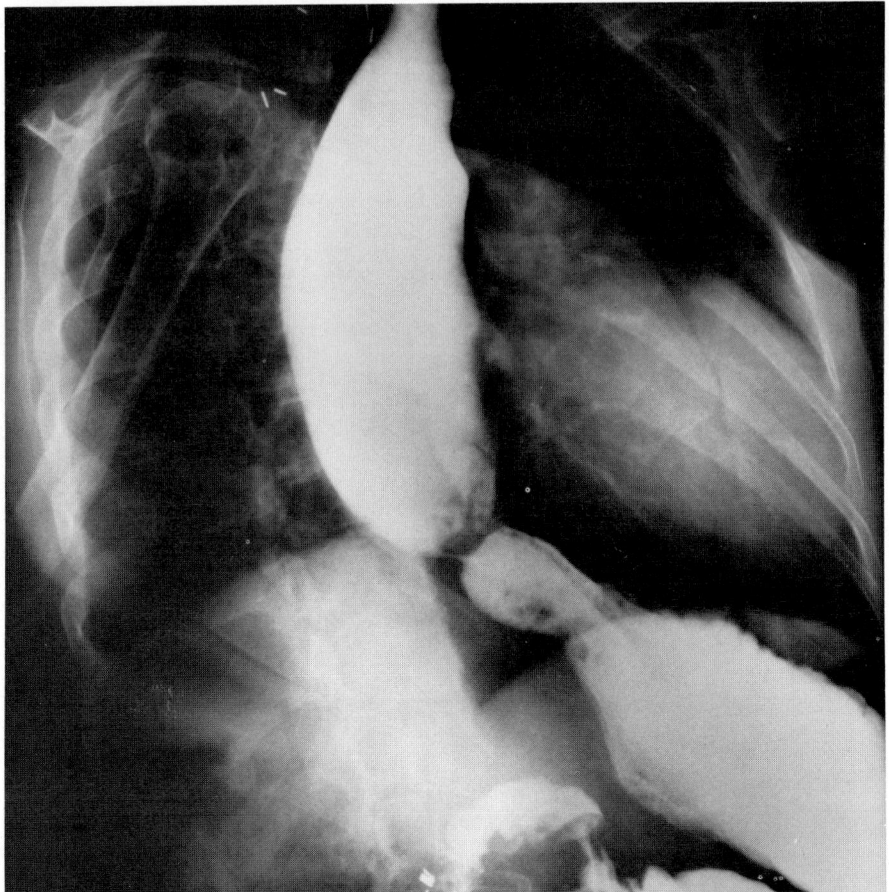

Figure 17.1. Barium Swallow: Patient with Scleroderma, Hiatal Hernia and Peptic Stricture
Radiologic study showed lack of effective peristalsis, a small hiatal hernia and free reflux. The peptic stricture is at the squamocolumnar junction and was indistinguishable endoscopically from a standard peptic stricture.

slight mechanical obstruction may give rise to major dysphagia. As will be shown later, the dysphagia resolves when mechanical obstruction is relieved by bouginage.

Investigation—Radiology

The barium esophagogram is not as accurate as manometry in the diagnosis of an adynamic esophagus. In one series of scleroderma patients, 84 per cent had manometric abnormalities but the radiologic studies were positive in only 70 per cent (12). Despite this limitation the radiologic examination gives more accurate information about other aspects of the disorder than do manometric studies and hence the two are complementary. Radiology detects the presence of a hiatal hernia, gastroesophageal reflux and the possible presence of a stricture (Fig. 17.1). It is also of value in excluding associated malignancy (16–18).

The most characteristic radiologic feature of scleroderma is esophageal atony—that is, loss of effective peristalsis in the lower two-thirds of the organ (13). This observation may be missed in the erect position and hence the patient should be observed prone or head down (19). The examiner will detect prolonged esophageal emptying times and may note slight esophageal dilatation and, associated with this, the presence of an air esophagogram (Fig. 17.2). The air esophagogram has been reported in up to 12.5 per cent on conventional chest x-rays (20, 21).

The other major radiologic feature is the high incidence of hiatal hernia and evidence of reflux and peptic esophagitis. The esophagitis may be severe and show evidence of pebbling (22) from chronic ulceration, or a

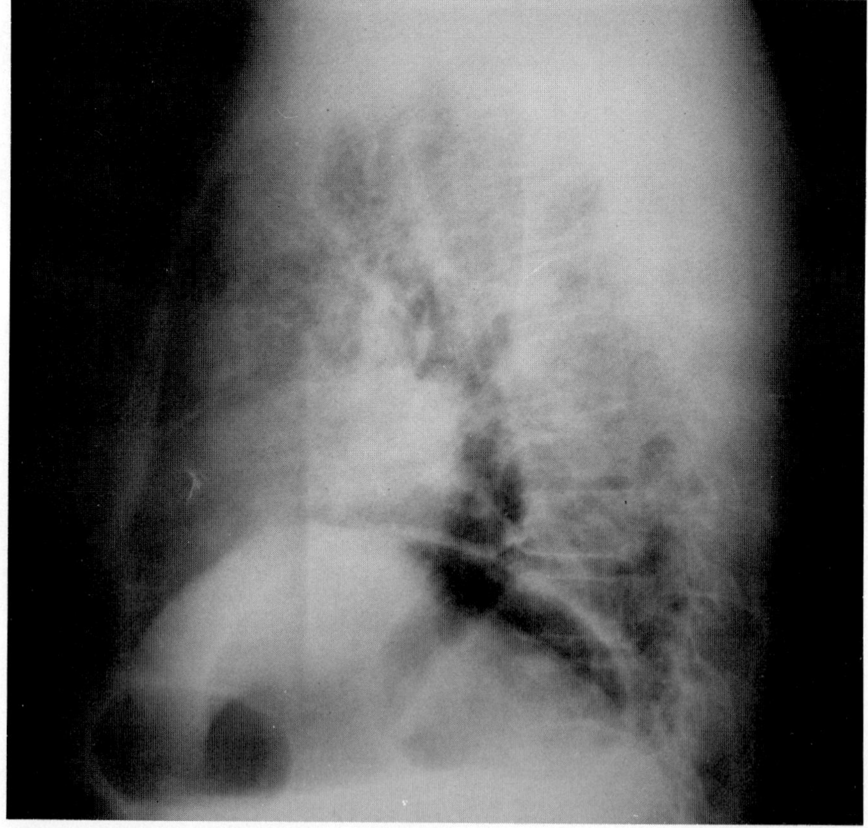

Figure 17.2. Scleroderma—Air Esophagogram
Air in the esophagus has diagnostic value. It appears in a number of disorders, most characteristically in achalasia. In scleroderma its presence indicates severe motor paralysis and the loss of esophageal propulsive force.

peptic stricture. Atypical and often multiple wide-mouthed esophageal diverticula have been reported in association with the sclerodermatous esophagus (23).

Advances in esophageal scintigraphy show delayed emptying of the esophagus. While this is radiologically obvious, scintigraphy allows quantitation of the defect (24).

Manometry

Manometry has proved to be the most accurate diagnostic tool in scleroderma and related disorders. The classic changes consist of a loss or marked diminution of esophageal motor function and severe disordered motor activity in the lower two-thirds of the esophagus, together with a loss of tone in the gastroesophageal junction (25–27). The degrees of motor loss vary and, indeed, in the early stages the examiner may encounter motor hyperactivity similar to that seen in diffuse spasm (14); however, the fully developed motor pattern is unmistakable (Fig. 17.3). Our own experience demonstrates the value of manometry, as the initial diagnosis of sclero-

derma was made at manometry in 13 of 26 patients and confirmed later by clinical evaluation.

The Mecholyl (3) test has been used in the diagnosis of scleroderma, but it does not produce any motor change. This lack of response has some differential diagnostic value because it helps to separate this disorder from achalasia.

The manometric disorder in dermatomyositis (28) has not been clearly delineated. Some workers report motor loss in the proximal (striated muscle) esophagus, and others total motor loss in the proximal and distal esophagus. This suggests that the disease process may involve both striated and smooth muscle.

In earlier studies the investigator did not often perform endoscopy in scleroderma because of the small size of the patients' mouths and technical difficulties attendant upon the safe passage of the esophagoscope. However, the introduction of the flexible esophagoscope has removed this barrier. The most valuable contribution of endoscopy is to assess the stage of esophagitis and detect stric-

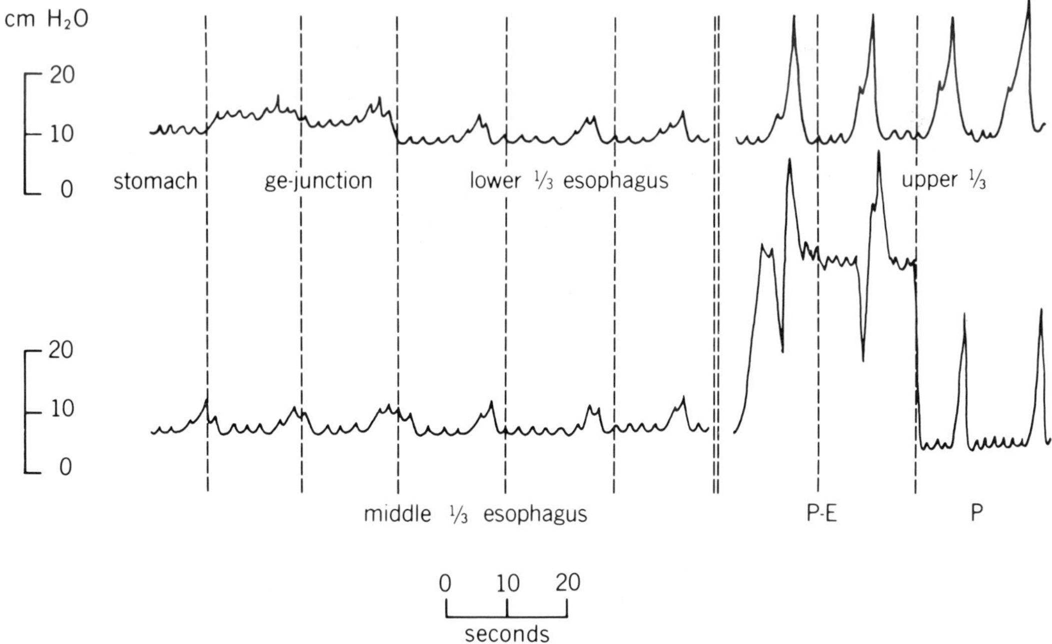

Figure 17.3. Manometric Pattern in Scleroderma
Characteristic motor features of scleroderma and related disorders are a marked reduction in gastroesophageal (ge) tone associated with low amplitude disordered motor activity in the lower two-thirds of the esophagus. In the upper third there is normal peristaltic motor activity. The pharynx (P) and cricopharynx (P-E) are normal.

ture. When encountered, areas of esophagitis should be biopsied to exclude malignancy.

Careful application of these investigative procedures permits an accurate assessment of esophageal damage in scleroderma and related disorders. Following complete evaluation, it is possible to make a rational plan for the management of the patient and his esophageal disease.

Unless he takes a careful history and does a systematic evaluation, even the conscientious physician may overlook the disease in these patients.

Case 1. Mrs. G., age 52, had had symptoms of reflux for 15 years. Three hiatal hernia repairs had failed to relieve her symptoms. When I saw her, this patient did not show any radiologic evidence of a recurrence of the hernia, but her symptoms and the radiologic signs were those of reflux. On manometry she had a typical adynamic esophagus, and only then did we recognize that this unfortunate woman had scleroderma with typical Raynaud's phenomenon and arthritis. Subsequently she underwent gastroplasty, which effectively controlled her reflux, and she remains free of these symptoms 3 years after operation

The esophageal disorder often is only one component of the disease under investigation, but it may be the dominant component. If the patient has advanced peptic esophagitis and stricture, he is in profound distress and this may be compounded by weight loss, aspiration pneumonia and secondary respiratory infection. He deserves careful evaluation and anticipation of these complications, so that through early treatment he can avoid the more extreme manifestations of the esophageal lesion.

References

1. Saladin, T. A., French, A. B., Zarafonetis, C. J., and Pollard, H. M.: Esophageal motor abnormalities in scleroderma and related diseases. Am. J. Dig. Dis., *11:* 522, 1966.
2. Code, C. F.: *An Atlas of Esophageal Motility in Health and Disease.* Charles C Thomas, Springfield, Ill., 1958.
3. Tuffanelli, D. L., and Winkelmann, R. K.: Systemic scleroderma; a clinical study of 727 cases. Arch. Dermatol., *84:* 359, 1961.
4. Stevens, M. B., Hookman, P., Siegel, C. I., Esterly, J. R., Shulman, L. E., and Hendrix, T. R.: Aperistalsis of the esophagus in patients with connective-tissue disorders and Raynaud's phenomenon. N. Engl. J. Med., *270:* 1218, 1964.
5. Krejs, G. J., Lobsiger, M. M., Rau, R., Bron, B. A., Uren, V. B., and Peter, P.: Esophageal function in progressive systemic sclerosis. Acta Hepatogastroenterol., (Stuttg.), *23:* 40, 1976.
6. Ehrmann, S.: Über die Beziehung der Sklerodermie zu den autotoxischen Erythemen. Wien. Med. Wochenschr., *53:* 1097, 1903.
7. Olsen, A. M., O'Leary, P. A., and Kirklin, B. R.: Esophageal lesions associated with acrosclerosis and scleroderma. Arch. Intern. Med., *76:* 189, 1945.
8. Rake, G.: On pathology and pathogenesis of scleroderma. Bull. Johns Hopkins Hosp., *48:* 212, 1931.
9. Treacy, W. L., Baggenstoss, A. H., Slocumb, C. H., and Code, C. F.: Scleroderma of the esophagus; a correlation of histologic and physiologic findings. Ann. Intern. Med., *59:* 351, 1963.
10. Winkelmann, R. K.: Classification and pathogenesis of scleroderma. Proc. Mayo Clin., *46:* 83, 1971.
11. Cohen, S., Fisher, R., Lipshutz, W., Turner, R., Myers, A., and Schumacher, R.: The pathogenesis of esophageal dysfunction in scleroderma and Raynaud's disease. J. Clin. Invest., *51:* 2663, 1972.
12. Bettarello, A., Brito, T., and Zaterka, S.: Progressive systemic sclerosis: II. Esophageal involvement; correlation between bind biopsy of the esophagus, acid drip test and radiology. Am. J. Dig. Dis., *12:* 808, 1967.
13. Fraser, G. M.: The radiological manifestations of scleroderma (diffuse systemic sclerosis). Br. J. Dermatol., *78:* 1, 1966.
14. Garrett, J. M., Winkelmann, R. K., Schlegel, J. F., and Code, C. F.: Esophageal deterioration in scleroderma. Mayo Clin. Proc., *46:* 92, 1971.
15. Henderson, R. D., and Pearson, F. G.: Surgical management of esophageal scleroderma. J. Thorac. Cardiovasc. Surg., *66:* 686, 1973.
16. Matzner, M. J., Trachtman, B., and Mandelbaum, R. A.: Coexistent carcinoma and scleroderma of esophagus. Am. J. Gastroenterol., *39:* 31, 1963.
17. Olsted, W. W., and Madewell, J. E.: The esophageal and small-bowel manifestations of progressive systemic sclerosis. A pathophysiologic explanation of roentgenographic signs. Gastrointest. Radiol., *1:* 33, 1976.
18. Johnson, R. B., and Monroe, L. S.: Carcinoma of the esophagus developing in progressive systemic sclerosis. Gastrointest. Endosc., *19:* 189, 1973.
19. Neschis, M., Siegelman, S. S., Rotstein, J., and Parker, J. G.: The esophagus in progressive systemic sclerosis; a manometric and radiographic correlation. Am. J. Dig. Dis., *15:* 443, 1970.
20. Dinsmore, R. W., Goodman, D., and Dreyfuss, J. R.: The air esophagram; a sign of scleroderma involving the esophagus. Radiology, *87:* 348, 1966.
21. House, A. J., and Griffiths, G. J.: The significance of an air oesophagogram visualized on conventional chest radiographs. Clin. Radiol., *28:* 301, 1977.
22. Clements, J. L., Abernathy, J., and Weens, H. S.: Corrugated mucosal pattern in the esophagus associated with progressive systemic sclerosis. Gastrointest. Radiol., *3:* 119, 1978.
23. Clements, J. L., Abernathy, J., and Weens, H. S.: Atypical esophageal diverticula associated with progressive systemic sclerosis. Gastrointest. Radiol., *3:* 383, 1978.
24. Tolin, R. D., Malmud, L. S., Reilley, J. E., and Fisher, R. S.: Exophageal scintigraphy to quantitate esophageal transit. Gastroenterology, *76:* 1402, 1979.
25. Dornhorst, A. C., Pierce, J. W., and Whimster, I. W.:

Oesophageal lesion in scleroderma. Lancet, *1:* 698, 1954.

26. Creamer, B., Andersen, H. A., and Code, C. F.: Esophageal motility in patients with scleroderma and related diseases. Gastroenterologia (Basel), *86:* 763, 1956.

27. Tatelman, M., and Keech, M. K.: Esophageal motility in systemic lupus erythematosus, rheumatoid arthritis, and scleroderma. Radiology, *86:* 1041, 1966.

28. Dornhorst, A. C., Harrison, K. N., and Pierce, J. W.: Observations on the normal esophagus and cardia. Lancet, *1:* 695, 1954.

CHAPTER 18

Treatment of Scleroderma

The symptoms of scleroderma were described in Chapter 17. A rational approach to therapy begins with the recognition of two features of this symptomatology. Firstly, the physician must recognize that an adynamic esophagus does not necessarily give rise to symptoms. Four of the 26 patients we studied were completely asymptomatic, and if all patients with scleroderma were studied an even higher proportion would be shown to be asymptomatic. Secondly, when the symptoms are present, they are due to gastroesophageal reflux. If these assumptions are correct (and much experience says they are), effective control of reflux should give good symptomatic relief.

Esophageal strictures developed in almost half of the 26 patients we studied—dramatic evidence of the severity of the reflux. These behaved like peptic strictures in that they developed at the squamocolumnar junction and on biopsy showed scar tissue and inflammation. Correction of the stricture by dilatation and control of the reflux have been shown to give effective relief of symptoms.

Medical Management

When a patient with an adynamic esophagus develops symptoms of reflux, he should be treated as early and as vigorously as possible to minimize the risk of stricture formation. Medical management includes strict dietary control and the liberal use of antacids. In this situation, antacids act to neutralize gastric acid and are unlikely to have any effect on sphincter tone. Metoclopramide (1) may be added to speed gastric emptying, but it is doubtful if the stomach and gastroesophageal sphincter respond to any form of drug therapy. Cimetidine should be added to treatment if the other measures fail. This will reduce gastric acidity and is effective in some

patients; however, it is not effective in healing established ulceration or stricture formation. Elevation of the head of the bed is important because in the patient with an adynamic esophagus the secretions tend to pool in the esophagus and increase local injury.

When a stricture does develop, the severity of the mechanical dysphagia is disproportionate to the degree of narrowing. Obstruction to food passage when the subject is erect is a function of the diameter of the esophageal lumen at the point of stricture, the bolus size and the force available to pass the bolus through the stricture (Fig. 18.1). In scleroderma, since there is no motor activity, the only effective propulsive force is gravity, so the bolus more readily impacts at the stricture. This feature is well illustrated by the following case.

Case 1. Mrs. B., age 56, presented with a hiatal hernia, scleroderma and an adynamic esophagus. We saw her early in our experience and performed a partial fundoplication gastroplasty. She was lost to follow-up for 2 years; however, when next seen her indigestion and heartburn had totally resolved but persistent dysphagia was present. Radiographic (Fig. 18.2) and endoscopic studies showed no evidence of stricture, but when a size #60 Fr Malloney bougie was passed, the organ gripped the bougie slightly. This mild degree of stricture was treated with bougienage and her dysphagia resolved completely. We have seen this situation— severe dysphagia in the presence of very mild stricture—on several occasions and in every patient it has responded well to this form of bougienage.

If medical management is to succeed in the presence of stricture it must include adequate (#60 Fr) dilatation as well as reflux control. Neglect or inadequate dilatation of the stricture allows the scar to mature to the point where indirect bougienage is no longer effec-

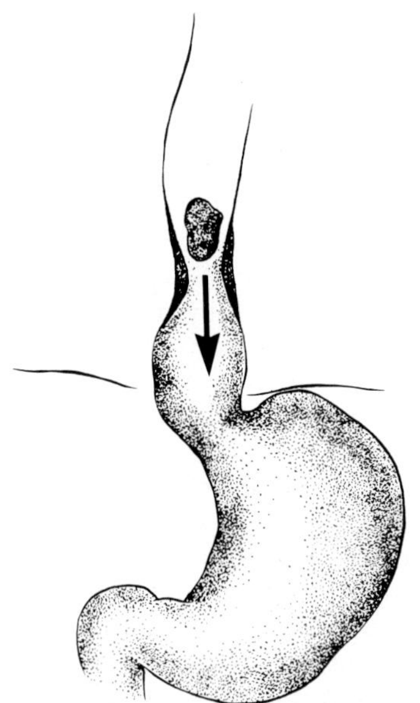

Figure 18.1. Dysphagia in Adynamic Esophagus
Food obstruction occurs early in scleroderma because the esophagus lacks motor power and descent of the bolus depends upon gravity alone. Obstruction will occur early and will develop as soon as bolus size is greater than luminal diameter. Motor power, when it is present, assists the passage of the bolus and delays the development of obstructive symptoms.

because often these patients are severely disabled and corticosteroid therapy may have altered their tissue resistance. Most authors believe that operative management should be reserved for those with major complications of the disease such as hemorrhage (2) or malignancy (3), and many recommend dilatation as the only effective method of control (4–6). However, increasing experience and increasing confidence in the results that can be achieved have persuaded me to recommend surgical repair to patients who do not respond to vigorous conservative management. The scleroderma in patients who are selected for surgery must be of a stable vari-

tive. Since it is difficult for the patient with scleroderma to achieve adequate nutrition at the best of times and since even slight narrowing gives rise to dysphagia, any stricture however slight must be treated carefully and thoroughly.

Most patients treated vigorously can continue on medical management. In a few patients, because they have a stricture that has been neglected or because they do not respond to drugs or diet, the symptoms of reflux progress to the stage where operation provides the only effective therapy.

Management of Severe Stricture

In scleroderma, the stricture may be severe when the patient is first examined, or it may progress despite intensive medical management and repeated bouginage. Finally, the spiral of symptoms may become unmanageable and require surgical intervention. The decision for operation is not made slightly

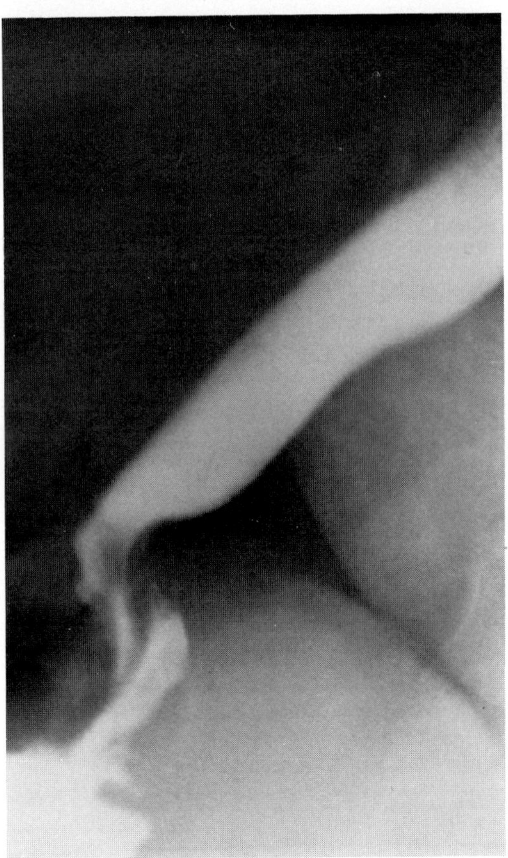

Figure 18.2. Dysphagia following Hiatal Hernia Repair
Mrs. B. (Case 1), who had had a modified Belsey hiatal hernia repair 2 years earlier, had persistent dysphagia. Radiologic study shows no evidence of a stricture, but, following passage of a #60 bougie, she has had total relief of her symptoms.

ety. This can be judged from its duration and the general continued activity of the patient. The presence of gastric, small or large bowel atony carries with it a poorer prognosis and in particular an atonic stomach increases reflux potential and is a contraindication to surgical intervention (7, 8).

Payne (9) approached the sclerodermatous esophagus using a complicated gastric resection and jejunal interposition (Fig. 18.3); other surgeons have used jejunal or colonic interposition without gastric resection (10–14). Standard hiatal hernia repair or the Thal-Nissen procedure has also been advocated (15, 16). All of these series are small and hence it is difficult to assess the long-term results of these surgical approaches.

The replacement procedures noted briefly here have several unsatisfactory features.

1. First, resection and bowel interposition is a major operation even in an other-

wise healthy patient and must impose a tremendous stress on the patient with scleroderma.

2. Second, as it advances, the sclerodermatous process may involve the small or large bowel that was used to replace the diseased esophagus.

3. Finally, if the interposed segments become atonic, they may lose their effectiveness; e.g., even in patients with normal bowel function, colon tortuosity and food retention may pose major problems.

Because of these defects in current procedures, we have oriented our approach to reflux control. Seventeen patients (17, 18) with a manometrically adynamic esophagus were treated surgically. Two of these patients have had a cricopharyngeal myotomy; however, one required reflux control 2 years later. Eleven patients have had a partial fundoplication gastroplasty (PFG) and 6 have had a total fundoplication gastroplasty (TFG). All patients treated surgically had dysphagia as a dominant symptom and 8 had a peptic stricture (Table 18.1).

Cricopharyngeal myotomy was used in two patients with dominant cricopharyngeal dysphagia secondary to reflux. One patient has been well controlled while the other, although free of symptoms for 2 years, then developed severe reflux and was treated by PFG.

Our results with PFG have been satisfactory and others have now reported similar results (18). Five of our patients have continued with reflux symptoms and although substantially improved, they require continued

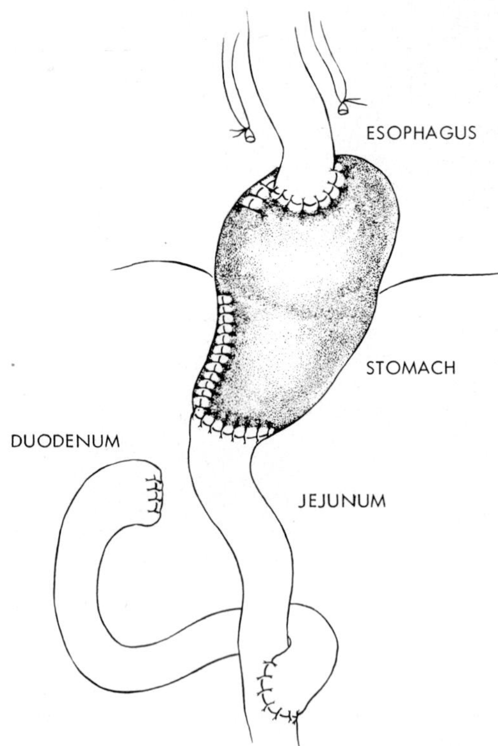

Figure 18.3. Esophageal Resection for Stricture in Scleroderma
Radical resection of the stricture and distal stomach with Roux-en-Y reconstruction has been suggested (9). This operation is a more formidable procedure than gastroplasty.

Table 18.1
Esophageal Symptoms in 17 Patients with Scleroderma Requiring Surgical Control of Reflux*

Heartburn	17	Eructation	8
Pain		Hiccough	1
Epigastric	13	Waterbrash	3
Retrosternal	17	Nausea	8
Precipitating factors		Vomiting	5
tors		Total dysphagia	17
Food	17	Mechanical	8
Posture	13	Motor	9
Reflux	12		
Aspiration	3		

* The symptoms in these 17 patients are similar to those encountered in patients with reflux; however, all patients had dysphagia as a significant problem.

medical management and 3 require intermittent bougienage. One of the patients, treated by PFG died from complications of aspergillosis unrelated to the operation. One patient has required conversion to a TFG because of severe reflux (Table 18.2).

Six patients have been treated by TFG. Five of these are now asymptomatic and eating normally. One had excellent relief for 3 years; however, she now has gastric and colonic atony, has redeveloped dysphagia and is physically deteriorating as a result of progression of her scleroderma.

Table 18.2
Results of Gastroplasty in Patients with Scleroderma*

	Excellent	Good	Poor
Partial fundoplication	5	4	2
Total fundoplication	5	1	0

* Using partial fundoplication, although most patients were improved, reflux was still present in 6 of 11 patients. With total fundoplication reflux was completely controlled.

TFG must be done with great care and the length of total fundoplication tailored to avoid overcompetence and dysphagia (Fig. 18.4). The gastroplasty tube is prepared in the usual fashion, cut 5 cm long over a #60 Fr bougie. Fundus of stomach is now approximated to the gastroplasty tube with interrupted sutures. Total fundoplication is restricted to 0.5 to 1 cm in length. Using this reduced length, reflux control can be achieved and dysphagia avoided. All of these patients retain the ability to eructate, and none have had difficulty with vomiting.

Case 2. Mrs. A., age 48, had disseminated lupus erythematosus, and developed severe heartburn and stricture formation. She had been treated earlier by medical management and bouginage. On one occasion her esophagus had been perforated, but this complication had been managed conservatively. At the time of initial consultation she had been in hospital for 9 weeks on vigorous conservative therapy but had continued to lose weight (25 pounds). She had had a myocardial infarction 1 year before and was known to have impaired renal function. Manometry and radio-

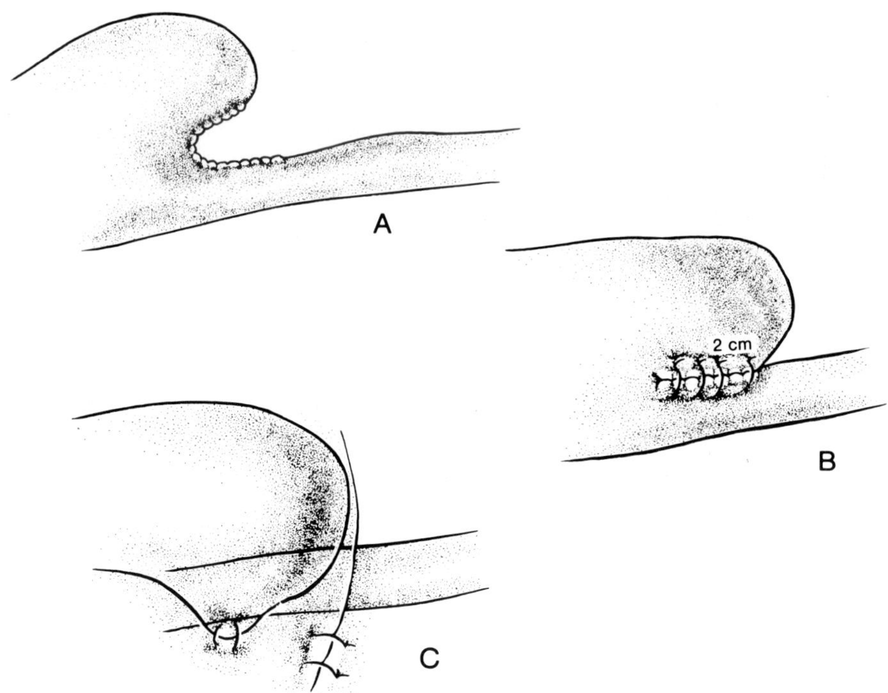

Figure 18.4. Modified Total Fundoplication Gastroplasty in Patients with Scleroderma
Total fundoplication gastroplasty is modified in patients with scleroderma. The gastroplasty tube is unchanged and fundus is sewn to gastroplasty tube plus distal 2 cm of esophagus. Completed fundoplication is reduced to ½ to 1 cm.

logic studies (Fig. 18.5) confirmed that she had an adynamic esophagus and an undilatable stricture. At operation the stricture was dilated through a gastrotomy with Hegar dilators and a gastroplasy

was done to control reflux. Now, 1 year after operation, she is eating a normal diet and has no residual dysphagia or heartburn (Fig. 18.6).

Case 3. Ten years earlier, Mrs. J., age 44, had had a vagotomy, pyloroplasty and transabdominal hernia repair for symptoms of severe reflux. Her symptoms improved temporarily. During this period the diagnosis of scleroderma had been made. Her reflux symptoms had returned and for the past 8 years had remained severe. Mrs. J. had severe heartburn with each meal and recognizable

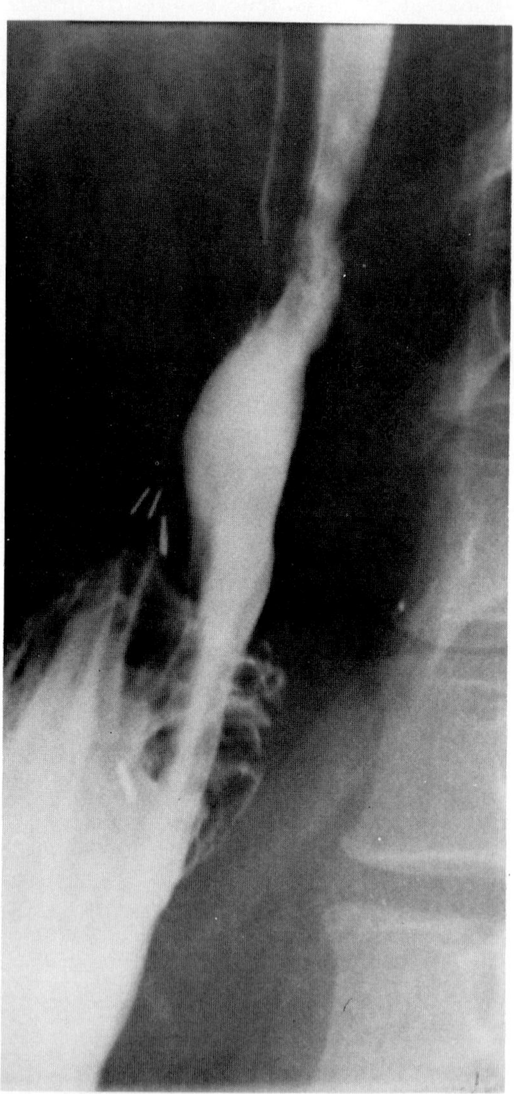

Figure 18.5. Barium Swallow in Scleroderma and Peptic Stricture
Mrs. A. (Case 2) had an adynamic esophagus that was demonstrated radiologically and manometrically. She had a severe peptic stricture and during a previous dilatation had sustained a local perforation. Clinical, radiological and endoscopic evolution showed severe reflux.

Figure 18.6. Barium Swallow following Gastroplasty
Mrs. A. (Case 2) postoperatively. This film shows an adequately dilated esophagus. The hernia was repaired around a gastroplasty tube and the patient had no residual clinical or radiologic reflux.

reflux to the throat. Most nights she aspirated gastric contents despite adequate bed elevation. In addition, she had had recurrent episodes of respiratory infection. Her dysphagia was extremely severe and she could swallow only liquids and foods of soft consistency such as custard. In the previous year she had lost 10 pounds and over the preceding 6 years her body weight had gradually declined from 130 to her present 95 pounds. Her previous program of medical management, which was judged to be adequate, included liberal antacids and intermittent bouginage to #40 Fr.

Manometric studies confirmed the presence of an adynamic esophagus. On radiologic examination she had evidence of an adynamic esophagus and a peptic stricture at the gastroesophageal junction. Endoscopy showed severe ulcerative esophagitis and confirmed the presence of the peptic stricture. Dilatation was attempted, but the stricture could be enlarged only to #50 Fr and, despite this enlargement, her dysphagia, although improved, remained severe.

At operation the stricture was dilated from below through a gastrotomy using Hegar dilators, and her reflux was controlled by a gastroplasty and a modified Belsey hernia repair. Her postoperative recovery was uneventful and she developed no complications. On two occasions within 3 months of operation, she required indirect dilatation with Malloney bougies, but since then has required no further therapy. Two years after operative repair she is free of symptoms and eats a normal diet.

Although the results of PFG have been satisfactory, reflux is present in many of these patients and for this reason a modified TFG with very short fundoplication is now considered the procedure of choice.

Case 4. Mrs. N., age 46, had slowly progressive scleroderma for 15 years. For 5 years dysphagia was a dominant symptom and she was able to take only very carefully chewed solids and drink liquids to wash the solids into her stomach (Fig. 18.7). Manometrically she had an adynamic esophagus and radiologically a tight, short stricture was present at the gastroesopageal junction.

Initial dilatation gave significant relief to her dysphagia; however, the stricture recurred. Total fundoplication gastroplasty has given complete symptomatic relief and 2 years following surgery she eats a normal diet (Fig. 18.8).

Case 5. Mrs. St.M., age 52, has had reflux symptoms for 10 years. She was treated by transabdominal hiatal hernia repair 7 years ago. Although her reflux symptoms were mostly controlled she had persistent severe cricopharyngeal dysphagia.

Although radiologically and endoscopically she

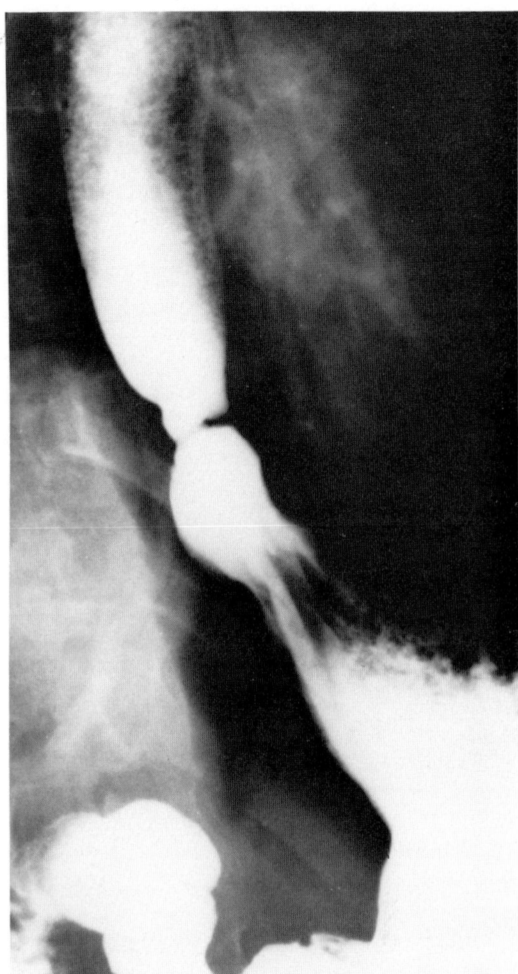

Figure 18.7
Mrs. N. (Case 4) has long standing scleroderma with reflux and a peptic stricture. The barium swallow shows a tight stricture with poor esophageal emptying.

has a recurrent hiatal hernia, her dominant symptom was cricopharyngeal dysphagia and aspiration while eating. Rather than repairing her hernia she has had a cricopharyngeal myotomy under local anesthesia with good relief of her dysphagia. Although rarely indicated, in the presence of reflux, when cricopharyngeal dysphagia is the dominant symptom this approach can be effective. The cricopharyngeal dysphagia is caused by motor incoordination and is secondary to reflux. Since the cricopharyngeus is striated muscle, it is unlikely to be involved by scleroderma.

These patients illustrate the problems encountered in advanced scleroderma. Many of those treated surgically are in lower risk categories and usually tolerate surgery well, but

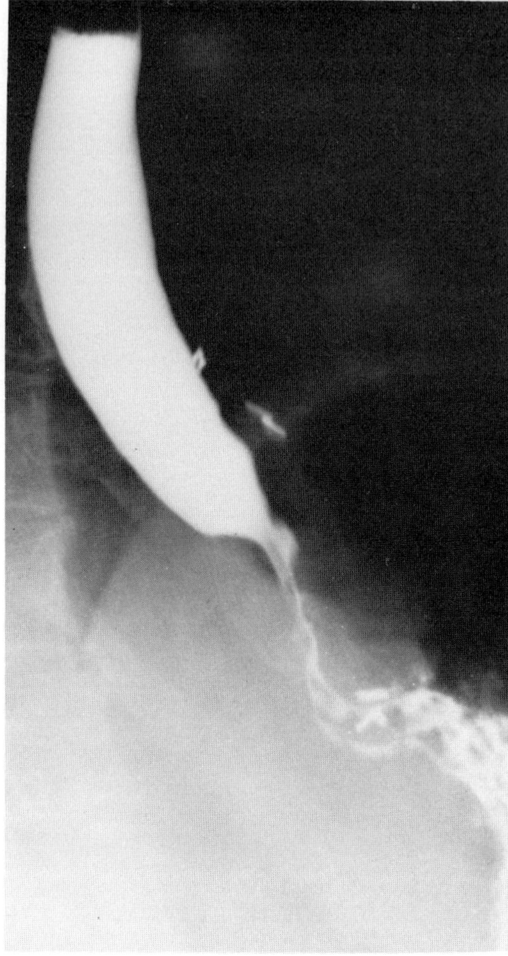

Figure 18.8
Mrs. N. was treated by dilatation, gastroplasty and shortened Nissen fundoplication. The barium swallow shows no residual obstruction. She eats a normal diet.

our experience with patients such as these demonstrate that even those with advanced disease can be salvaged and restored to excellent swallowing function. In terms of its stress, gastroplasty in the scleroderma patient is comparable to a standard hiatal hernia repair and is more likely to be tolerated than resection and bowel interposition. With effective control of reflux the stricture eventually resolves satisfactorily.

Medical management is undoubtedly the treatment of choice in the reflux esophagitis associated with scleroderma and similar collagen diseases. This program should be pursued vigorously and may include bouginage of associated strictures. If medical measures fail, an operation aimed at the correction of reflux and adequate stricture dilatation can give lasting relief of symptoms.

References

1. Stanciu, C., and Bennett, J. R.: Metoclopramide in gastroesophageal reflux. Gut, *14:* 275, 1973.
2. Berliner, S. D., and Burson, L.: Esophageal hemorrhage in scleroderma. Am. J. Gastroenterol., *46:* 477, 1966.
3. Matzner, M. J., Trachtman, B., and Mandelbaum, R. A.: Coexistent carcinoma and scleroderma of esophagus. Am. J. Gastroenterol., *39:* 31, 1963.
4. Olsen, A. M., O'Leary, P. A., and Kirklin, B. R.: Esophageal lesions associated with acrosclerosis and scleroderma. Arch. Intern. Med., *76:* 189, 1945.
5. Bockus, H. L.: *Gastroenterology*, ed. 2. W. B. Saunders Co., Philadelphia, 1963.
6. D'Abreu, A. L.: *Clinical Surgery of the Thorax.* Butterworths, London, 1965.
7. Winkelmann, R. K.: Classification and pathogenesis of scleroderma. Mayo Clin. Proc., *46:* 83, 1971.
8. Azouz, E. M., and Lapointe, A.: The roentgen spectrum of progressive systemic sclerosis. Mod. Med. Can., *31:* 23, 1976.
9. Payne, W. S.: Surgical treatment of reflux esophagitis and stricture associated with permanent incompetence of the cardia. Mayo Clin. Proc., *45:* 553, 1970.
10. Perdue, G. D., and Morris, A. J.: Surgical manifestations of scleroderma. Surg. Gynecol. Obstet., *115:* 745, 1962.
11. Merendino, K. A., and Thomas, G. I.: The jejunal interposition operation for substitution of the esophagogastric sphincter; present status. Surgery, *44:* 1112, 1958.
12. Akiyama, H., Kogure, T., and Itai, Y.: Esophageal reconstruction for stenosis due to diffuse scleroderma. Utilizing blunt dissection of esophagus. Arch. Surg., *107:* 470, 1973.
13. Hochman, R. B.: Neuromotor disorders of the esophagus. Primary Care, *3:* 41, 1976.
14. Brindley, G. C., Jr.: Surgical management of strictures of the lower thoracic esophagus. Am. Surg., *41:* 94, 1975.
15. O'Leary, J. P., Hollenbeck, J. I., and Woodward, E. R.: Surgical treatment of esophageal stricture in patients with scleroderma. Am. Surg., *41:* 131, 1975.
16. Langdon, D. E., and Lindberg, E. F.: Scleroderma and esophageal hiatal hernioplasty. Minn. Med., *56:* 643, 1973.
17. Henderson, R. D., and Pearson, F. G.: Surgical management of esophageal scleroderma. J. Thorac. Cardiovasc. Surg., *66:* 686, 1973.
18. Orringer, M. B., Dabich, L., Zarafonetis, C. J., and Sloan, H.: Gastroesophageal reflux in esophageal scleroderma; diagnosis and implications. Ann. Thorac. Surg., *295:* 120, 1976.

The Pharyngoesophageal Junction

CHAPTER 19

Disorders of the Pharyngoesophageal Junction

The term pharyngoesophageal (PE) junction is used to describe the pharynx, cricopharynx and the upper third of the esophagus. It is desirable to consider disorders of these organs together because disease in any one area tends to express itself in common symptoms and, in addition, many disorders involve the pharyngoesophageal junction as a unit. The symptoms are similar because diseases of the junctional area present most often with dysphagia due to a reduction in the amplitude of pharyngeal motor waves, to an elevation in tone or failure of relaxation in the cricopharynx, to disordered motor activity in the upper esophagus, or to motor incoordination. The tendency for diseases to involve the entire pharyngoesophageal junction is related to its common muscular composition, because this zone, unlike the lower esophagus, consists of striated muscle and, as such, is subject to myogenic and neurogenic disorders of a type not seen in smooth muscle organs.

Classification of Pharyngoesophageal Disorders

Pharyngoesophageal motor problems can be classified in a manner similar to that used in the lower esophagus. By far the most frequent cause of pharyngoesophageal symptoms is hiatal hernia, which is present in at least 90 per cent of all patients seen with symptoms localized to the upper esophagus. This disorder may be regarded as secondary, because it appears to be related directly to the injury produced by pharyngoesophageal reflux (Table 19.1).

Primary disorders, although much rarer, represent a large number of interesting neurogenic and myogenic problems, including myotonia as a pure myogenic disorder, myasthenia gravis as a disorder of the myoneural junction, and a group of central and peripheral neurogenic diseases.

Some of the pharyngoesophageal disorders are of unknown etiology and these include cricopharyngeal bars and cricopharyngeal diverticula. Although muscular incoordination has been recognized in these disorders, the cause of this is undetermined.

When faced with a diagnostic decision involving the pharyngoesophageal junction the physician must remember to exclude mechanical forms of obstruction. Carcinoma must always be considered, and, in addition, various webs and bony prominences should be carefully searched for and excluded.

Psychogenic disorders should also be included in the differential diagnosis. Globus hystericus is well recognized as a psychogenic form of food obstruction, but this diagnosis can be made only after exclusion of the various motor and mechanical problems.

These various pharyngoesophageal problems have certain symptoms in common and an understanding of these general symptoms gives the clues necessary to plan further investigation.

General Symptoms

Pain associated with pharyngoesophageal disorders is usually mild. It is present in disorders associated with motor spasm and is characteristic of a cricopharyngeal bar or of the secondary motor disturbance of hiatal hernia. The discomfort is nonspecific, is often described as a lump in the throat or a collar-like tightness around the neck, and occasionally is referred to the jaws and ears. The pain may be intermittent, but often persists as a

Table 19.1
Disorders of Pharyngoesophageal Junction*

I. Motor Disorders
  1. Primary
    A. Myogenic
      a. Myotonia
      b. Thyrotoxic
    B. Neurogenic
      a. Congenital: Riley-Day syndrome
      b. Acquired central:
        (1) Strokes
        (2) Bulbar poliomyelitis
      c. Acquired peripheral:
        (1) Recurrent laryngeal
        (2) Nerve injury or neuritis
    C. Myoneurogenic: myasthenia gravis
  2. Secondary
    A. Endogenous: gastroesophageal reflux
    B. Exogenous: lye burn
  3. Secondary—reflux associated
    A. Cricopharyngeal bar
    B. Cricopharyngeal diverticulum
II. Non-Motor Disorders
  1. Mechanical
    A. Carcinoma
    B. Stricture
    C. Bony spur
  2. Psychogenic: Globus hystericus

* Primary disorders are related to myogenic, neurogenic or myoneurogenic disease. Secondary disorders are related to injury, either from the refluxed bolus or from an exogenous source such as ingested lye. The disorders (#3) associated with reflux are specific problems which have investigative findings suggesting an etiology in common with the cricopharyngeal dysphagia on gastroesophageal reflux.

constant discomfort over long periods. When present as a constant discomfort, it can give rise to much distress. The pain is not always associated with dysphagia and occasionally swallowing gives some relief.

Dysphagia, the most common symptom, has several characteristics which merit emphasis. Obstruction may occur with either liquids or solids, but more commonly with both. This obstruction is recognized within 1 second of swallowing and the patient can localize it to the cricopharynx. Coughing and choking are due to forward spillage of the food bolus to the larynx. These symptoms may be present in almost any pharyngoesophageal obstruction. The regurgitation of food through the nose, which indicates more extensive muscular weakness, occurs almost

exclusively in patients with primary neurogenic or myogenic disorders (Fig. 19.1).

Other systemic symptoms should be carefully elucidated because they may help to characterize the disease process. Often this correlation of the pharyngoesophageal disorder with the patient's other symptoms, such as gastroesophageal reflux or symptoms of generalized neurologic and myogenic disease, is most helpful in establishing the diagnosis.

Secondary Motor Disorders— Gastroesophageal Reflux

Pharyngoesophageal dysphagia is common in patients with a gastroesophageal reflux (1–3), but despite the frequency of its occurrence the etiologic mechanism has not been established. Indeed debate continues as to whether

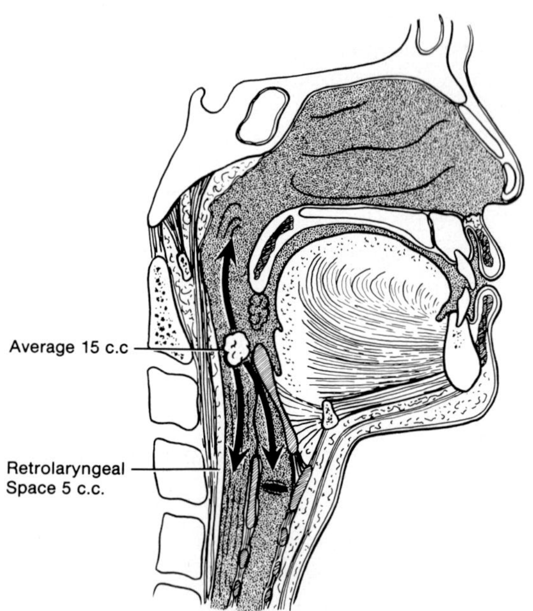

Figure 19.1. Cricopharyngeal Dysphagia
This patient, who has phryngoesophageal dysphgia due to a neurologic abnormality, has associated weakness of the soft palate and hence poor control of the food bolus as it descends through the pharynx. Thus food may spill forward into the trachea or may pass into the nasopharynx and be regurgitated through the nose. When the bolus is halted by an obstruction, in patients with normal pharyngeal and nasopharyngeal motor power, it can spill forward to the larynx, but only rarely will it go up through the nasopharynx.

food truly obstructs at the pharyngoesophageal level, or whether the obstruction occurs distally in the esophagus and only the discomfort is referred to the neck. In disorders such as peptic stricture or achalasia, where obstruction is known to be in the distal esophagus, the sensation of food sticking may be referred proximally to the pharyngoesophageal junction. Proximal referral may also occur in patients with a gastroesophageal reflux and motor obstruction; however, it can clearly be shown that some of these patients have true pharyngoesophageal motor obstruction. Coughing and choking associated with pharyngoesophageal obstruction indicate a high-level obstruction with forward spillage of the food bolus to the larynx. It can be shown experimentally that when food obstruction distends the midesophagus, the cricopharyngeus develops secondary spasm. This phenomenon may account for the reference of obstructive symptoms to the cricopharynx and may even account for some patients developing actual cricopharyngeal obstruction secondary to distal esophageal disease.

A simple confirmatory test can be used to document the level of obstruction. The patient is given a solid bolus to swallow (a 1-cm marshmallow) and the time is measured from swallowing to food obstruction. The patient indicates the exact time of swallowing and the location of obstruction, and allows timing of obstruction by pointing with his finger. If obstruction occurs within 1 second of swallowing, the block is at the pharyngoesophageal level, whereas if obstruction is recognized in 4 to 8 seconds, it is in the distal esophagus. Occasionally, when food obstructs 4 to 8 seconds after a swallow, patients point to the pharyngoesophageal junction and this is taken to indicate distal obstruction with proximal reference of the symptom.

Pharyngoesophageal obstruction was confirmed by timing a marshmallow bolus in 50 patients with gastroesophageal reflux (4,5). Thirteen had no obstruction; 20 localized the obstruction to the pharyngoesophageal junction within 1 to 2 seconds of the swallow; 10 localized it to the gastroesophageal junction after 4 to 6 seconds; 7 had combined pharyngoesophageal and gastroesophageal obstruction at 1 to 2 and then at 4 to 5 seconds. One patient reported gastroesophageal junctional

obstruction at 4 seconds, then at 6 seconds he described the sensation of obstruction at the cricopharynx. In all the patients except this last, the localization and timing of obstruction corresponded and indicated that the obstruction produced the symptoms and that the patient accurately identified the site.

The pathogenesis of the pharyngoesophageal dysphagia accompanying gastroesophageal reflux is obscure, but probably the refluxed bolus pools in the upper esophagus when it reaches the cricopharyngeal sphincter. Here the gastric juice irritates the esophagus, and the inflammation so produced induces motor changes and dysphagia. The process is most likely to occur at night when the patient is horizontal, and this may account for the frequent symptomatic improvement following bed elevation. This hypothesis is partly supported by the occasional finding of proximal esophageal inflammation at endoscopy. An alternate explanation which may well account for symptoms in some patients is reflex cricopharyngeal spasm secondary to distal obstruction.

Motor changes have been described, but these remain controversial. Using a nonperfused manometric catheter system, Hunt and colleagues (6) described elevations in the cricopharyngeal pressures, and more recently Watson and Sullivan (7) confirmed these findings using perfused catheters in patients with "globus." Winans (8) has shown that pharyngoesophageal pressures may vary with the position of the motility catheters in relationship to the cricopharyngeus. This and similar observations raise doubts concerning the validity of described pressure variations.

Because up to the present no one has clearly delineated the mechanism responsible for pharyngoesophageal dysphagia, we carried out an extensive analysis of the pharyngoesophageal junction in a series of patients with gastroesophageal reflux. We analyzed manometric tracings made in 52 patients with gastroesophageal reflux and 10 normal subjects (4) using high-speed recording techniques (1 cm per second paper speed). Analysis was performed only on those patients in whom a complete cricopharyngeal and pharyngeal study was obtained. (With practice it is possible to obtain a satisfactory tracing in the majority of patients.) Figure 19.2 shows the individual components of the pharyngeal and cricopharyngeal motor waves. The amplitude, velocity and duration were measured for the pharyngeal motor wave (P_2), the preceding low amplitude wave (P_1) and the basal pharyngeal pressure (P). Cricopharyngeal pressure (PE) was measured and we noted the presence of a small preceding contraction (ΔPE), the relaxation of the cricopharynx (R) and its contraction phase (C_1). We also measured cricopharyngeal contraction and the duration of its elevation above basal pressure (C_2).

This analysis demonstrated only one significant difference between the normal subjects and the patients with a gastroesophageal reflux. Some of the refluxing patients (20 of 52) showed incoordination (Fig. 19.3), and the pharyngeal motor wave (P_2) was seen to arrive at the cricopharynx (PE) during the period when cricopharyngeal pressure was elevated above baseline (C_2). The normal subjects did not exhibit this abnormality, which we considered represented muscular incoordination. Since the pharyngeal motor wave was normal in amplitude, duration and velocity, this motor change probably represents premature contraction of the cricopharynx.

Following completion of our analysis, the findings were compared with the patient's history to determine whether the presence or absence of incoordination could be correlated with historic evidence of dysphagia, coughing and choking. Seven of the 20 patients with incoordination had major pharyngoesophageal dysphagia (occurring with every meal); 7 had minor dysphagia (occurring less frequently) and 6 had no dysphagia. None of the 32 patients with normal coordination had major dysphagia, 8 had minor dysphagia and 24 had no dysphagia. Nine of the 20 with

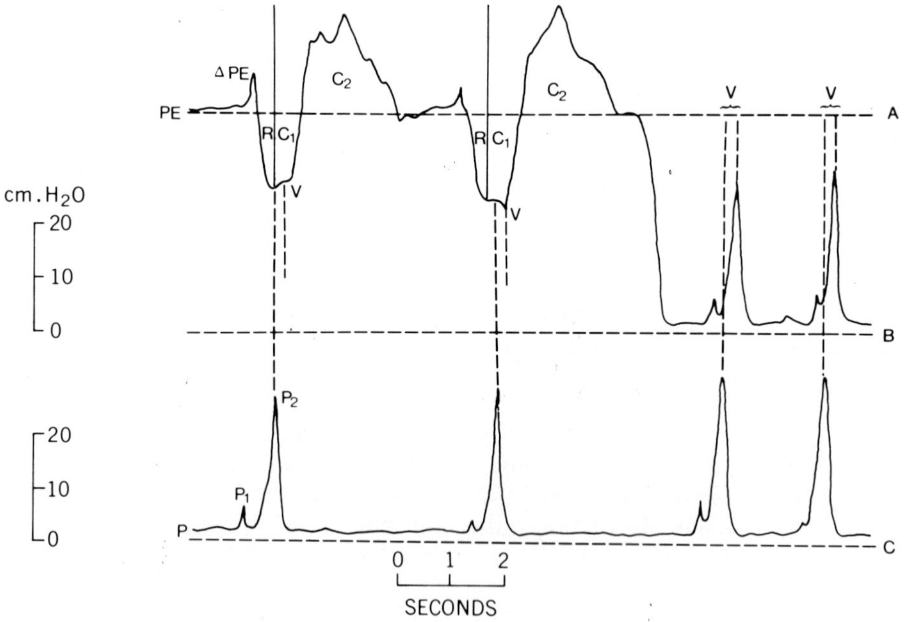

Figure 19.2. Coordinate Pharyngoesophageal Junction
Lines B and C are atmospheric pressure and line A is the average cricopharyngeal pressure. PE is cricopharyngeal pressure. ΔPE is a small preceding contraction wave. R is relaxation from basal PE pressure. C_1 is the contraction back to PE pressure and C_2 is contraction above basal pressure. P is pharyngeal pressure above atmospheric pressure in line C. P_1 is a small preceding pharyngeal motor wave and P_2 is the main pharyngeal motor wave. V is the time interval between motor waves recorded 2.5 cm apart by separate pressure catheters. In this study cricopharyngeal pressure is normal, and cricopharyngeal relaxation and contraction are also normal. The pharyngeal motor wave P_2 coordinates with cricopharyngeal relaxation. This tracing, in which motor function is normally coordinated, should be contrasted with tracings from the incoordinate esophagus (Fig. 19.3).

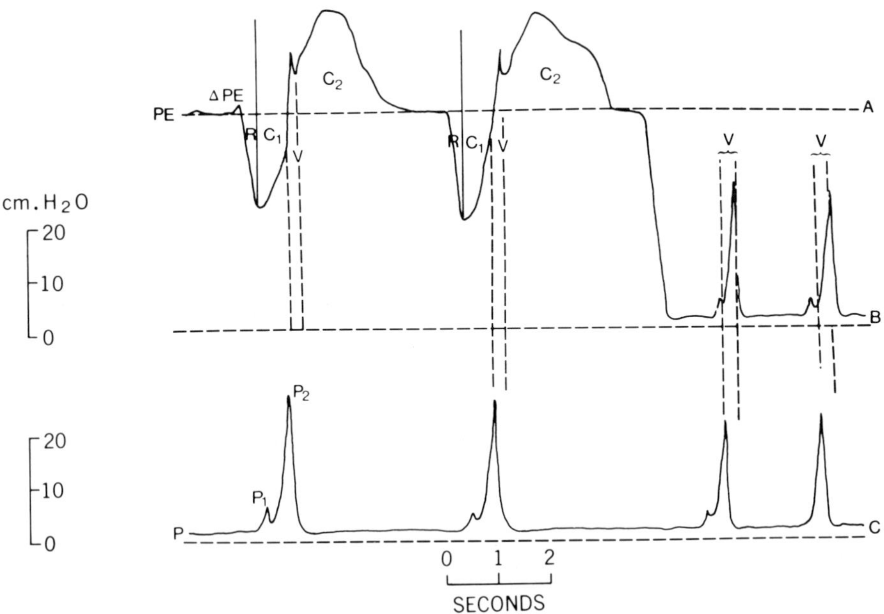

Figure 19.3. Uncoordinate Pharyngoesophageal Junction
Symbols used in this figure are the same as in Figure 19.2. Here the pharyngeal motor wave produces a peak of pressure which coordinates with the contraction phase of cricopharyngeus (C_2). The incoordination seen in this figure appears to be due to premature contraction (C_1) in the cricopharynx.

incoordination had a history of coughing and choking with swallowing, and only 2 of 32 with normal coordination gave this history.

This correlation between symptoms and incoordination was supported further by a study of 10 asymptomatic volunteers. None of these had symptoms of reflux or dysphagia, and all had normal pharyngeal and cricopharyngeal coordination. These observations in the asymptomatic volunteers and in those with gastroesophageal reflux are contrary to the findings of Hunt and colleagues (6) and of Watson and Sullivan (7). This incoordination in the presence of a normal tone in the cricopharyngeus is identical to the abnormality Ellis and colleagues (9) described in patients with a cricopharyngeal diverticulum and points to a possible common etiology.

Medical Management of Pharyngoesophageal Dysphagia and Gastroesophageal Reflux

For most patients, pharyngoesophgeal dysphagia is only one of their symptoms, but it will respond with the others to diet, bed elevation, the liberal use of antacids and,

when necessary, to metachlopremide and cimetidine. Occasionally this symptom is severe and does not respond, despite improvement in the patient's general symptoms. The most important single element in treatment appears to be bed elevation, and this suggests that reflux, proximal pooling of the reflux and upper esophageal irritation are the chief agents in the etiology of pharyngoesophageal dysphagia.

Case 1. Mr. B., age 45, had had severe pharyngoesophageal dysphagia for 6 years. His physician had noted a small hiatal hernia, but had disregarded this because of the severity and dominance of the pharyngoesophageal symptoms. One year of psychiatric care had not altered his symptoms. After referral, the consultant added to his management only elevation of the head of his bed; with this he had complete remission of his symptoms.

Most patients present with the whole spectrum of reflux symptoms, and pharyngoesophageal dysphagia is one symptom of varying intensity. General medical management gives satisfactory control of these symptoms but does not necessarily stop all reflux. Persistence of minor pharyngoesophageal symptoms may be due to some continuance of reflux. Surgical correction of reflux is aimed at the total correction of reflux, and for this reason studies of surgical patients give a better indication of the responsiveness of pharyngoesophageal symptoms to reflux control.

Pharyngoesophageal Dysphagia and Surgical Correction of Reflux

Henderson and colleagues (4) have now completed a further study which allows the evaluation of the effects of surgical correction of reflux on the symptom of pharyngoesophageal dysphagia. In this study, 200 consecutive patients with symptomatic reflux were evaluated by history (Table 19.2), radiology, endoscopy and manometry. Because medical management failed to control their symptoms, the reflux was corrected surgically in all, and each patient has been followed for 9 to 30 months. Before operation they had a characteristic distribution of symptoms. Fifty per cent (100 patients) had pharyngoesophageal dysphagia that varied in severity from mild and intermittent (minor dysphagia) to that which appeared with each meal (major dysphagia). The symptoms in 20 of the 100 patients were classified as major, and those in 80 were classified as minor because of their intermittency.

Since the correction of reflux, all of these

Table 19.2
Symptoms in 200 Patients with Reflux*

Symptom	Occurrence
Heartburn	99.5
Reflux	87
Aspiration	31.5
Nausea and vomiting	79
Dysphagia total	79.5
Mechanical	6
Gastroesophageal motor	67.5
Pharyngoesophageal motor	50
Pharyngoesophageal plus aspiration	23

* Half of these 200 patients had pharyngoesophageal motor dysphagia and almost half of these (46) had the coughing and choking characteristic of aspiration. When those with pharyngoesophageal dysphagia and those without were compared, no significant difference was noted in the frequency of reflux symptoms.

patients have been followed clinically and their symptoms have been evaluated. During follow-up, of the 100 patients who did not have pharyngoesophageal dysphagia originally, 9 developed minor degrees of dysphagia—food sticking less than once per day. This symptom was so mild that it could not have been recognized except during direct questioning. Of the 100 with pharyngoesophageal dysphagia before operation, 10 had residual dysphagia; in 8, this was very mild and was similar to those symptoms already described in the patients without preoperative dysphagia. In 2 other patients major pharyngoesophageal dysphagia persisted with coughing and choking on aspiration. Both these patients had major symptoms before operation, suggesting that approximately 10 per cent of those with major pharyngoesophageal dysphagia will not respond to operative correction of reflux.

In a total experience of 490 hiatal hernia repairs, 9 patients (1.8 per cent), including the 2 mentioned previously, had major pharyngoesophageal dysphagia that failed to respond to surgical correction. Eight of the 9 have now had a cricopharyngeal myotomy, which was performed at least 6 months after the hernia repair; all have had satisfactory relief of their dysphagia and none have symptoms suggesting aspiration of food.

This and similar experience is important, because it demonstrates the necessity of recognizing pharyngoesophageal dysphagia. Before operation I now advise patients with severe symptoms that their pharyngoesophageal dysphagia may not be corrected by reflux control, and that the additional minor procedure of cricopharyngeal myotomy will be necessary if this symptom persists.

Case 2. Dr. E., a 55-year-old physician, had had typical heartburn and associated major pharyngoesophageal dysphagia for 20 years. On radiologic examination he had a small hiatal hernia with demonstrable reflux. At endoscopy there was no evidence of esophageal ulceration, but manometry showed a mild associated motor abnormality. As conservative management did not control his symptoms, he was submitted to a transthoracic Belsey repair. His other symptoms were much improved, but the pharyngoesophgeal dysphagia remained as severe as before.

This man was one of the first patients we had investigated with this disorder; hence, it was difficult to determine why the repair failed to correct his pharyngoesophageal dysphagia. Three years after the Belsey repair, he underwent a pharyngoesophageal myotomy and was rewarded by an immediate improvement in his swallowing. Before the myotomy he required 1 hour to eat his meal, and had great difficulty if he attempted to eat and carry on a conversation simultaneously. Any distraction produced spasms of coughing and choking. At the time of writing (3 years after myotomy) he eats normally without any trace of dysphagia.

The dysphagia which these patients describe can be extremely severe as the following case will illustrate.

Case 3. Mrs. H. had had pharyngoesophageal dysphagia with associated coughing and choking of aspiration for 17 years (5). Both solids and liquids became obstructed with almost every meal. Her fear of choking was so great that she could not eat in company and could not eat even with her own family. Any distraction during eating produced obstruction and aspiration. She had mild symptoms of heartburn and occasionally had recognizable reflux to the throat. Radiologically, manometrically, and endoscopically she had a hiatal hernia. Conservative management of her hernia had not altered her symptoms. Surgical correction of the hiatal hernia produced immediate and continued relief. During the 3 years since operation she has continued to eat normally and has no recognizable food obstruction.

Dr. E. had severe dysphagia which did not respond to operative correction of reflux, whereas the second patient, Mrs. H., who had symptoms that were even more severe, did respond. At present I am unable to predict the quality of improvement that will be obtained in the individual patient. For this reason, when discussing the procedure with the patient, I describe this dilemma frankly.

We now have good reason to believe that a degenerative process is present in the cricopharyngeus and that this change is most likely secondary to the damaging effects of reflux. In 16 patients muscle biopsies of cricopharyngeus have been studied by light and electron microscopy.

The cricopharyngeal biopsies showed on light microscopy minimal changes. However on electron microscopy 12 out of 16 biopsies examined revealed marked disruption of the normal architecture of myofibrils. There are numerous mitochondria with some aberrant forms and an increase in glycogen. Nemaline rods were seen in many fibers in each biopsy, both in the subsarcolemmal regiona and along the Z bands. In cases where the nemaline rods were numerous, paraffin sections stained with phosphotungastic and hematohylin (PTAH) showed the rods as multiple small red elongated bodies (Fig. 19.4). The presence of these ultrastructural changes clearly indicates the organic nature of the pathologic process occurring in these patients (10–12). Materal obtained from the cricopharyngeus of patients dying with metastatic cancer did not show any nemaline rods.

Surgical Management—Poor Risk Patient

A few patients with pharyngoesophageal dysphagia have very severe symptoms but may be so disabled from other systemic disease that the risk of surgical correction of the hernia is prohibitive. In three such patients I performed only pharyngoesophageal myotomy and relieved the dysphagia. These patients continue to need intensive medical management of their hernias and, in particular, must sleep with the head of the bed elevated to protect their tracheobronchial tree from reflux and night aspiration.

Case 4. Mr. G., age 73, was known to have a hiatal hernia for 10 years and because of age and poor respiratory function had been treated conservatively. Over the previous year he had developed dominant pharyngoesophageal dysphagia with frequent episodes of coughing and choking during swallowing. He failed to respond to vigorous conservative management and had had a severe exacerbation in his chronic bronchitis. He was so debilitated that he had to have intravenous alimentation for 3 weeks before he was transferred for surgical management. Because of his severely compromised respiratory function, a pharyngoesophageal myotomy was performed under local anesthesia. His dysphagia completely resolved, the episodes of aspiration ceased and his respiratory symptoms improved markedly. He has maintained this improvement for 3 years, has gained 20 pounds and is now physically active.

This man illustrates the extreme debility occasionally seen in these patients and shows how cricopharyngeal myotomy can improve the dysphagia. This limited approach is used only under unusual circumstances and, when used, must be supported by continued con-

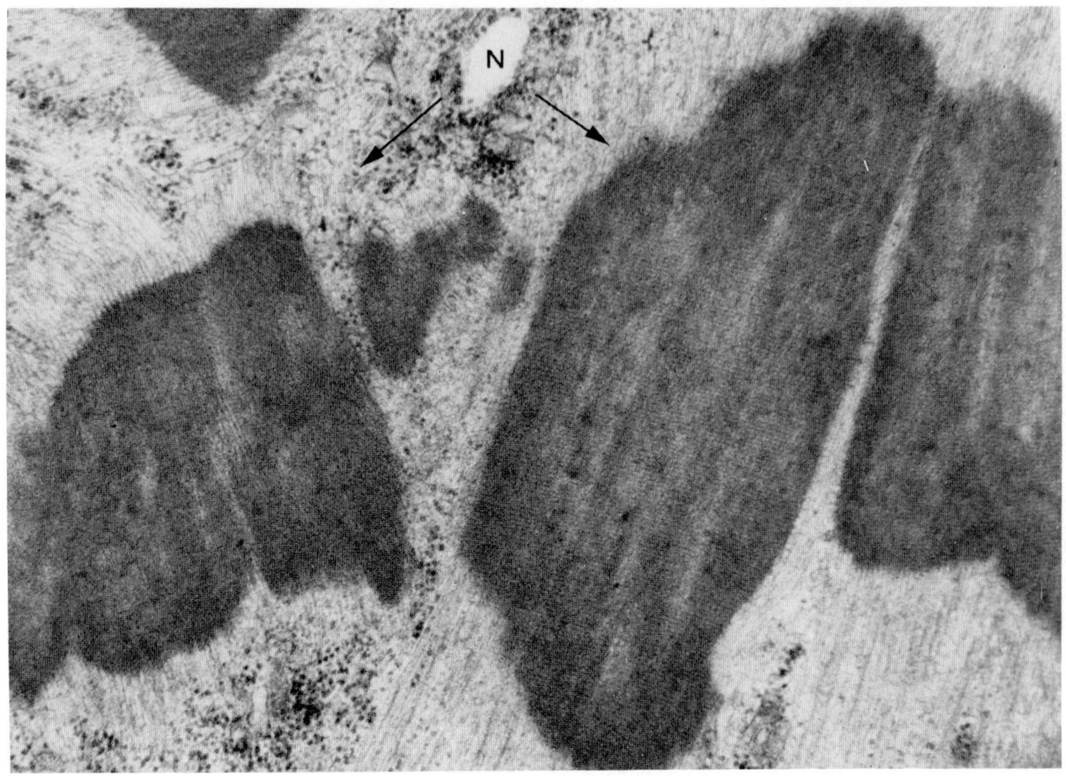

Figure 19.4
Electron microscopic studies of the cricopoharyngeal muscle have shown the presence of nemaline rods (N) along the myofibrils. These rods indicate the presence of muscle degeneration and are proof of the presence of significant pathology, accounting for the symptom of cricopharyngeal dysphagia (×38232).

servative care with particular attention to bed elevation to control reflux and night aspiration.

Pharyngoesophageal Diverticulum and Disorders Associated with Reflux

Ludlow in 1769 (13) first described obstruction to the passage of the food bolus by a pharyngoesophageal pouch. The pathogenesis of this diverticulum remains obscure, although it is now attributed to abnormalities of the cricopharyngeus muscle, which are said to produce obstruction and proximal diverticular formation. The diverticulum forms at the junction of the pharynx and cricopharynx, through a weakened zone between the oblique and transverse fibers of the cricopharyngeus muscle. This weakened zone, which is present in 30 per cent of cadavers

(14), extends farther to the left of the midline than the right—a finding which explains the tendency for the pouch to develop on the left side (Fig. 19.5).

Initially, manometric studies in patients with pharyngoesophageal diverticulum were considered to be normal (15), but Ellis and colleagues (9) have demonstrated incoordination between pharyngeal contraction and cricopharyngeal relaxation. This incoordination is similar to that which we have described in patients with a hiatal hernia. With incoordination the peak of pharyngeal contraction comes after maximal cricopharyngeal relaxation, and for this reason there is a constant pressure barrier between pharynx and cricopharynx (Fig. 19.6). The formation of a pulsion diverticulum at the upper margin of the cricopharyngeus has been attributed to this increase in local pressure.

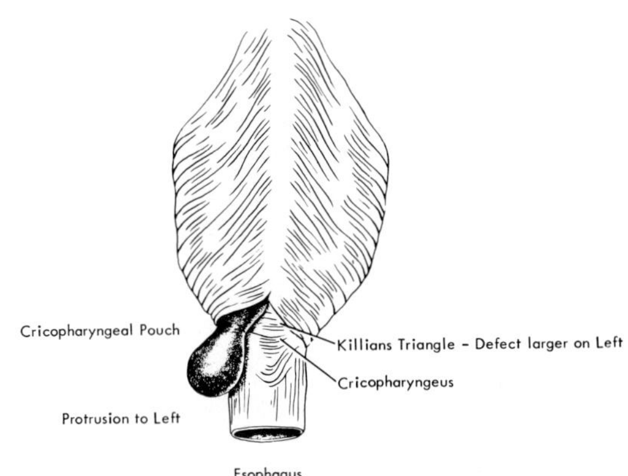

Figure 19.5. Pharyngoesophageal Diverticulum
There is an anatomical defect between the pharyngeal musculature and the cricopharyngeus. This defect is more prominent on the left, which accounts for the frequency of diverticulum protrusion to this side.

Almost all patients with a pharyngoesophageal diverticulum also have radiologic evidence of a hiatal hernia or of gastroesophageal reflux. During acid barium studies on these patients the barium column is thrust upward against the closed cricopharynx (16), producing local irritation and promoting muscle spasm. Similarly, reflux at night may pool immediately below the cricopharynx and produce irritation and spasm. Manometrically, we have not been able to demonstrate true spasm, but the incoordination described by Ellis and colleagues (4,9) may represent a response to acid irritation of the cricopharynx. Pharyngoesophageal dysphagia is a common symptom in patients with reflux and a diverticulum may result when reflux triggers cricopharyngeal incoordination in the presence of a weakened Killian's triangle.

Pharyngoesophageal diverticulum is rare under age 40 and tends to occur more frequently in males than in females (17). A few congenital diverticula (18) have been reported and Groves (19) has described a rare familial incidence of pharyngoesophageal diverticulum.

Symptoms and Investigation

Symptoms in patients who have pharyngoesophageal diverticulum are related to the accumulation of food in the diverticulum and to obstruction to the passage of food (20). While the subject is eating, turbulence in the pouch may produce a gurgling sound that may be embarrassing socially. The dysphagia varies in intensity and may be punctuated by episodes of total obstruction when a large bolus of food lodges in the pouch. The coughing and choking, which may occur during swallowing, are due to obstruction and forward spillage. Aspiration may occur while swallowing and also at night from spillage of retained pouch content. During its course, this disorder may be complicated by aspiration pneumonia and lung abscess.

Occasionally a carcinoma (21) may develop in a long-standing pharyngoesophageal diverticulum and more rarely still, ulceration (22) or bleeding (23) has been reported from the diverticulum.

Dysphagia is the most common and usually the presenting symptom. Although in most patients the diverticulum is the major cause of dysphagia, in patients with a small diverticulum dysphagia may be equally profound

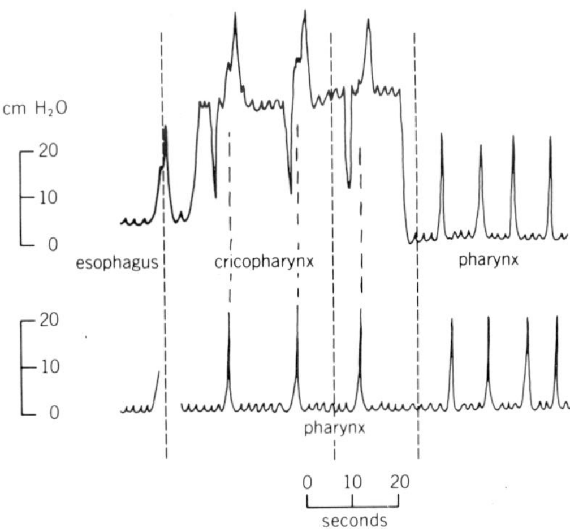

Figure 19.6. Cricopharyngeal Diverticulum
An incoordination between pharyngeal contraction and cricopharyngeal relaxation has been noted in patients with a cricopharyngeal diverticulum. The pharyngeal contraction wave reaches its peak of pressure shortly after completion of cricopharyngeal relaxation. This imbalance results in a residual pressure gradient from pharynx to cricopharynx. The motor defect is similar to the defect we encountered in 20 of 52 patients with gastroesophageal reflux.

and must in part be related to cricopharyngeal incoordination.

Case 5. Mrs. S., age 72, had a long history of cricopharyngeal dysphagia and a previous history of gastroesophageal reflux treated surgically. She initially presented with a left lower lobe aspiration pneumonia.

Despite surgical correction of her hiatal hernia, the dysphagia persisted. Radiologically she had a very small diverticulum (Fig. 19.7) and manometrically the cricopharyngeus was incoordinate. Because of symptom severity she required a cricopharyngeal myotomy under local anesthesia. She has had excellent symptomatic relief and is eating normally. The diverticulum was not visualized and was not treated.

The diverticulum in this patient was too small to produce food obstruction and the severe dysphagia was secondary to cricopharyngeal incoordination.

The investigation of a patient suspected of harboring a pharyngoesophageal diverticulum includes radiologic studies and endoscopy. Manometry is of some interest because it may show an abnormal motor pattern, but it has much less diagnostic value. The diagnosis of a pharyngoesophageal diverticulum depends upon the radiologic demonstration of a diverticulum protruding posteriorly in the midline or to the left (Fig. 19.8). Usually this diagnosis is made easily, and the chief purpose of radiography is to exclude other causes of dysphagia at the cricopharyngeal level. Occasionally a plain film will show an airfluid level in a large diverticulum (Fig. 19.9).

During radiologic evaluation, the examiner should take care to assess the distal esophagus because of the high incidence of associated reflux. Endoscopy should be carried out with great care because the esophagoscope may enter and perforate the diverticulum. Endoscopy is valuable in excluding malignancy and in assessing the distal esophagus for evidence of reflux.

As noted earlier, manometry is of considerable theoretical interest, but contributes little to the diagnosis.

Treatment

Operation is the treatment of choice in a symptomatic pharyngoesophageal diverticulum (24) because there are no effective conservative measures. If the patient has significant dysphagia and associated aspiration, his condition is likely to show progressive deterioration unless it is corrected surgically. Since the operation can be carried out simply under local anesthesia, age and general debility are rarely a contraindication in patients (25) with severe symptoms.

The two-stage resection procedure (26), popularized by Lahey, has produced good results. However, it entails two separate anesthetics, considerably technical difficulty (related to the scar formation encountered at the time of the second stage) and considerable risk of fistula formation. For these reasons, a one-stage approach has been used more widely in recent years. The one-stage procedure carries an operative mortality and a fistula rate of less than 1 per cent (26). Long-term follow-up of results is satisfactory. After simple pouch excision, Einarsson and Hallén (27) have reported recurrence of the diverticulum, and Bingham (28), has described continued dysphagia despite pouch removal. Because of these problems, most surgeons now prefer to combine pouch excision or suspension with cricopharyngeal myotomy (9, 29–31).

Operative Treatment

Operative treatment can be carried out under either a local or general anesthetic. An oblique cervical incision is made along the anterior border of the sternomastoid muscle, which is reflected laterally, and dissection is carried medial to the carotid sheath. The omohyoid muscle and the inferior thyroid artery are divided after identification of the recurrent laryngeal nerve. Usually the pouch is easily found lying on the cervical vertebrae. If the pouch is difficult to identify, a bougie can be gently introduced into it from the mouth or packing can be inserted. Once identified, the pouch is fully mobilized and tacked to the anterior cervical ligament with interrupted silk sutures. The operation is completed by performing a lateral myotomy which extends from a point 0.5 cm into the pharynx, through the cricopharynx and into the upper 2 or 3 cm of esophagus (Fig. 19.10). Once the myotomy is complete I dissect the muscle laterally and place a catgut suture in the anterior muscle bundle to hold this bundle forward and to avoid fusion of the myotomy. A Penrose drain is inserted and the wound is drained through a separate stab incision. The drain is used to minimize the risk of hematoma as this interferes with the return of adequate swallowing. The wound is closed.

These patients can be started on fluids

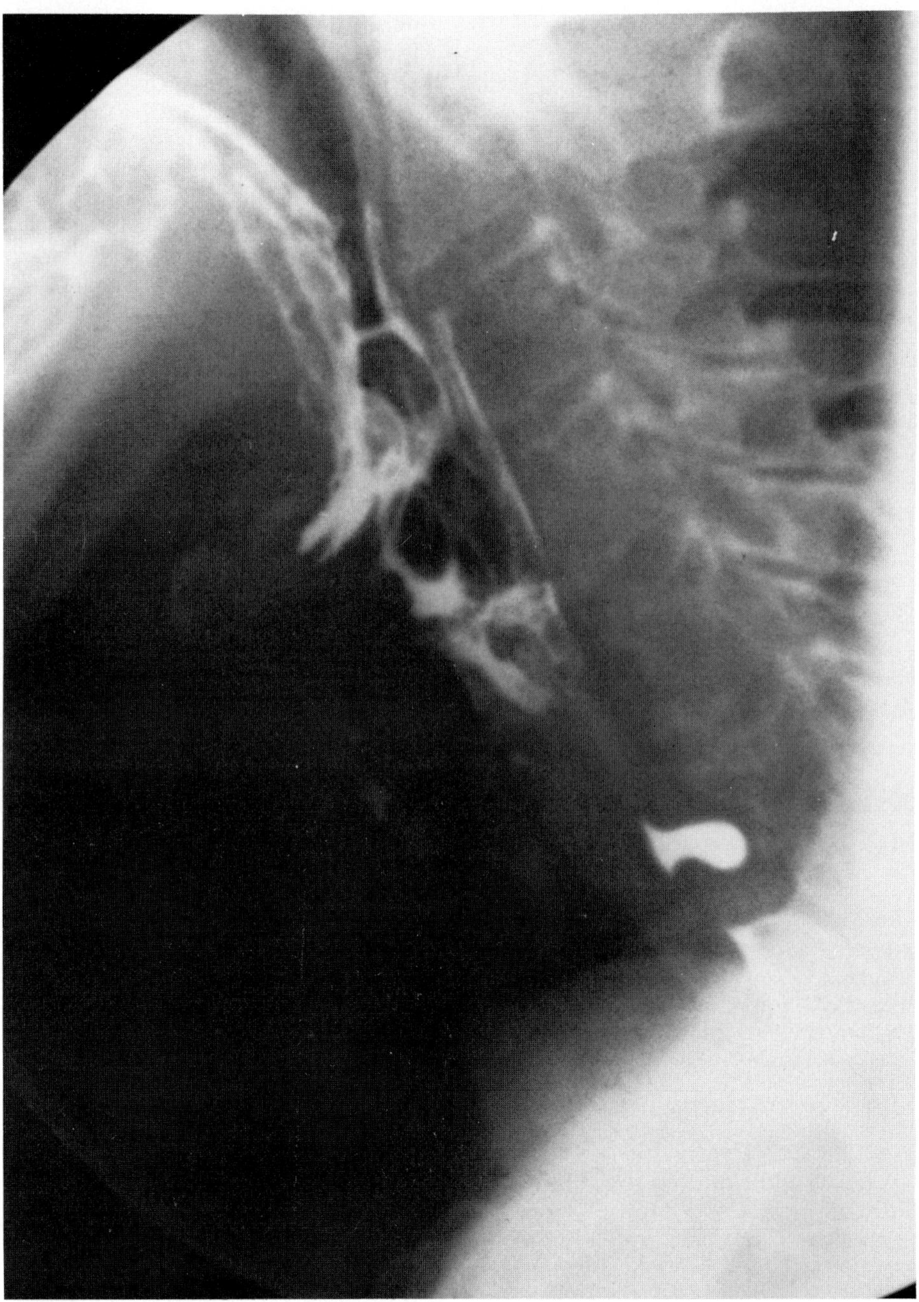

Figure 19.7
Mrs. S. (Case 5) has profound cricopharyngeal dysphagia and a diverticulum. The diverticulum radiologically is small and cannot be considered the source of obstruction. Cricopharyngeal myotomy alone has given effective symptomatic relief.

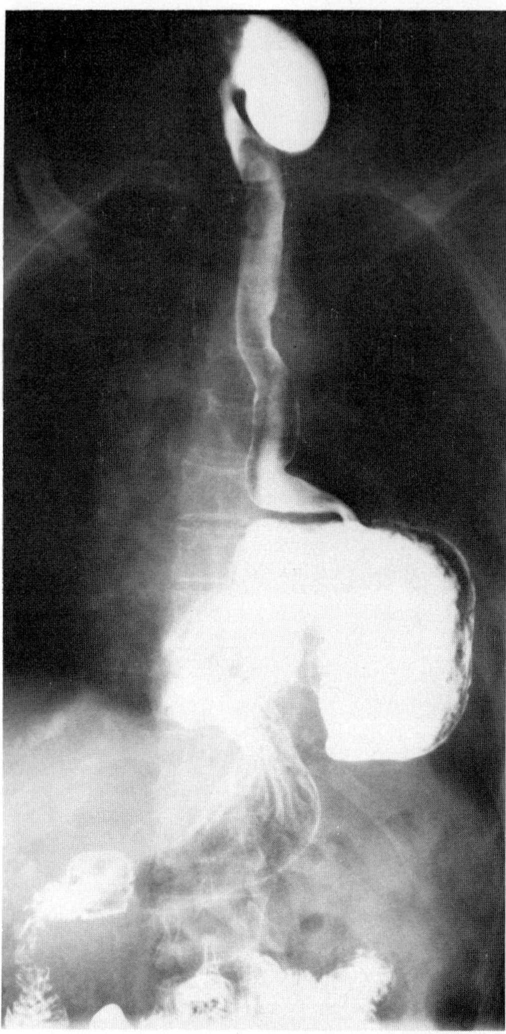

Figure 19.8. Radiologic Cricopharyngeal Diverticulum
Classic radiologic appearance is a dependent diverticulum, of variable size, tending to be to the left of the mid-line. A hiatal hernia is almost always associated. In this patient the diverticulum is of moderate size and protrudes to the left. The hiatal hernia is very large.

within 48 hours and can eat a soft diet by the time of discharge in 4 to 5 days.

Endoscopic Surgery for Pharyngoesophageal Diverticulum

Dohlman and Mattsson (32) have described an endoscopic method in which they divide the wall between the pharyngoesophageal pouch and the diverticulum. This method uses a specially designed endoscope with a blade fitting the esophagus and a blade in the pouch (Fig. 19.11). The wall between pouch and esophagus is coagulated and divided by a diathermy knife. They reported a 7 per cent recurrence rate in almost 100 cases. Although this recurrence rate is higher than for myotomy and diverticulopexy, the operation can be repeated with no added technical problems or risk. Dohlman himself recommended this procedure for aged and debilitated patients.

Cricopharyngeal Bar

Occasionally patients presenting with pharyngoesophageal dysphagia have recognizable radiologic abnormalities of the cricopharyngeus muscle. These abnormalities, unfortunately, are not specific to the disorder and may occur in patients with no recognizable symptoms. In radiologic studies of asymptomatic subjects, 4 to 5 per cent have a recognizable cricopharyngeal bar (33). In some this bar is associated with dysphagia, but the bar itself is not conclusive evidence of a disease process (Fig. 19.12) (34).

When cricopharyngeal muscle spasm presents without an associated diverticulum, the patient complains of dysphagia, often with an associated collar-like tightness in the neck. Usually radiologic studies will show a prominence of the cricopharyngeal muscle and often a "radiologic" hiatal hernia. Manometry demonstrates a very high cricoesophageal pressure—occasionally greater than 200 cm of water. At operation there is recognizable hyperplasia of the cricopharyngeus, and myotomy brings effective relief (35). A truly hyperplastic cricopharyngeus is very rare.

Primary Motor Disorders of Pharyngoesophageal Junction

In the first part of this chapter the cricopharyngeal muscle disorders discussed were secondary to or associated with gastroesophageal reflux. The only detectable abnormality lies in the cricopharyngeus muscle or in related diverticula. Since these patients have normal pharyngeal and soft palate function, the point of obstruction is at the cricopharyngeus and for this reason cricopharyngeal

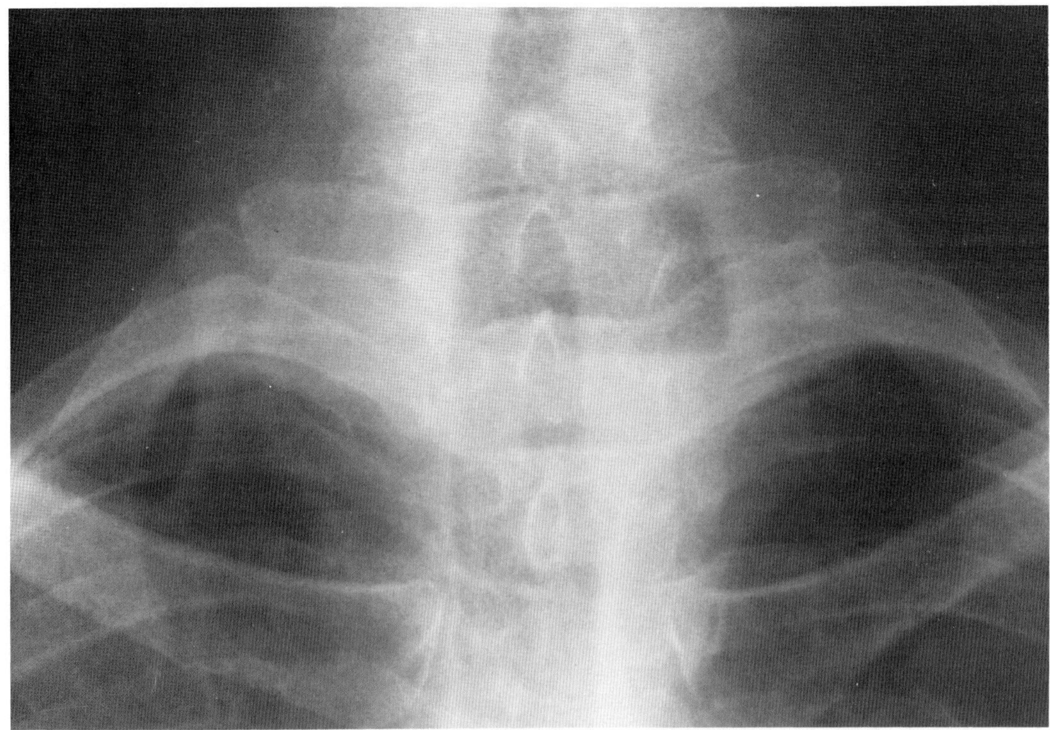

Figure 19.9
Radiograph of the chest in a patient with a cricopharyngeal diverticulum. Note the air-fluid level in the large diverticulum in the upper mediastinum.

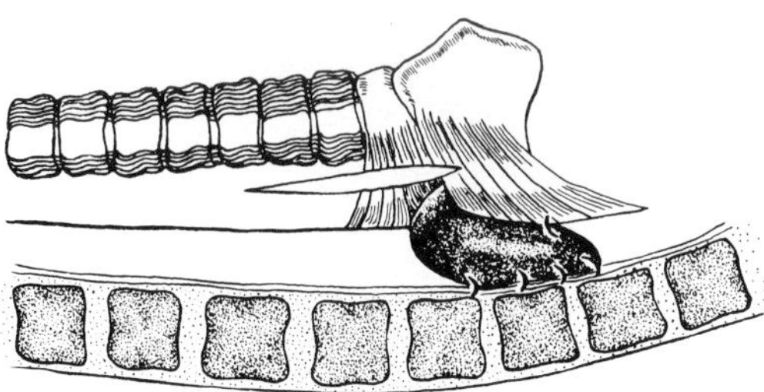

Figure 19.10. Cricopharyngeal Myotomy
Operative procedure exposes the cricopharyngeal muscle using an oblique incision along the anterior margin of the sternomastoid muscle. With the muscle exposed, the myotomy is performed, extending from pharynx, through cricopharynx and 2 to 3 cm into the proximal esophagus.

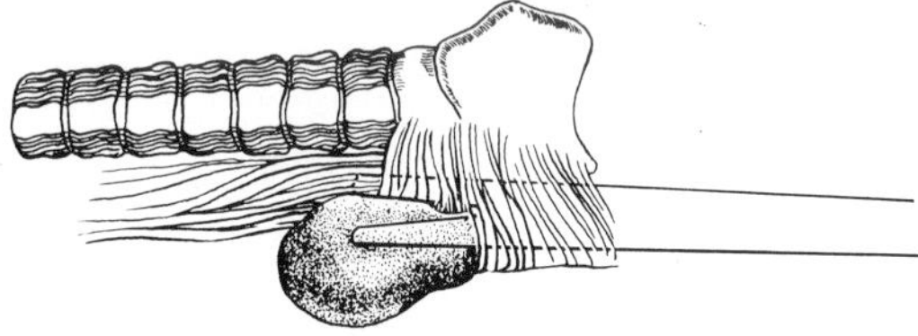

Figure 19.11
The Dohlman procedure uses specially designed instruments to expose the posterior aspect of the esophagus and anterior aspects of the cricopharyngeal diverticulum. Electrocautery is used to divide the cricopharynx in this location.

myotomy is successful in the majority of patients requiring surgery.

With primary motor disorders the abnormality is related to neurogenic, myoneurogenic or myogenic abnormalities and often the entire upper one-third of esophagus, cricopharyngeus, pharynx and soft palate are involved. The investigation and treatment of these disorders is a challenge and requires considerable experience and careful use of radiology, manometry and endoscopy before a decision is made as to the likelihood of success by surgical myotomy.

It is important at this time to look at the forces active in controlling the swallowed

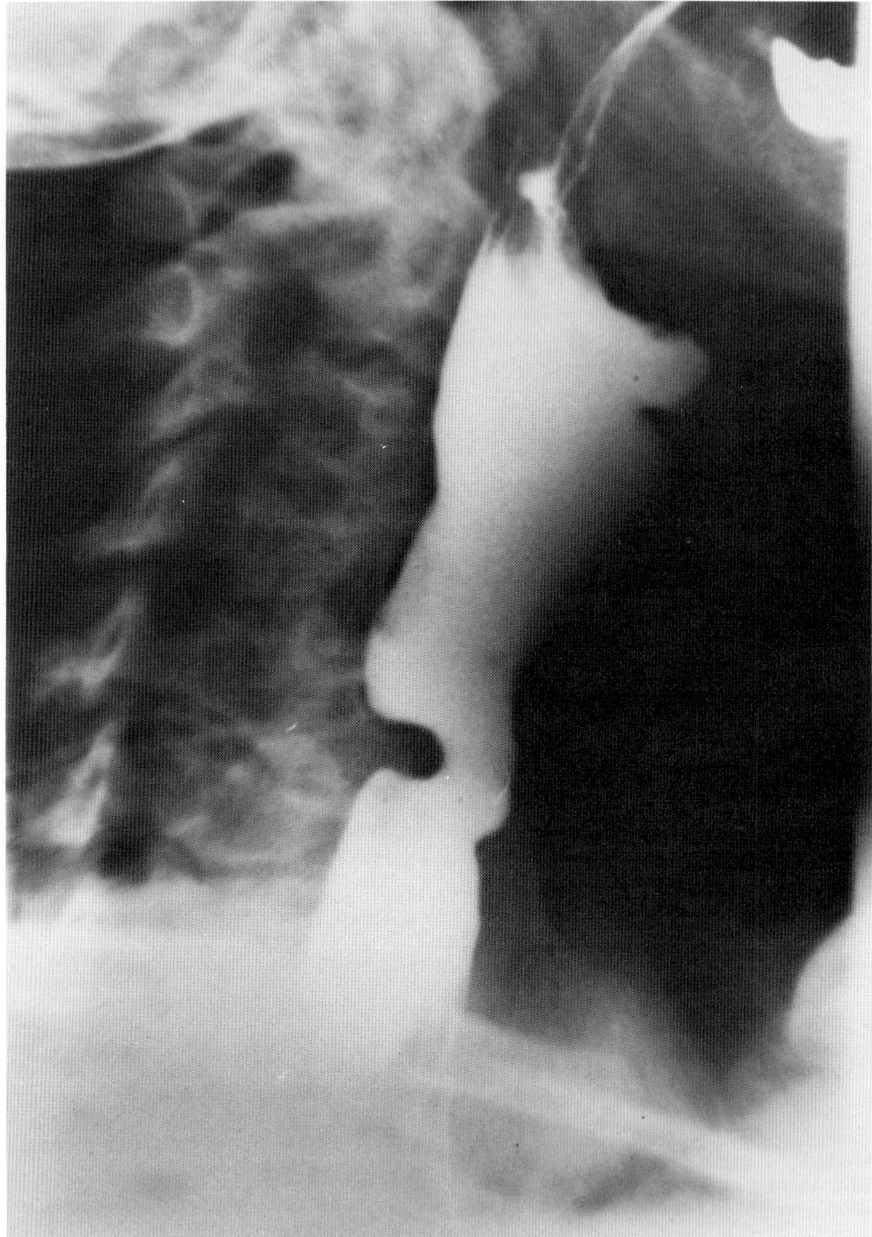

Figure 19.12. Cricopharyngeal Bar on Barium Swallow
Radiologically a cricopharyngeal bar can be detected in 5 to 6 per cent of normal subjects. This bar is also noted in patients with cricopharyngeal muscle spasm.

food bolus. Descent of the bolus is initiated by the thrust of the tongue and by gravity then its descent and directional control is dependant upon the motor power of the pharynx. Coordinated cricopharyngeal relaxation allows passage of food into the upper esophagus.

History is important to recognize the systemic manifestations of disorders which affect the pharyngoesophageal junction. Also by history, the presence of tracheal aspiration or the more specific symptom of nasal regurgitation is important. Nasal regurgitation strongly suggests soft palate involvement.

Radiology may help in demonstrating pharyngeal delay, occasionally shows nasal regurgitation (Fig. 19.13), and often will document tracheal aspiration.

Manometry is of critical importance in deciding whether cricopharyngeal myotomy will be of value. When the pharynx and cricopharynx are both paralyzed, myotomy is of no value. Myotomy is successful only when it obliterates a cricopharyngeal pressure barrier produced by incoordination, poor relaxation or relative hypertonicity. This type of detailed manometric evaluation is technically difficult; however, the information obtained is invaluable.

The problem of Parkinsonism illustrates well the necessity of careful evaluation.

Case 6. Mrs. H., age 78, had profound cricopharyngeal dysphagia with nasal regurgitation and tracheal aspiration. She developed recurrent episodes of respiratory infection. There was a known hiatal hernia with relatively mild reflux symptoms; however, conservative management of reflux did not relieve her dysphagia.

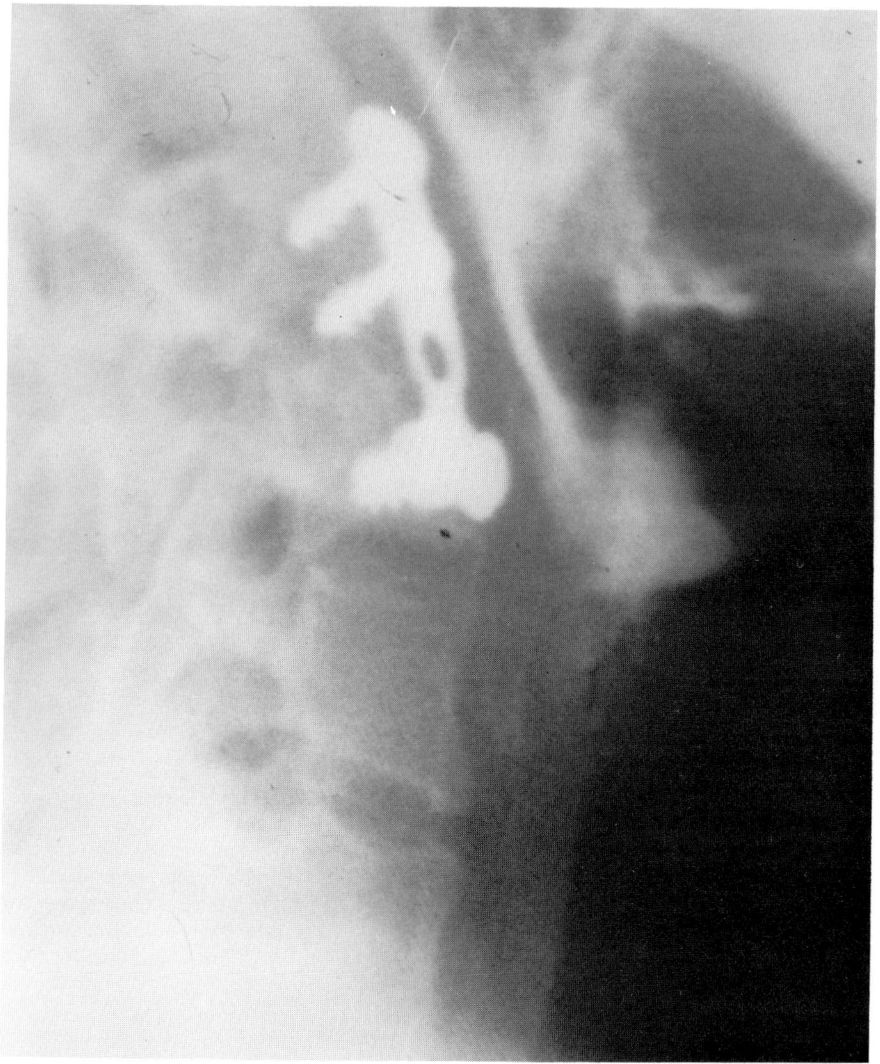

Figure 19.13
Mrs. K. (Case 7) has a paralyzed pharynx and soft palate, together with spinal deformity from neurofibromatosis. Nasal regurgitation and tracheal aspiration occur with swallowing. Nasal regurgitation is present in this radiologic study.

Radiologically food obstruction was present at the cricopharyngeal junction, and tracheal aspiration of barium occurred. Manometric studies showed reduced, but present, pharyngeal motor waves and a normal tone cricopharyngeus with incoordinate relaxation. She appeared to be an ideal candidate for cricopharyngeal myotomy. Myotomy was carried out under local anesthesia, and there was an immediate improvement, however, the patient still had intermittant tracheal aspiration. Although the clinical result was satisfactory, complete relief was not obtained and this failure was due to Parkinsonian tongue movements which prevented the patient initiating the full thrust of the swallowing mechanism. It is important to consider all aspects of the swallowing mechanism before proceeding to myotomy.

Case 7. Mrs. K., age 30, has Von Recklinghausen's disease. Neurofibromatous masses had been removed from her left carotid chain on three occasions, and she had developed dysphagia following each procedure. Gradual recovery had taken place; however, following a cervical spine fusion she developed dysphagia and tracheal aspiration of such severity that a feeding gastrostomy had to be inserted.

Radiology confirmed the presence of both tracheal and nasopharyngeal spillage and very little radiopaque material entered her esophagus.

Manometry showed a low tone cricopharyngeus (25 cm of water) with poor relaxation and absent pharyngeal motor waves. Again myotomy was considered likely to be of value. Following myotomy the patient continued to have severe tracheal aspiration. Radiologic studies showed most of the meal to pass directly into the esophagus and were substantially better than before myotomy. Clinically the aspiration remained severe. Reviewing the radiologic studies it was recognized that with spinal deformity food was dropping directly into the trachea and the esophagus was partially occluded behind the curve of the cervical spine (Fig. 19.14). This anatomic defect in the presence of a paralyzed pharynx directed food onto the vocal cords and detracted from the effects of her myotomy. In the presence of a paralyzed pharynx food has to be able to drop directly into the esophagus under the influence of tongue thrust and gravity.

These two patients illustrate the difficulty of obtaining good results from surgical myotomy in the presence of an atonic pharynx.

Cricopharyngeal Achalasia

The term "cricopharyngeal achalasia" suggests loss of relaxation and a condition similar to achalasia of the gastroesophageal junction.

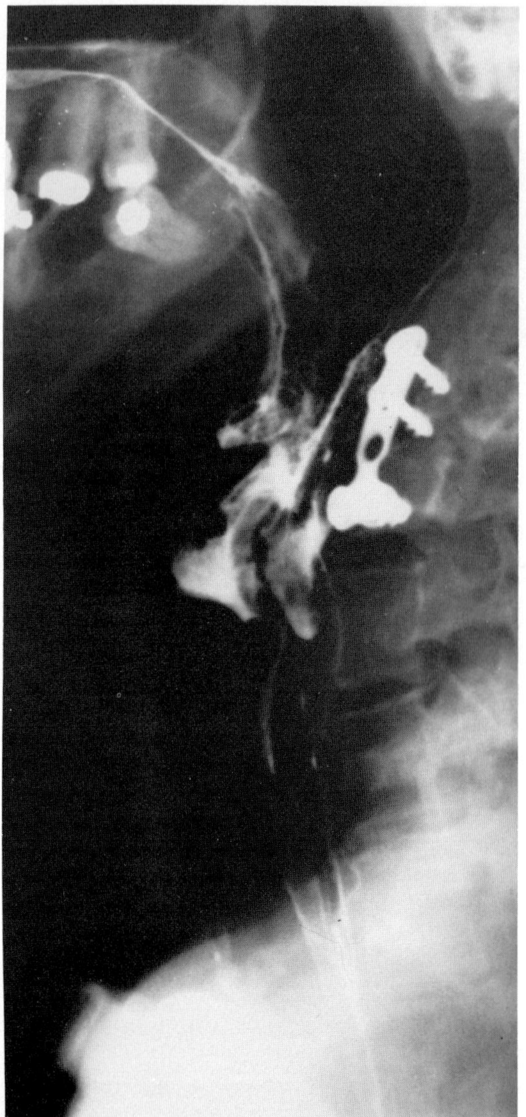

Figure 19.14
Mrs. K. (Case 7) has a marked forward curve of the cervical spine secondary to bony destruction by neurofibromatosis. She has had an anterior spinal fusion. Her pharynx is paralyzed. Because of the shape of her spine the gravitational descent of her food bolus carries it directly into her larynx and produces tracheal aspiration.

Although this term is used in the literature, such loss of relaxation has not been substantiated manometrically (28).

Unless a specific syndrome can be defined in which the cricopharyngeus can be shown to have lost its ability to relax, this term should be discontinued.

Cricopharyngeal Incoordination

Utian and Thomas (36) and Mitchell and Armanini (37) have done radiologic studies on two children with incoordination of the cricopharynx. One child died and at autopsy had no ganglia in the upper third of his esophagus, suggesting a neurogenic basis for the dysphagia and a possible relationship to achalasia of the cardia. As far as I know, the literature contains no other reports of the condition and clearly further study is necessary before it can be accepted as a separate entity.

Myoneurogenic Disorders

Myasthenia gravis is characterized by failure of impulse transmission at the myoneurogenic junction in skeletal muscle. Skeletal muscles such as those of the pharnyx, cricopharynx, upper esophagus, muscles of mastication and those of voluntary deglutition are involved in this disorder (38). When the disorder is not adequately controlled by drug therapy, dysphagia may become a significant problem. Characteristically the dysphagia is more severe when the patient is tired, e.g., at the end of a meal and at the end of the day. Because they do not chew food adequately and swallow effectively, these patients may cough and choke and may regurgitate food through the nose. This symptom does not indicate a motor obstruction but rather relative paralysis associated with an inability to close off the nasopharynx and the larynx.

Manometric studies show a failure of the pharyngeal, cricopharyngeal and proximal esophageal motor power (Fig. 19.15) which does not present as an obstruction but as an inability to control the early stages of food passage through the pharynx. Myotomy of the cricopharynx is not indicated; instead attention should be focused on drug therapy which will improve the patient's general muscle strength (39).

Case 8. Mr. J., age 76, has a hiatal hernia and peptic stricture which is being treated by bouginage to #60 Fr approximately every 3 months. His stricture produces dysphagia only when he is tired and when drugs fail to control his myasthenia.

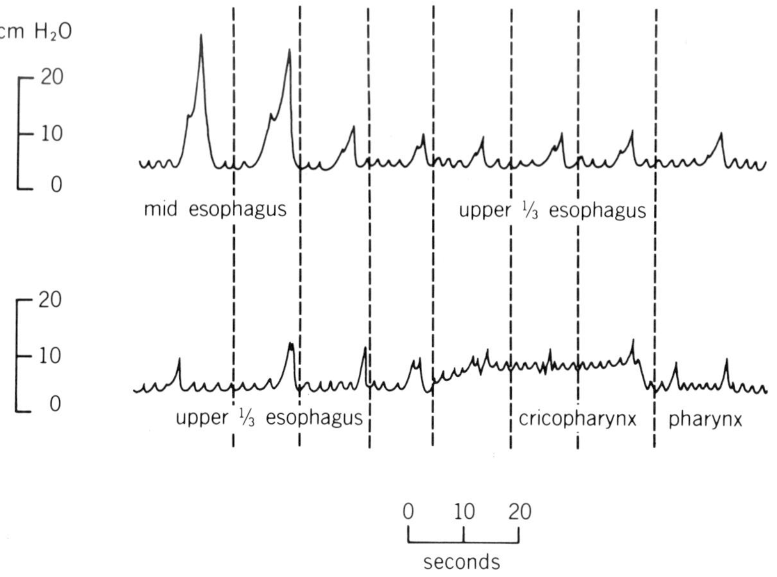

Figure 19.15. Manometric Disorder of Myasthenia Gravis
On manometric examination, the lower two-thirds of the esophagus are normal in the myasthenic patient. There is a marked diminution in the amplitude of proximal esophageal motor waves and a reduction in the tone of the cricopharyngeus. Pharyngeal motor waves are weak or absent. The site of this motor weakness corresponds to the striated muscle in the upper esophagus, cricopharynx and pharynx.

Under normal circumstances he has no recognizable disturbance of pharyngoesophageal function and he can chew and swallow his food well. Recently he was acutely ill with a ruptured appendix. During his illness, his drug program did not provide effective control and he was unable to chew and swallow his food. During this time he coughed and choked with swallowing and had nasal regurgitation.

In this particular patient, who had mild and well-controlled myasthenia, the dysphagia was usually noticeable only when he was unable to chew his food adequately. When his myasthenia temporarily exacerbated, the more common pharyngoesophageal symptoms developed.

Myogenic Disorders

Myotonia

This disorder presents with general weakness of the muscles of mastication, voluntary deglutition and the muscle groups in the upper pharynx and esophagus (40). Symptoms of ineffective swallowing, namely, nasal regurgitation with coughing and choking, stem from an inability to control the pharyngeal descent of the food bolus.

The manometric changes in this disorder are similar to those seen in myasthenia gravis. The motor defect is present at all times and does not vary with fatigue. In addition, these patients usually have generalized skeletal muscle symptoms.

Case 9. Mrs. S., age 44, who had had two hiatal hernia repairs over the previous 10 years, presented with a 2-year history of pharyngoesophageal dysphagia. Her dysphagia was constant and was associated with coughing and choking and with nasal regurgitation of food.

Radiologic and endoscopic studies had failed to show any abnormality. Manometrically she had a marked reduction in proximal esophageal motor power, no recognizable function of the cricopharyngeus and markedly diminished pharyngeal motor power. Because of these findings she was referred to the neurologist, who recognized that she suffered from myotonia. In retrospect, she had noted some muscle weakness and had given up square-dancing because she could not release her partner's hand—this delay in release of the hand grip is, of course, characteristic of myotonia.

Oculopharyngeal Muscular Dystrophy

The dysphagia encountered in this rare disorder is similar to that described in myasthenia and myotonia (40–42). Manometric studies show decreased amplitude of the pharyngeal motor wave together with abnormal coordination and relaxation of the cricopharyngeal sphincter (43, 44). Electromyographic studies confirm that this is a primary muscle disorder. Radiologic studies have shown nasal regurgitation and aspiration. The dysphagia may be quite profound.

We had the opportunity to carry out manometric studies on three patients with oculopharyngeal muscular dystrophy. Two had only mild pharyngoesophageal symptoms and were manometrically normal; the third had severe pharyngoesophageal dysphagia, a history of coughing and choking on swallowing, and a progressive weight loss. The amplitude of the pharyngeal motor wave was reduced but the cricopharyngeus and upper esophagus were normal. In the last patient, pharyngoesophageal myotomy produced a marked symptomatic improvement, a return to normal eating habits and a moderate weight gain (45).

This disorder is rare, and more cases must be studied before the motor defect can be adequately categorized.

Other myopathies, such as thyrotoxic myopathy, also have been said to produce dysphagia.

Neurogenic Disorders

Central Neurologic Defects

Various central neurologic lesions may produce esophageal motor dysfunction, but the frequency and significance of these have not been established. Cricopharyngeal and pharyngeal disorders have been described in amyotrophic lateral scleroses (46, 47), progressive supranuclear opthalmoplegia (48), Arnold-Chiari malformation (49), Parkinsonism and a variety of other central neurologic problems (50, 51).

Bulbar poliomyelitis may result in paralysis of the pharynx with preservation of the cricopharynx (52, 53). Although now rare, this specific motor abnormality can produce severe motor obstruction (Fig. 19.16). Relief of obstruction can be obtained by cricopharyngeal myotomy, which by reducing cricopharyngeal tone allows food to pass freely into the upper esophagus. Myotomy removes cricopharyngeal tone, but leaves the patient with pharyngeal paralysis. Poor control of a swal-

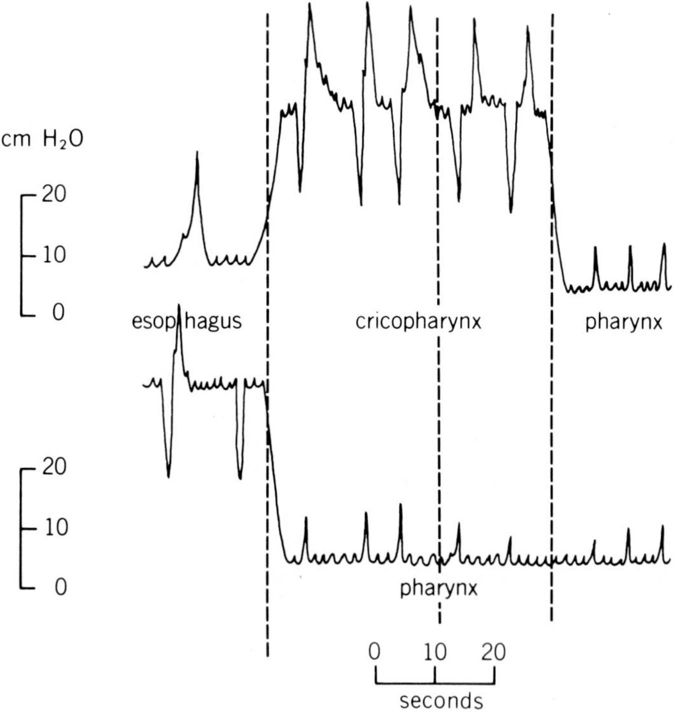

Figure 19.16. Manometric Disorder of Bulbar Poliomyelitis
Manometric pattern in poliomyelitis indicates that esophageal motor function is normal and that the cricopharyngeus has been preserved. However, there is marked reduction in the amplitude of pharyneal motor waves and because of this the cricopharyngeus becomes a major pressure barrier and causes dysphagia.

lowed bolus may still produce forward spillage and provoke coughing and nasal regurgitation. Despite these limitations, patients are otherwise usually much improved.

Case 10. Mr. B., age 43, had bulbar poliomyelitis at the age of 13 years. He made an excellent recovery and had only minor weakness of his shoulder muscles. However, dysphagia remained as his dominant complaint, and persisted unaltered into adult life. This symptom occurred with all his meals and was present with both liquids and solids. He coughed and choked frequently during his meals and occasionally had nasal regurgitation. Despite these symptoms he led a normal life, maintained his weight well and worked at heavy manual labor. Radiologic study did show a prominent cricopharyngeus. Manometrically he had markedly reduced pharyngeal motor power, but the cricopharynx and upper esophagus were normal. Myotomy of the cricopharyngeus has given total relief of his symptoms.

This patient coped with his motor dysfunction well, but suffered for many years with an unpleasant symptom that eventually was relieved com-

pletely by myotomy. Manometric study delineated the point of obstruction and allowed precise surgical correction of the disorder.

Congenital Central Neurologic Defects

Several congenital defects have been described as giving rise to pharyngoesophageal dysphagia including congenital suprabulbar (53) paresis and the Riley-Day syndrome (54). Most of these abnormalities are rare and incompletely studied. The Riley-Day syndrome, was first described in 1949 (54). Approximately half of these patients have a defect in swallowing. They develop a dilated atonic esophagus with poor emptying in the horizontal position (55). A pharyngeal abnormality has also been described; although they can form a pharyngeal bolus of food, they cannot propel the bolus through the cricopharynx. Aspiration is common, and many of these patients develop secondary respiratory infections (56, 57).

To date, assessment of these patients has

been limited to direct observation, history and radiology. Manometric studies would be illuminating and might point the way to more effective management of their esophageal complaints.

Peripheral Nerve Disorders

Recurrent laryngeal nerve (RLN) palsy may occur secondary to such malignancies as bronchogenic carcinoma, or may follow viral neuritis or accidental division of the RLN during neck surgery. When it occurs, this disorder produces simultaneously vocal cord paralysis and pharyngoesophageal dysphagia (58). The dysphagia reflects damage to the nerve supply of the cricopharyngeal muscle, which is derived in part from the recurrent laryngeal nerve.

Case 11. Mr. L., age 66, had a left pneumonectomy for bronchogenic carcinoma. His left RLN was resected because it was involved in nodes that had adhered to the aorta. After operation he developed marked voice changes and severe pharyngoesophageal dysphagia with coughing and choking (Fig. 19.17). Soon after he developed severe bronchopneumonia which did not respond well to physiotherapy and antibiotics. His diet was reduced to clear liquids and his infections cleared. When he was started on solids he again aspirated and his pneumonia recurred. A cricopharyngeal myotomy performed under local anesthesia subsequently gave effective relief of his symptoms. He could eat normally without aspiration and his pulmonary infections cleared. We followed up this patient for an additional 6 months, during which he had no further dysphagia.

I examined 15 patients with bronchogenic carcinoma in whom the RLN was sectioned by the cancer. We also studied 3 other RLN patients, 2 with nerve damage from thyroid resection and 1 with a viral neuritis. Eleven of 15 cancer patients developed pharyngoesophageal dysphagia; and of these, 8 coughed and choked with swallowing and 3 developed significant respiratory infections which did not respond to conventional therapy. These 3 were submitted to cricopharyngeal myotomy and achieved effective relief of dysphagia and improvement in their respiratory symptoms. (It should be emphasized that the pneumonectomized patient is particularly vulnerable to aspiration because the lungs are already damaged by parenchymal disease and by the trauma of surgery.)

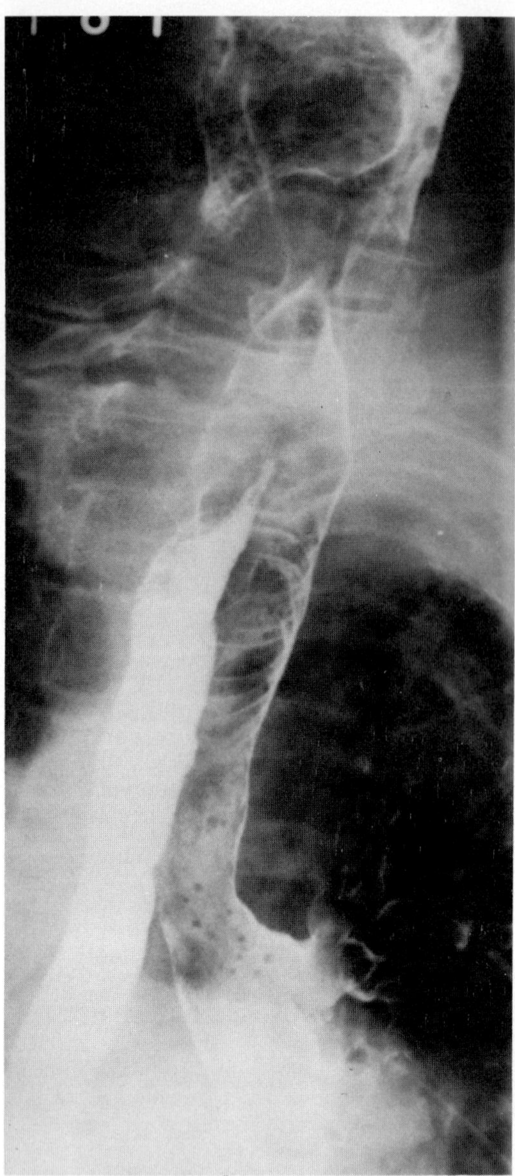

Figure 19.17. Radiologic Aspiration in Rercurrent Laryngeal Nerve Paralysis
Mr. L. (Case 11) had a left pneumonectomy with resection of his left recurrent laryngeal nerve. The barium swallow demonstrates aspiration with spillage of the barium into the tracheobronchial tree.

Of the 10 RLN patients who had radiologic studies, 2 aspirated barium during the examination. We found no evidence of esophageal obstruction either radiologically or at endoscopy. Manometric studies in 8 of these patients showed minor pharyngoesophageal abnormalities but did not show a specific defect that would account for the dysphagia. Two of the 10 had hiatal hernia.

It is important to recognize RLN damage following pneumonectomy, because if it goes unrecognized it may produce progressive respiratory infection and progressive damage to the remaining lung.

Differential Diagnosis of Pharyngoesophageal Motor Dysfunction

The differential diagnosis must always include mechanical forms of obstruction. Upper esophageal webs and strictures occur occasionally, and obstruction may also be due to bony spurs in the cervical spine, or to ossification of adjacent ligaments (59, 60). At all times one must exclude malignancy (21), and failure to recognize this possibility and adequately exclude it can lead to major tragedy.

Case 12. Mr. H., age 52, presented with a long history of mild heartburn interrupted by a 3-month history of cricopharyngeal dysphagia. His dysphagia was severe and he was referred for radiologic studies. Radiology showed the presence of a hiatal hernia; however, no abnormality was detected at the cricopharyngeus (Fig. 19.18). Manometric examination again showed a hiatal hernia but was otherwise nonspecific.

Endoscopy was done as part of evaluation recognizing the difficulties in cricopharyngeal radiology. The fiberoptic scope passed easily to duodenum, and his hiatal hernia was demonstrated. Upon withdrawal of the endoscope minor mucosal granularity was noted but could not be biopsied effectively. Rigid endoscopy and biopsy was necessary and at this time a squamous carcinoma was confirmed at the cricopharyngeal level.

He was treated with radiotherapy and following recurrence had a pharyngolaryngectomy and LeQuesne gastropharyngeal anastomosis. He had good palliation for 1½ years but died from recurrent disease.

Case 13. Mrs. Y., age 76, was seen for evaluation of recurrent respiratory infections and hemoptysis. Her problems dated back 10 years. Only on functional enquiry did she mention profound cricopharyngeal dysphagia with frequent aspiration. No abnormality was found in the tracheobronchial tree apart from inflammation. Radiologically a high and tight web (Fig. 19.19) was found immediately below the cricopharyngeus, and a second stricture at the gastroesophageal junction. Endoscopy and biopsy excluded malignancy.

Direct dilatation was unsuccessful because of the density of the scar tissue.

Surgical resection of her cervial stricture with plastic reconstruction was necessary to remove her upper stricture and 6 weeks later her lower stricture was dilated. She is now eating without recognizable obstruction, no longer aspirates and has noted a substantial reduction in cough and sputum production.

Both of these patients illustrate the difficulties which may be encountered in recognizing problems at the cricopharyngeal level. In the case of Mr. H. the diagnosis was missed until his malignancy was noted endoscopically. With Mrs. Y., her respiratory symtpoms were secondary to aspiration; however, this component of her history was only obtained on direct questioning and could easily have been missed. Other problems must be considered in differential diagnosis.

"Globus hystericus" is a term commonly applied to psychogenic dysphagia. Although this form of dysphagia can be psychogenic, most patients so labeled have an organic basis for their dysphagia. Recognition and appropriate treatment of the cause will result in gratifying improvement in their symptoms. In one review of 85 patients given the diagnosis "globus hystericus," 75 per cent had demonstrable organic disease (61). In another review of 440 patients, 79 per cent had organic disease and 62 per cent of these had a hiatal hernia (62). Therefore the symptom of this sensation, a "lump" in the throat, must be investigated thoroughly to exclude organic and remediable disease.

Although pharyngoesophageal dysfunction is usually secondary to gastroesophageal reflux, each patient should be evaluated fully before a specific diagnosis can be made. As a minimum, this investigation requires history and radiology, but many patients also need manometric studies and endoscopy to completely elucidate their problem.

On history alone the presence of reflux symptoms strongly suggests that the disorder is secondary; however, reflux may be associated with pharyngoesophageal pouches and bars and my coexist with myogenic or neurogenic disorders. Nasal regurgitation, if present, strongly suggests a neurogenic, myogenic or myoneurogenic disorder.

Manometric studies are of great value in the recognition of these various primary dis-

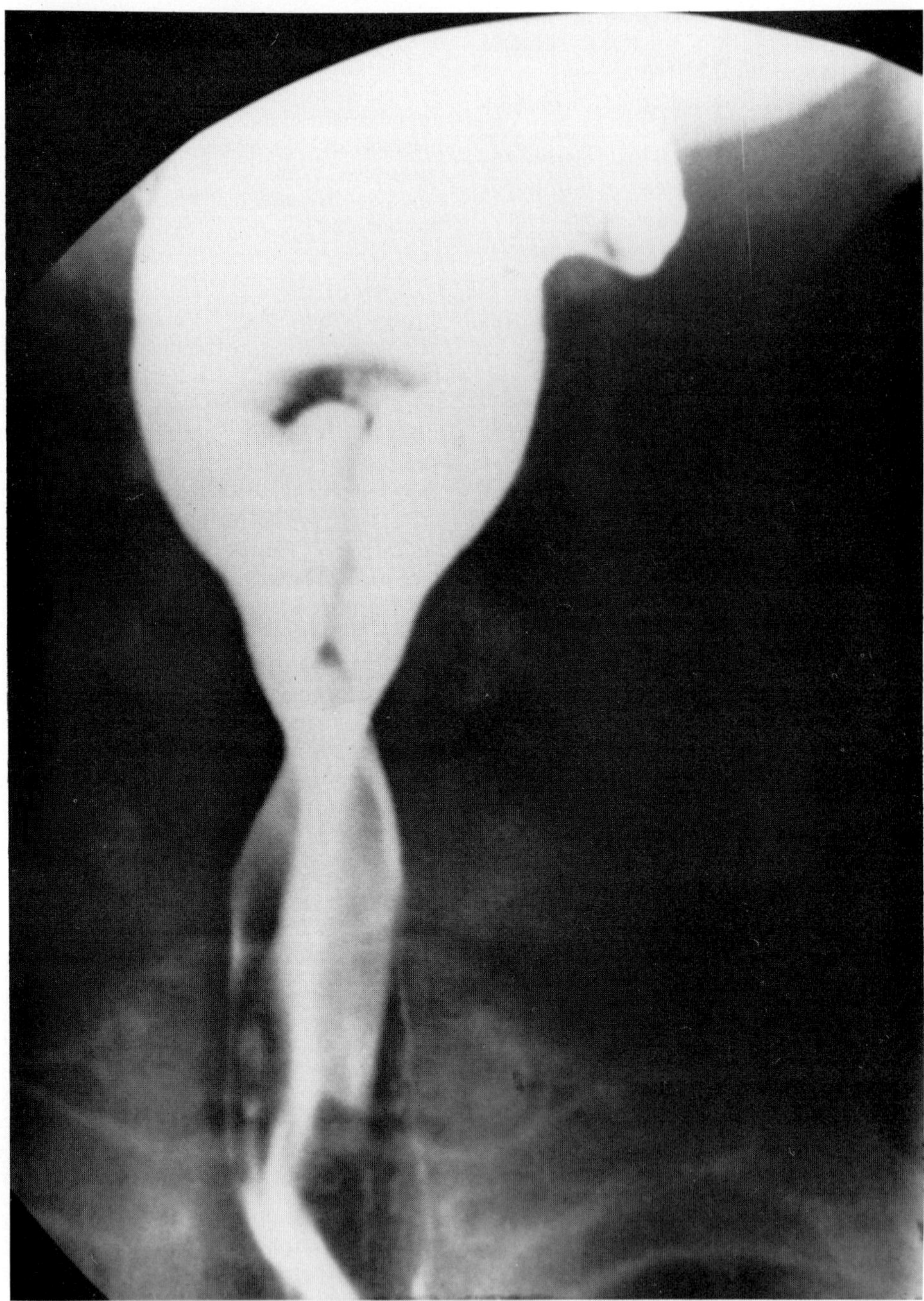

Figure 19.18
Mr. H. (Case 12) had a hiatal hernia with reflux and severe cricopharyngeal dysphagia. Radiologically his pharyngoesophageal junction was normal. Endoscopically a small squamous cell carcinoma was present.

orders. Manometry also may help in localizing the level of obstruction and allowing an adequate prediction of the effects of cricopharyngeal myotomy. Endoscopy makes a valuable contribution to assessment, particularly when it is desirable to exclude mechanical obstruction from the differential diagnosis.

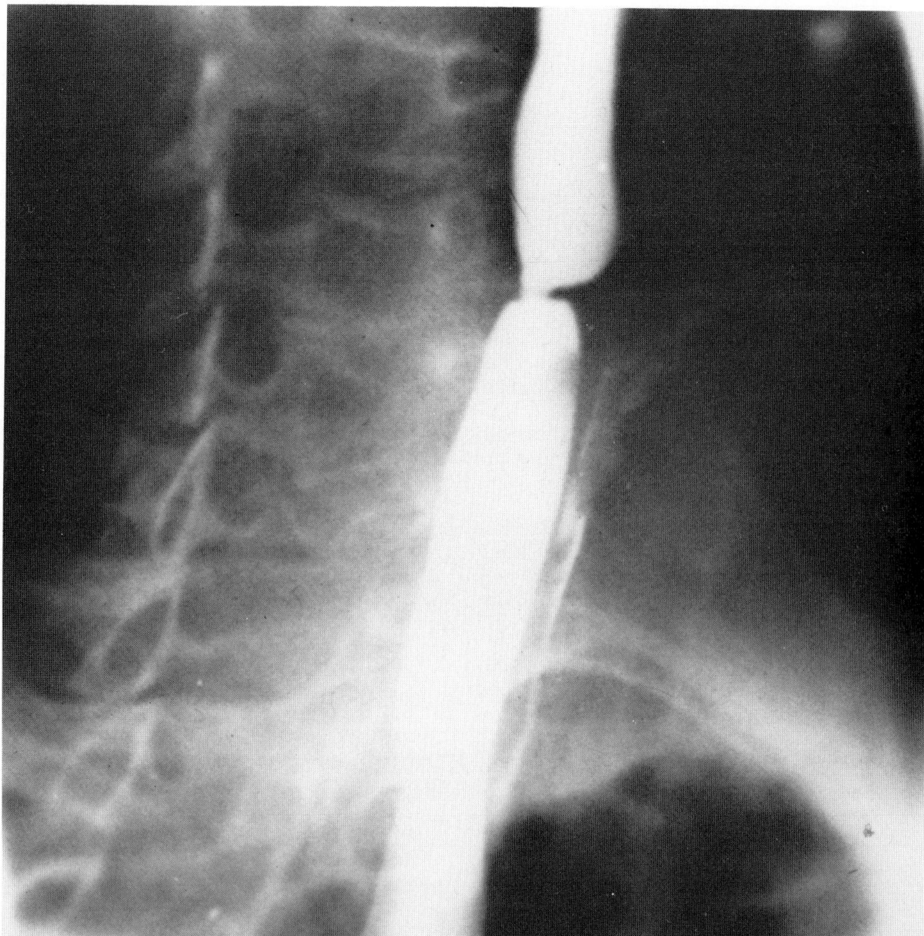

Figure 19.19
Mrs. Y. (Case 13). This patient had a hiatal hernia with reflux and severe cricopharyngeal dysphagia. A stricture was present in the cervical esophagus.

In most patients, careful evaluation permits the physician to arrive at a specific diagnosis and so recommend or carry out definitive therapy.

References

1. Henderson, R. D., and Pearson, F. G.: Surgical management of esophageal scleroderma. J. Thorac. Cardiovasc. Surg., *66:* 686, 1973.
2. Welch, R. W., Luckmann, K., Ricks, P. M., and Drake, S. T.: Manometry of the normal upper esophageal sphincter and its alterations in laryngectomy. J. Clin. Invest. *63:* 1036, 1979.
3. Weisbrodt, N. W.: Neuromuscular organization of esophageal and pharyngeal motility. Arch. Intern. Med., *136:* 524, 1976.
4. Henderson, R. D., Woolf, C., and Marryatt, G.: Pharyngoesophageal dysphagia and gastroesophageal reflux. Laryngoscope, *86:* 1531, 1976.
5. Henderson, R. D., and Marryatt, G.: Aspiration and gastroesophageal reflux. Can. J. Surg., *21:* 351, 1978.
6. Hunt, P. S., Connell, A. M., and Smiley, T. B.: The cricopharyngeal sphincter in gastric reflux. Gut, *11:* 303, 1970.
7. Watson, W. C., and Sullivan, S. N.: Hypertonicity of the cricopharyngeal sphincter; a cause of globus sensation. Lancet, *2:* 1417, 1974.
8. Winans, C. S.: The pharyngoesophageal closure mechanism; a manometric study. Gastroenterology, *63:* 768, 1972.
9. Ellis, F. H., Jr., Schlegel, J. F., Lynch, V. P., and Pyne, W. S.: Cricopharyngeal myotomy for pharyngo-esophageal diverticulum. Ann. Surg., *170:* 340, 1969.
10. Henderson, R. D., and Marryatt, G.: Cricophayngeal myotomy as a method of treating cricopharyngeal dysphagia secondary to gastroesophageal reflux. J. Thorac. Cardiovasc. Surg., *74:* 721, 1977.
11. Hanna, W., and Henderson, R. D.: Nemaline rods

in cricopharyngeal dysphagia. Am. J. Clin. Pathol., In press, 1980.

12. Shy, G. M., Engel, W. K., and Somers, J. E.: Nemaline myopathy; a new congenital myopathy. Brain, *86:* 793, 1963.

13. Ludlow: A case of obstructed deglutition from a preternatural dilation of, and bag formed in the pharynx. Medical Observations and Inquiries, Society of Physicians, London, *3:* 85, 1769.

14. Perott, J. W.: Anatomical aspects of hypopharyneal diverticula. Aust. N.Z. J.Surg., *31:* 307, 1962.

15. Kodicek, J., and Creamer, B.: A study of pharyngeal pouches. J. Laryngol. Otol., *75:* 406, 1961.

16. Delahunty, J. E., Margulies, S. I., Alonso, W. A., and Knudsen, D. H.: The relationship of reflux esophagitis to pharyngeal pouch (Zenker's diverticulum). Laryngoscope, *81:* 570, 1971.

17. Shallow, T. A., and Clerf, L. H.: One stage pharyngeal diverticulectomy; improved technique and analysis of 186 cases. Surg. Gynecol. Obstet., *86:* 317, 1948.

18. Brintnall, E. S., and Kridelbaugh, W. W.: Congenital diverticulum of posterior hypopharynx simulating atresia of esophagus. Ann. Surg., *131:* 564, 1950.

19. Groves, L. K.: Pharyngoesophageal diverticulum in each of three sisters; report of cases. Cleve. Clin. Q., *35:* 207, 1968.

20. Clgett, O. T., and Payne, W. S.: Surgical treatment of pulsion diverticula of the hypopharynx; one-stage resection in 478 cases. Dis. Chest, *37:* 257, 1960.

21. Fischer, M. J., and Bond, J. F.: Carcinoma in a pharyngoesophageal diverticulum. J. Thorac. Cardiovasc., Surg., *53:* 500, 1967.

22. Shirazi, K. K., Daffner, R. H., and Gaede, J. T.: Ulcer occurring in Zenker's diverticulum. Gastrointest. Radiol., *2:* 117, 1977.

23. Som, M. L., and Deitel, M.: Carcinoma in a large pharyngoesophageal diverticulum. Arch. Surg., *94:* 35, 1967.

24. Finney, G. G., Jr., and Gaertner, R. A.: Surgical treatment of pharyngo-esophageal diverticula. South. Med. J., *57:* 375, 1964.

25. Hiebert, C. A.: Surgry for cricopharyngeal dysfunction under local anesthesia. Am. J. Surg., *131:* 423, 1976.

26. Lahey, F. H., and Warren, K. W.: Esophageal diverticula. Surg. Gynecol. Obstet., *98:* 1, 1954.

27. Einarsson, S., and Hallén, O.: On the treatment of esophageal diverticula. Acta Otolaryngol. (Stockh.), *64:* 30, 1967.

28. Bingham, D. L.: Cricopharyngeal achalasia. Can. Med. Assoc. J., *89:* 1071, 1963.

29. Belsey, R.: Functional disease of the esophagus. J. Thorac. Cardiovasc. Surg., *52:* 164, 1966.

30. Butcher, R. B., and Larrabee, W. F.: Surgical treatment of hypopharyngeal (Zenker's) diverticulum. Arch. Otolaryngol., *105:* 254, 1979.

31. Silver, C. E., and Fell, S. C.: Repair of pharyngoesophageal diverticulum by resection with myotomy and muscle closure. Surg. Gynecol. Obstet., *147:* 599, 1978.

32. Dohlman, G., and Mattsson, O.: The endoscopic operation for hypopharyngeal diverticula; a roentgencinematographic study. Arch. Otolaryngol., *71:* 744, 1960.

33. Seaman, W. B.: Cineroentgenographic observations of the cricopharyngeus. A.J.R., *96:* 922, 1966.

34. Parrish, R. M.: Cricopharyngeus dysfunction and acute dysphagia. Can. Med. Assoc. J., *99:* 1167, 1968.

35. Sutherland, H. D.: Cricopharyngeal achalasia. J. Thorac. Cardiovasc. Surg., *43:* 114, 1962.

36. Utian, H. L., and Thomas, R. G.: Cricopharyngeal incoordination in infancy. Pediatrics, *43:* 402, 1969.

37. Mitchell, R. L., and Armanini, G. B.: Cricopharyngeal myotomy; treatment of dysphagia. Ann. Surg., *181:* 262, 1975.

38. Kramer, P., Atkinson, M., Wyman, S. M., and Ingelfinger, F. J.: The dynamics of swallowing; II. Neuromuscular dysphagia of pharynx. J. Clin. Invest., *36:* 589, 1957.

39. Schwab, R. S., and Viets, H. R.: Roentgenoscopy of pharynx in myasthena gravis before and after prostigmine injection. A.J.R., *45:* 357, 1941.

40. Schotland, D. L., and Rowland, L. P.: Muscular dystrophy. Features of ocular myopathy, distal myopathy and myotonic dystrophy. Arch. Neurol., *10:* 433, 1964.

41. Victor, M., Hayes, R., and Adams, R. D.: Oculopharyngeal muscular dystrophy; a familial disease of late life characterized by dysphagia and progressive ptosis of the eyelids. N. Engl. J. Med., *267:* 1267, 1962.

42. Bergman, A. B., and Lewicki, A. M.: Complete esophageal obstruction from cricopharyngeal achalasia. Radiology, *123:* 289, 1977.

43. Bender, M. D.: Esophageal manometry in oculopharyngeal dystrophy. Am. J. Gastroenterol., *65:* 215, 1976.

44. Hurwitz, A. L., Duranceau, A., and Haddad, J. K.: *Disorders of Esophageal Motility,* vol. XVI, Major Problems in Internal Medicine. W. B. Saunders Co., Philadelphia, 1979.

45. Dayal, V. S.: Cricopharyngeal myotomy for dysphagia in oculopharyngeal muscular dystrophy. Arch. Otolaryngol., *102:* 115, 1976.

46. Fischer, R. A., Ellison, G. W., Thayer, W. R., Spiro, H. M., and Glaser, G.: Esophageal motility in neuromuscular disorders. Ann. Intern. Med., *63:* 229, 1965.

47. Lebo, C. P., and Norris, F. H.: Cricopharyngeal myotomy in amyotrophic lateral sclerosis. Laryngoscope, *86:* 862, 1976.

48. Schleider, M. A., and Nagurney, J. T.: Progressive supranuclear ophthalmoplegia. J.A.M.A., *237:* 994, 1974.

49. Glendell, H. M., McCallum, J. E., and Reigel, D. H.: Cricopharyngeal achalasia associated with Arnold-Chiari malformation in childhood. Childs Brain, *4:* 65, 1978.

50. Calcaterra, T., Kadell, B. M., and Ward, P. H.: Dysphagia secondary to cricopharyngeal muscle dysfunction, surgical management. Arch. Otolaryngol., *101:* 726, 1975.

51. Kaplan, S.: Paralysis of deglutition, post-poliomyelitis complication treated by section of cricopharyngeus muscle. Ann. Surg., *133:* 572, 1951.

52. Kaplan, S.: Paralysis of the swallowing mechanism following bulbar poliomyelitis; surgical restoration of function. Arch. Otolaryngol., *65:* 495, 1957.

53. Weitz, R., Varsano, I., Geifman, M., et al: Cricopharyngeal achalasia associated with congenital suprabulbar paresis. Helv. Paediatr. Acta., *3:* 271, 1976.

54. Riley, C. M., Day, R. L., Greeley, D. M., and Langford, W. S.: Central autonomic dysfunction with defective lacrimination; report of 5 cases. Pediatrics, *3:* 468, 1949.
55. Linde, L. M., and Westover, J. L.: Esophageal and gastric abnormalities in dysautonomia. Pediatrics, *29:* 303, 1962.
56. Margulies, S. I., Brunt, P. W., Donner, M. W., and Silbiger, M. L.: Familial dysautonomia; a cineradiographic study of the swallowing mechanism. Radiology, *90:* 107, 1968.
57. Kilman, M. J., and Goyal, R. K.: Disorders of pharyngeal and upper esophageal sphincter motor function. Arch. Intern. Med., *136:* 592, 1976.
58. Henderson, R. D., Boszko, A., and van Nostrand, A. W. P.: Pharyngoesophgeal dysphagia and recurrent laryngeal nerve palsy J. Thorac. Cardovasc. Surg., *68:* 507, 1974.
59. Butler, E. C., and Tarsitano, J. J.: Dysphaga and ossified stylohyoid ligament; report of a case. Laryngoscope, *79:* 499, 1969.
60. Ratnesar, P.: Dysphagia due to cervical exostosis. Laryngoscope, *80:* 469, 1970.
61. Slater, E.: Diagnosis of "hysteria." Br. Med. J., *1:* 1395, 1965.
62. Malcomson, K. G.: Globus hystericus vel pharyngis (a reconnaissance of proximal vagal modalities). J. Laryngol. Otol., *82:* 219, 1968.

Esophageal Diverticula and Mixed Motor Disorders

CHAPTER 20

Esophageal Diverticula

Although relatively rare, esophageal diverticula present an interesting group of disorders with varying etiology and symptoms (Fig. 20.1). In 1840 Rokitansky (1) divided diverticula into traction and pulsation types, and this provided a classification which is still useful in defining their nature and location. Traction diverticula are associated with adjacent scar tissue, which by its adherence to the surface of the esophagus produces a traction force which tents the esophageal wall (2). Since the scar adheres to the surface of the diverticulum, the outpouching contains all the layers of the esophageal wall.

Pulsion diverticula are a local "blowout" of esophageal mucosa. They may be produced by intermittent increases in esophageal pressure associated with local weakness in the esophageal wall that allows the mucosa to escape between the muscle layers.

All esophageal diverticula do not fit this simple classification; some show no local scar that would have produced traction and occasionally there is no evidence of increased intraluminal pressures to produce the required pulsion force. Occasionally, diverticula may be congenital and represent an esophageal reduplication, and many diverticula defy adequate classification.

The three major groups described in the

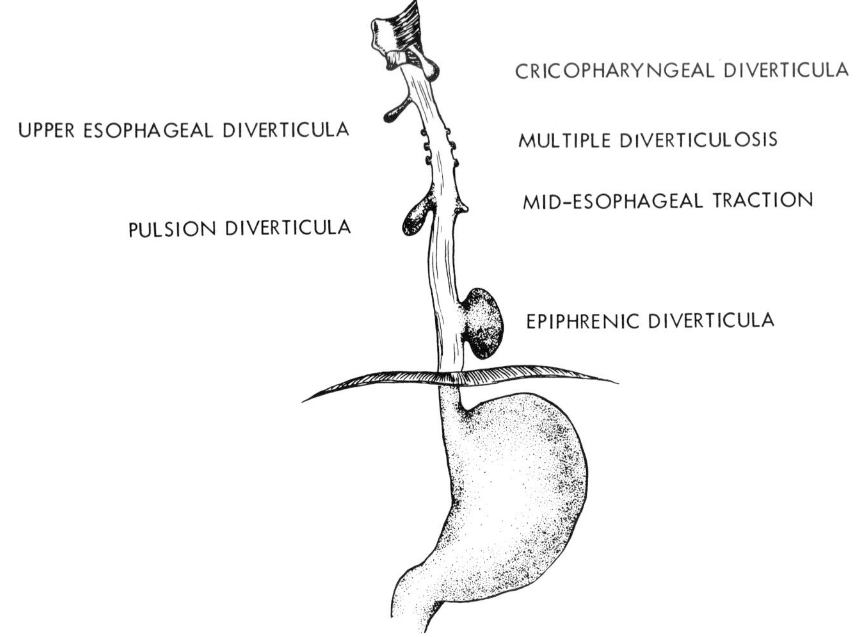

Figure 20.1. Esophageal Diverticula
The four major categories of diverticula are: 1) cricopharyngeal; 2) midesophageal: A) traction, B) pulsion; 3) epiphrenic, and 4) multiple diverticulosis. This figure also illustrates a lateral wall upper esophageal diverticulum.

literature are the cricopharyngeal diverticula, midesophageal diverticula and epiphrenic diverticula, although others have been described, such as upper one-third esophageal diverticula and multiple diverticula (diverticulosis) of the esophagus. The cricopharyngeal diverticula are of a typical pulsion type (3). With swallowing, pharyngeal and cricopharyngeal incoordination produces an increase in pressure immediately above the cricopharynx, and a "blowout" diverticulum develops through the weak posterior wall of the lower pharynx. This mucosal sac is devoid of the outer muscle layers of the pharynx. Chapter 19 provides a more detailed description of these diverticula.

Epiphrenic diverticula may develop in the lower one-third of the esophagus (4). These too are of a pulsion type and are related to increased intraluminal esophageal pressure and to a weakness of the esophageal wall. Epiphrenic diverticula do not have esophageal musculature in their walls.

Traction diverticula tend to appear in the midesophagus close to the subcarinal tracheobronchial lymph nodes. These are usually tent-shaped, and their walls contain the normal elements of the esophageal wall. As the surgeon examines each of these diverticula more closely, he sees that the Rokitansky description, while applicable to some, does not explain all of their features.

Epiphrenic Diverticula

The epiphrenic diverticulum is a rare but important abnormality. It is located in the distal esophagus, usually within 2 to 3 cm of the gastroesophageal junction. It varies in size from a few centimeters to grapefruit size. The term "pulsion diverticulum" is applied to it because of its spherical or pear-shaped configuration. Its walls are lined by mucosa, submucosa and muscularis, and there is some fibrous tissue on its surface.

In most series, over 50 per cent of epiphrenic diverticula are associated with motor abnormalities (4), and this association—motor abnormalities, a mucosal lining and the spherical shape—led to its classification as a pulsion diverticulum.

Habein and colleagues (5) have classified the motor abnormalities associated with these diverticula as diffuse spasm (DES) in 13 per

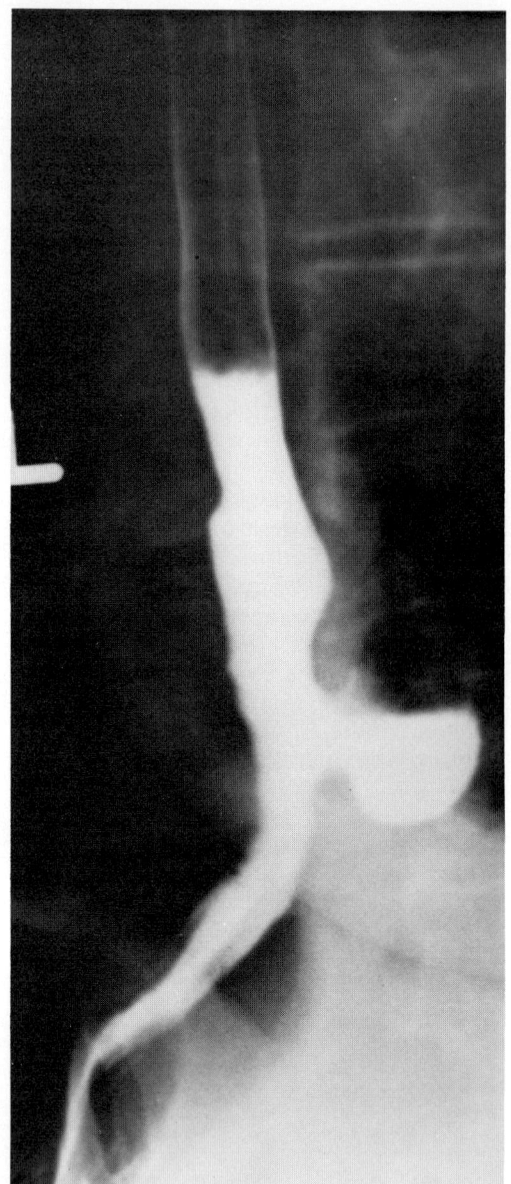

Figure 20.2
Mrs. W. (Case 1) presented with midretrosternal pain and dysphagia. Radiologically she had an epiphrenic diverticulum of moderate size associated with esophageal motor spasm. This patient shows the typical radiologic features.

cent, achalasia in 3 per cent, and those characteristic of hiatal hernia in 22 per cent. In a later series of 160 cases, Allen and Clagett (6) reported an incidence of DES of 24 per cent, achalasia of 10 per cent and hiatal hernias of

34 per cent. Some of the patients in Allen and Clagett's series were considered to have more than one disorder.

Symptoms

The symptoms produced by a diverticulum vary with the type of associated motor abnormality. Some patients may have no symptoms or minimal symptoms, and the diverticulum may be an incidental radiologic finding. In patients with associated DES, achalasia or a hiatal hernia, the symptoms follow the usual pattern for these disorders. The diverticulum may produce food obstruction, but the contribution of the diverticulum to the dysphagia cannot be determined from history. A review of the results of early surgical treatment (7), where the diverticulum was excised without correcting associated motor problems, suggests that in many of the patients the symptoms persisted following surgery, and that a significant part of the presenting symptoms was related to the associated motor disorder and not to the diverticulum.

Investigation

The choice of investigation, viz., radiology, manometry and endoscopy, and the mode of therapy depend on the presenting symptoms. If these symptoms are severe, full evaluation is mandatory, because management depends on the recognition of the associated pathology.

Radiology

The radiologic appearance is usually specific (Fig. 20.2), but one must be careful to exclude a sigmoid achalasia or local esophageal perforation (8). In patients with previous esophageal surgery a diverticulum may protrude at the site of muscle wall injury (9). The diverticulum protrudes from the esophageal lumen, usually with a wide base of attachment. The maximum diameter of the diver-

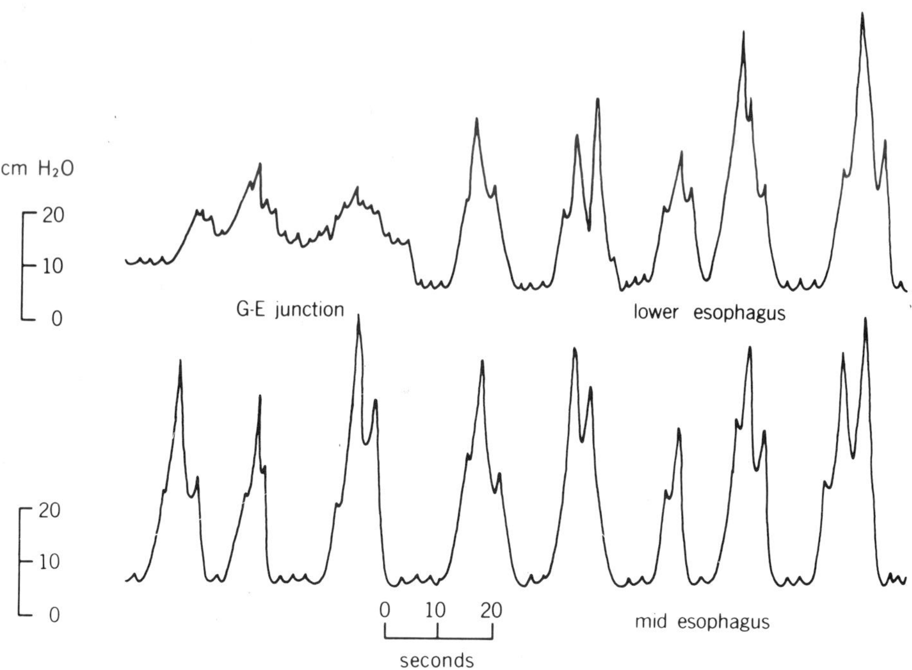

Figure 20.3. Epiphrenic Diverticulum and Primary Diffuse Spasm
Manometrically Mrs. W. (Case 1) had a low-tone gastroesophageal (G-E) junction which still relaxed in response to deglutition. The esophageal motor waves in the body of the organ were disordered, of high amplitude and often multiphasic. Peristalsis was present in the upper one-third of the esophagus. These findings support the diagnosis of an epiphrenic diverticulum with diffuse spasm.

ticulum varies from a few centimeters up to 20 to 30 cm. Radiographic examination permits some evaluation of the obstruction by observing the passage of liquids and solids and by observing whether old food products are retained. Careful inspection may detect ulceration within the diverticulum, and malignancy is occasionally found (6).

During the radiologic study care must be taken to detect or exclude the presence of a hiatal hernia, achalasia or DES (10). Often motor spasm will be recognized but will be difficult to categorize, and in this group of patients manometric evaluation is mandatory.

Esophageal Manometry

Occasionally it is difficult to obtain full manometric evaluation because the catheters may lodge in the diverticulum and will not pass into the distal esophagus. When full evaluation is possible, as it usually is with perseverence, the main object is to detect and record the secondary disordered motor activity of a hiatal hernia, or a primary motor abnormality of DES or achalasia. In my series of 51 patients treated surgically for diffuse spasm, 3 have had epiphrenic diverticula.

The combination of history, radiology and manometry usually allows a specific diagnosis and gives the examiner enough information to plan definitive therapy. Endoscopy is a useful addition because it allows assessment of the pouch and the detection of associated pathology. This procedure excludes malignancy with a high degree of accuracy (11). In some patients it is difficult to pass the endoscope into the distal esophagus; however, with care and experience full evaluation is usually possible.

Treatment

Medical management is limited to the amelioration of symptoms. A careful dietary and antacid regimen may benefit associated gastroesophageal reflux. Achalasia and DES usually do not respond to conservative management. Surgical treatment is not mandatory and should be reserved for those who have significant major symptoms which do not respond to medical treatment.

Early surgical approaches excised the diverticulum but made no attempt to correct the underlying motor disorder. Several small

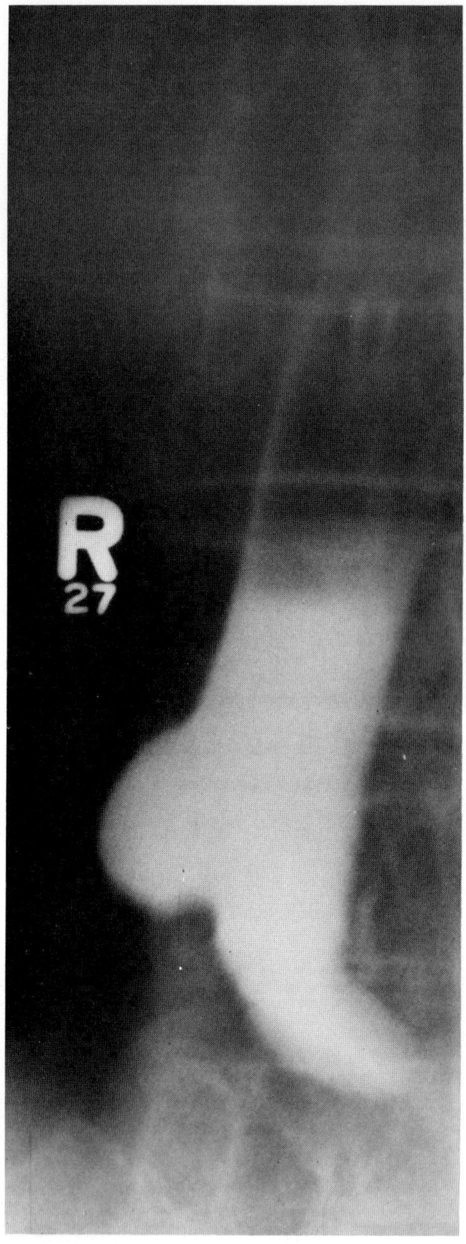

Figure 20.4
Mr. S. (Case 2) has a small radiologic epiphrenic diverticulum and a hiatal hernia with reflux. His dominant symptoms were those of reflux; he had no significant dysphagia.

series reported fistula formation or persistent dysphagia in up to 50 per cent of cases (7).

In those selected for operation, the guiding principles are now well established. It is vital that full evaluation be completed before surgery, because the choice of operation depends on the recognition of the associated motor abnormality and its specific type. For example, all patients do not require a myotomy; this should be reserved for those with DES or achalasia.

Three types of procedure may be planned following evaluation. If the patient has gastroesophageal reflux it should be corrected and the diverticulum excised. If the patient has DES or achalasia, the diverticulum is excised and the motor disorder corrected by an appropriate myotomy (12–14). In this situation it is important that all defects be recognized before operation, because the precise categorization of the motor abnormality is based chiefly on preoperative evaluation and assessment.

The following case histories illustrate the value of preoperative evaluation.

Case 1. Mrs. W., age 60, presented with symptoms of reflux and with a clear history of night aspiration. In addition, she had major food obstruction at the gastroesophageal junctional level. Her episodes of aspiration were magnified by severe asthma, which was not controlled by drug therapy.

Radiologically she had a hiatal hernia with free reflux (Fig. 20.2). She also had a 20-cm epiphrenic diverticulum, but no evidence of food retention in the diverticulum.

Manometric studies showed a severe, high-amplitude type of disordered motor activity (DMA) (Fig. 20.3) unlike the low-amplitude DMA commonly seen in association with a hiatal hernia. Peristalsis in the proximal esophagus was normal and the cricopharynx and pharynx were also normal. She was considered to have an epiphrenic diverticulum, hiatal hernia and DES.

At thoractomy the large diverticulum was excised. The esophageal muscle was hyperplastic and on direct palpation showed typical and marked spasm. Extended myotomy was done and the hiatal hernia was repaired. In the 4 years since operation she has remained well and has had no significant residual esophageal symptoms.

Case 2. Mr. S., age 30, presented with gastroesophageal reflux and typical epigastric and retrosternal burning discomfort. He had only occasional and mild gastroesophageal dysphagia.

The radiograph showed a 10-cm epiphrenic diverticulum, a 6-cm hiatal hernia and gastroesophageal reflux (Fig. 20.4). On manometry the motor changes were slight and of low amplitude (Fig. 20.5).

Because of failure of conservative management, the hiatal hernia was repaired and the diverticulum excised. The esophageal wall was normal to palpation. Because of the lack of objective evidence of achalasia or DES, he did not have a myotomy. His postoperative course has been excellent and he remains free of symptoms 3 years later.

These two cases illustrate the wide variance in associated pathology and show how the procedure of choice can be selected before operation. The first patient had DES and needed a myotomy to relieve dypshagia. The

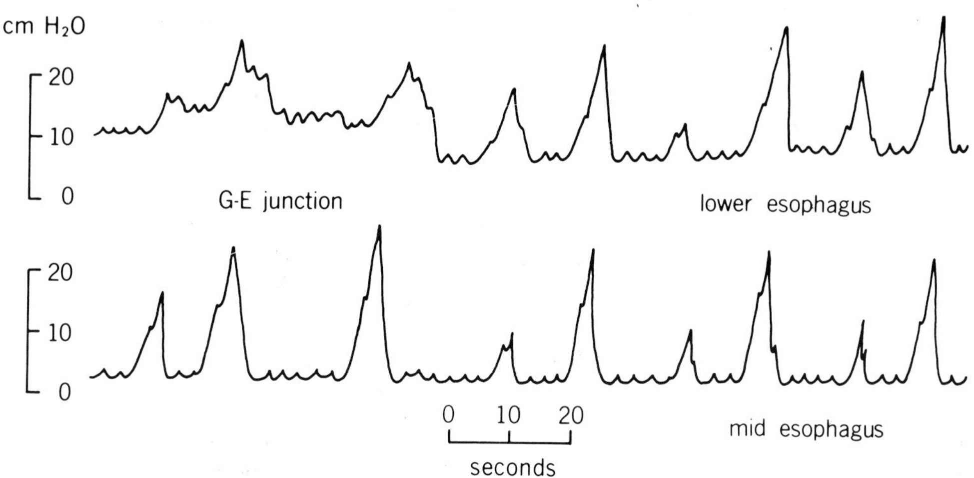

Figure 20.5. Epiphrenic Diverticulum and Hiatal Hernia
Manometrically Mr. S. (Case 2) had a totally respiratory negative gastroesophageal (G-E) junction and a slight degree of low-amplitude disordered motor activity. These findings are in keeping with a hiatal hernia.

second patient had only a hiatal hernia, and correction of reflux with excision of the diverticulum effectively controlled his dysphagia. Achalasia in my experience is very rarely associated with an epiphrenic diverticulum.

Midesophageal Diverticula

Most commonly these diverticula are of the traction type and the esophageal wall is tented outward, suggesting that it is fixed by scar to adjacent lymph nodes. The diverticula are made up of the normal esophageal wall. Their relationship to scar fixation has not been firmly established, and when they are examined at operation, most do not show any fixation (2). Certainly scar fixation can cause traction diverticula, and this presumably was etiologically more common when tuberculosis was rampant (15).

These diverticula are usually found accidentally during radiologic examination (16) and of themselves give rise to only minor symptoms. Occasionally when inflamed they can produce dysphagia and odynophagia. Authors have described fistulous communication from traction diverticula to the tracheobronchial tree and to the vascular system (16, 17). Recently recurrent laryngeal paralysis has also been noted (18).

Although the bulk of midesophageal diverticula are of the tented traction type, some "pulsion" diverticula do occur. Kaye (19) described such diverticula in 12 patients, 6 of whom had associated motor abnormalities— DES in 5 and achalasia in 1. The remaining 6 patients had minor unclassifiable motor abnormalities. This association of diffuse spasm and a pulsion type of midesophageal diverticulum is not as rare as previously considered, and I have personal experience with 5 such cases, 3 of whom have required surgical correction.

In evaluating midesophageal diverticula the primary assessment is historical. If symptoms are slight, usually these patients can be followed and treated conservatively. Where symptoms are more severe and persistent, full evaluation is necessary before selecting therapy. Again radiology, manometry and endoscopy are the main modes of investigation. Radiology allows accurate localization and characterization of diverticular shape and size. Motor abnormalities may be recognized and, if present, indicate the need for further study. In the traction diverticulum, manometry will show little abnormality; associated motor problems are more common in the pulsion type. Endoscopy is valuable in excluding alternate diagnoses and in detecting inflammation or ulceration.

Treatment, which is reserved for the few patients who have significant and persistent symptoms, ranges from simple excision of the diverticulum to excision and myotomy to correct the motor disorder.

The following case histories illustrate the range of diagnostic and therapeutic problems encountered in these patients.

Case 3. Dr. W., a 35-year-old physician, suddenly developed midretrosternal pain on swallowing, which persisted for 24 hours and then subsided. Thereafter it recurred intermittently but with diminished severity over the next 4 years. His symptoms throughout remained mild and did not require treatment. Radiologic study demonstrated a small midesophageal diverticulum (Fig. 20.6), and no further evaluation or treatment was considered necessary.

Case 4. Mrs. P., age 76, had a 10-year history of painful dysphagia which had become much more severe in the previous 6 months. All solids produced pain, dysphagia and regurgitation, and she had reduced her intake to liquids and semisolids. Even with this diet, she had considerable pain at each meal and she reduced her oral intake further. She lost 20 pounds over this 6-month period. The radiograph (Fig. 20.7) showed a midesophageal pulsion diverticulum with an ulcer at its base. She had, in addition, a small hiatal hernia. The manometric changes were compatible with a hiatal hernia and gastroesophageal reflux, but the dominant esophageal motor waves were peristaltic (Fig. 20.8). Endoscopy showed a large pulsion diverticulum with a central ulcer crater. Because of the severity of her symptoms the diverticulum was treated by local excision. No attempt was made to repair her hernia, because we did not believe she could stand the trauma of a major procedure. She tolerated local excision well, and 6 months later eats a normal diet.

These case histories illustrate the two ends of the spectrum of midesophageal diverticula. It should be emphasized that the great majority of diverticula in this zone do not require surgical correction.

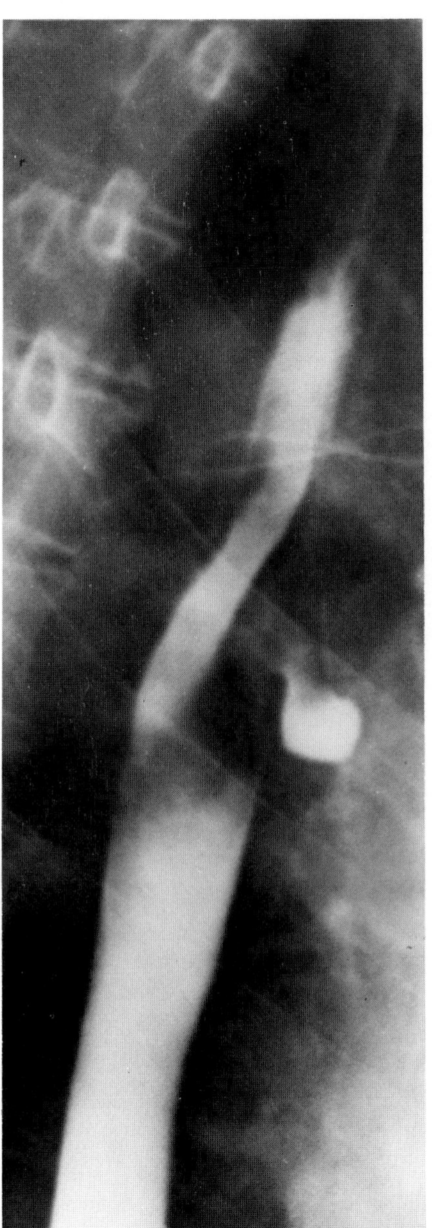

Figure 20.6. Midesophageal Traction Diverticulum.
Radiograph of Dr. W. (Case 3) illustrates a typical midesophageal traction diverticulum which is tented laterally from the esophagus at the subcarinal level. These outpouchings usually do not produce symptoms and are often an incidental radiologic finding. There are no calcific lymph nodes.

Case 5. Mrs. McS., age 50, was admitted to hospital for investigation of chest pain. She had had recurrent episodes of midesophageal pain going to her back and left shoulder. The pain had been present for 3 years but was becoming more severe. It usually came on spontaneously, but was occasionally aggravated by exercise and by midesophageal dysphagia.

Cardiologic studies including an exercise cardiogram and coronary angiography were normal. Radiologically, a small midesophageal pulsion diverticulum was present, and the esophageal wall was measured and found to be 6 mm thick. Manometry demonstrated a high-amplitude motor disorder characteristic of DES (Fig. 20.9). Acid perfusion studies exactly reproduced her chest pain. This woman has been treated conservatively by diet and long-acting nitrites, but continues to have symptoms. She has elected to continue with medical management.

This case demonstrates the combination of a pulsion type of midesophageal diverticulum associated with a primary motor disorder.

Case 6. Mrs. F., age 58, had a 2-year history of dysphagia which had progressively increased in severity and now was disabling with a 15-pound weight loss and increasing general debility. She had rheumatoid arthritis and was consuming enteric-coated aspirin necessary to maintain her joint function.

Radiologic studies demonstrated a midesophageal pulsion diverticulum with a stricture immediately below the outflow of the diverticulum (Fig. 20.10). Manometry indicated the presence of diffuse spasm and a hiatal hernia. She was treated by dilatation to #60 Fr. The stricture was in squamous lined midesophagus. Her symptoms, although improved by dilatation, were still severe and it was elected to proceed to surgery. At operation the diverticulum was excised, an extended myotomy performed and reflux control gained by a modified Nissen fundoplication with only ½ to 1 cm of total fundoplication. Now, 1 year following surgery, she is asymptomatic. This combination of a midesophageal pulsion diverticulum, diffuse spasm and a midesophageal web stricture is unusual; however, I have treated one other patient with identical findings and this woman has also done well following surgery. My impression is that these unusual strictures are due to swallowed irritants producing a local burn at the outflow of the diverticulum. In Case 6, this patient used enteric aspirin and in the presence of stasis this may produce erosions and ultimately stricture formation.

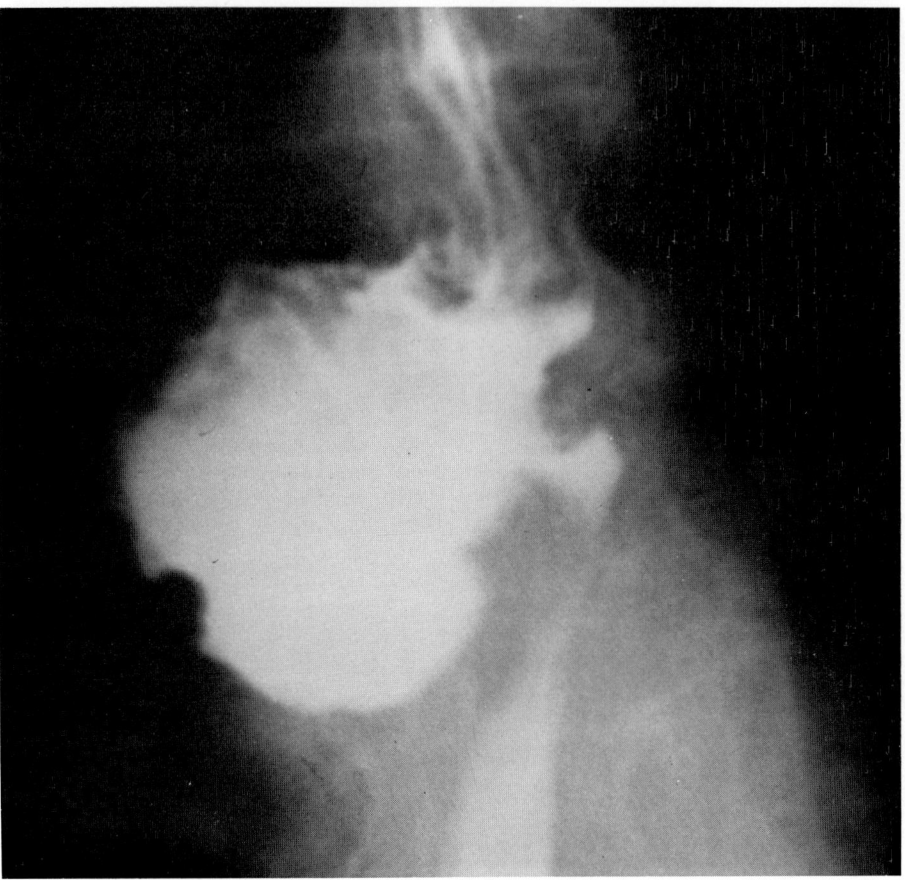

Figure 20.7. Non-traction Diverticulum of Midesophagus
Mrs. P. (Case 4) presented with severe dysphagia. The diverticulum visualized on the radiograph was large and ulcerated. At operation there was no evidence of granulomatous adherence. The patient had an associated hiatal hernia with a slight secondary motor disorder.

Intramural Diverticulosis

This rare disorder, which consists of multiple, small (1 to 3 mm) diverticula scattered throughout the esophagus (Fig. 20.1) was first described by Mendl and colleagues in 1960 (20). These patients can present in any age group (21), and most present with dysphagia, the cause of which is uncertain even though associated motor spasm and high esophageal strictures have been reported in this disorder (22–25). *Candida albicans*, which has been cultured from esophageal specimens in several of these patients, may predispose to spasm (26) and stricture formation (27). At present treatment is confined to management of complications, e.g. dilatation of strictures and treatment of the monilia infection by nystatin (Mycostatin). The most established form of treatment is dilatation and in the limited number of reported cases this is moderately effective (28).

Multiple Esophageal Diverticula

Intramural diverticulosis must not be confused with multiple esophageal diverticula. Both are very rare conditions, however, quite distinct. I have now seen 2 patients, one with four diverticula and one with six diverticula scattered throughout the body of the esophagus. There are rare reports of similar diverticula (29) and also reports of unusual diverticula associated with an adynamic esophagus in patients with scleroderma (30).

In one of the patients, Case 7, Mr. A., age 53, the initial presentation was at another hospital. At that time he gave a history of occasionally wakening at night choking on undigested food. He had surgical removal of his largest diverticulum which was epiphrenic. I saw him only for management of postoperative problems which spontaneously

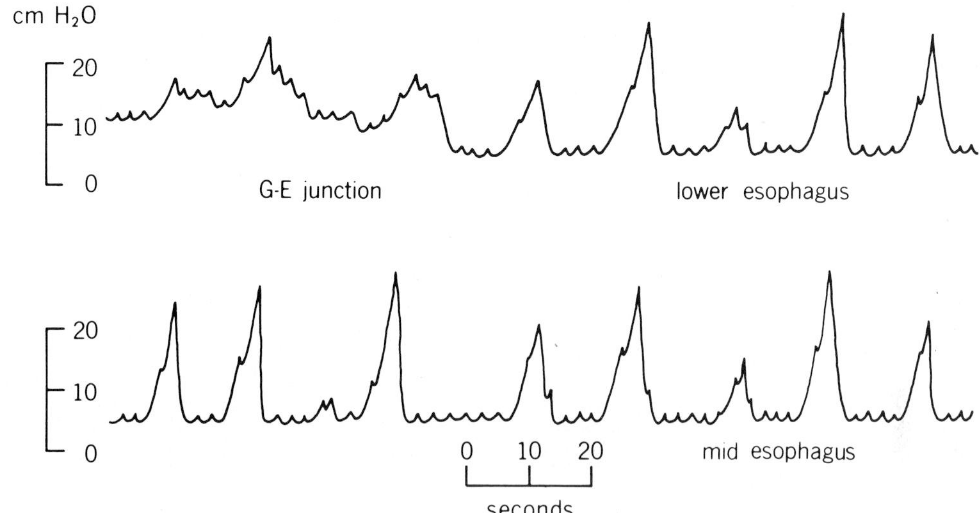

Figure 20.8. Midesophageal Pulsion Diverticulum and Hiatal Hernia
Mrs. P. (Case 4) has a midesophageal pulsion diverticulum with an associated hiatal hernia. Manometry showed only a slight degree of secondary disordered motor activity. These findings confirm the diagnosis of hiatal hernia and exclude the presence of a primary motor disorder. G-E, gastroesophageal.

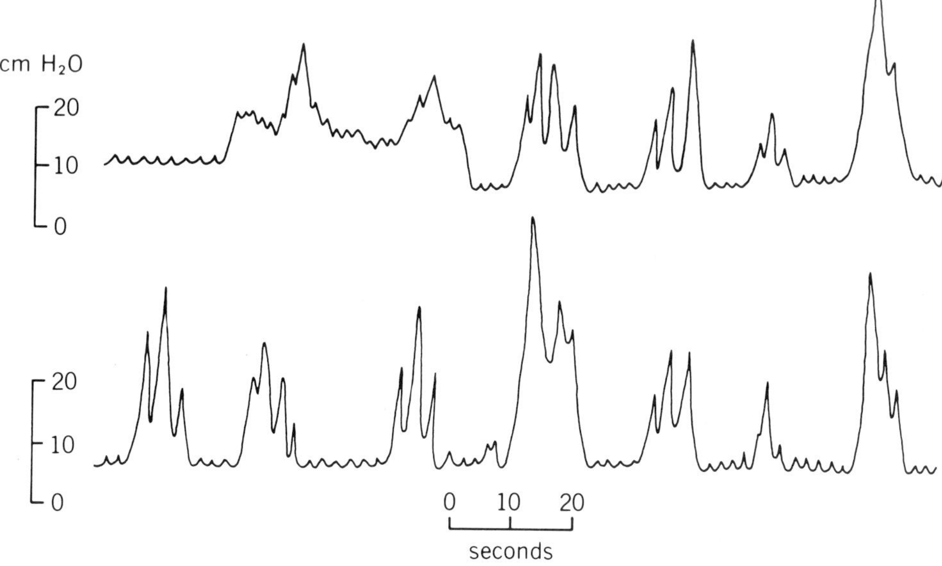

Figure 20.9. Hiatal Hernia, Midesophageal Diverticulum and Diffuse Spasm
Mrs. McS. (Case 5) has a midesophageal diverticulum and a hiatal hernia with associated reflux. She has a severe motor disorder that was characterized manometrically as DES. In the distal two-thirds of the esophagus this tracing shows high-amplitude multiphasic motor waves of prolonged duration similar to those seen in Figure 20.3.

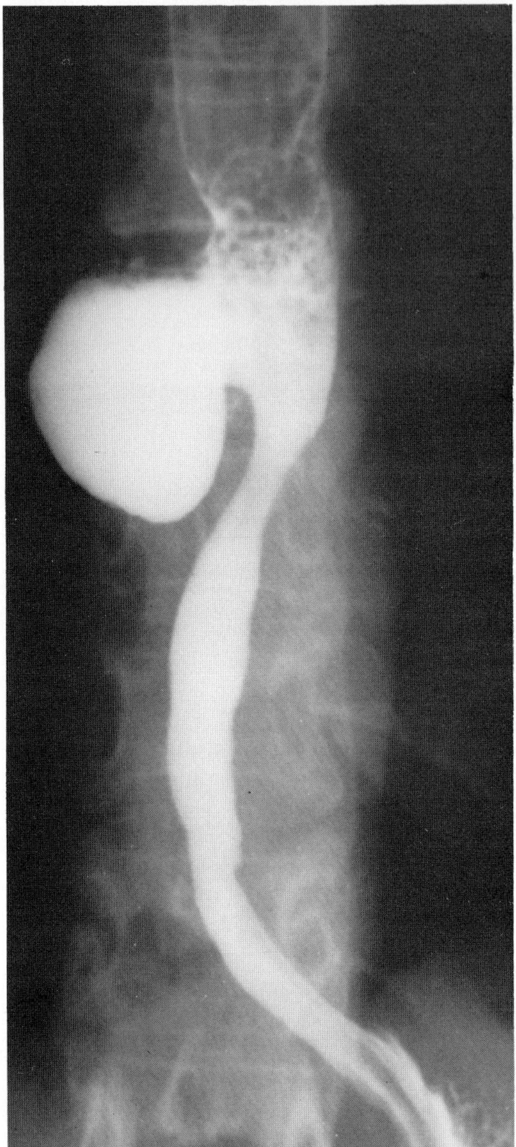

Figure 20.10
Mrs. F. (Case 6) has a midesophageal pulsion diverticulum, a hiatal hernia with reflux and DES. This narrow zone immediately below the diverticulum is a fixed stricture in squamous line esophagus.

resolved. He is now asymptomatic and has no significant manometric disorder. No further treatment is necessary (Fig. 20.11).

My other patient with multiple diverticula has minor heartburn symptoms, no evidence of a primary motor disorder and requires only minimal antacid medication for effective control.

Other rare diverticula of the esophagus do not conform to the usual classic descriptions. The following case histories illustrate two such diverticula.

Case 8. Mr. Z., age 48, had a lateral esophageal diverticulum below the level of the cricopharyngeal muscle (Fig. 20.12), which was associated with a hiatal hernia, reflux and aspiration. The origin of this diverticulum and its relationship to his symptoms are uncertain. He described a constant discomfort in his throat and pain radiating to his right ear. Manometric evaluation did not

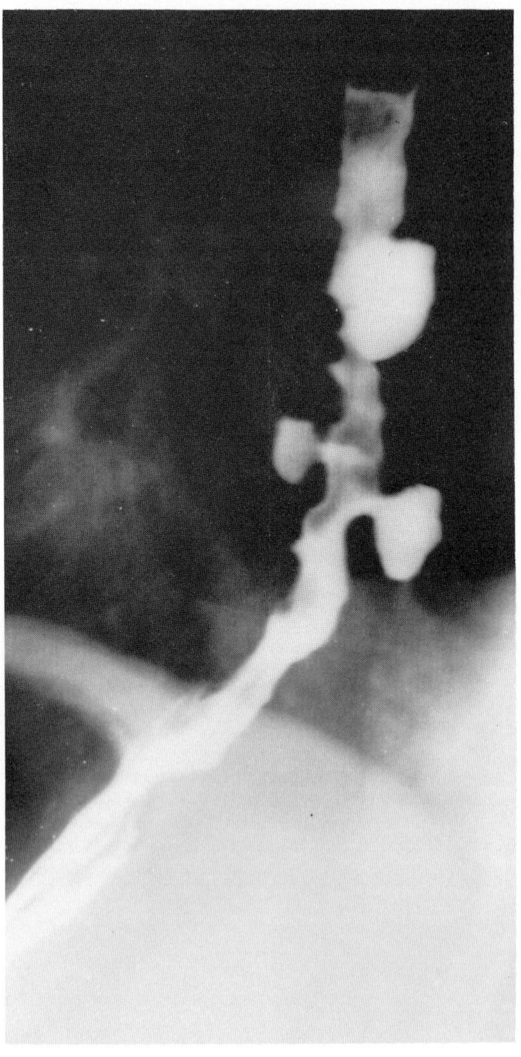

Figure 20.11
Mr. A. (Case 7) had 6 esophageal diverticula. One was excised by another surgeon and three are visible in the present x-ray.

show any motor abnormality, and, in particular, showed no motor changes at the pharyngoesophageal junction. The mouth of the diverticulum was seen at endoscopy, but there was no evidence of inflammation. His symptoms and, in particular, the discomfort in his throat and right neck were relieved by diverticulopexy, cricopharyngeal myotomy and correction of his hiatal hernia.

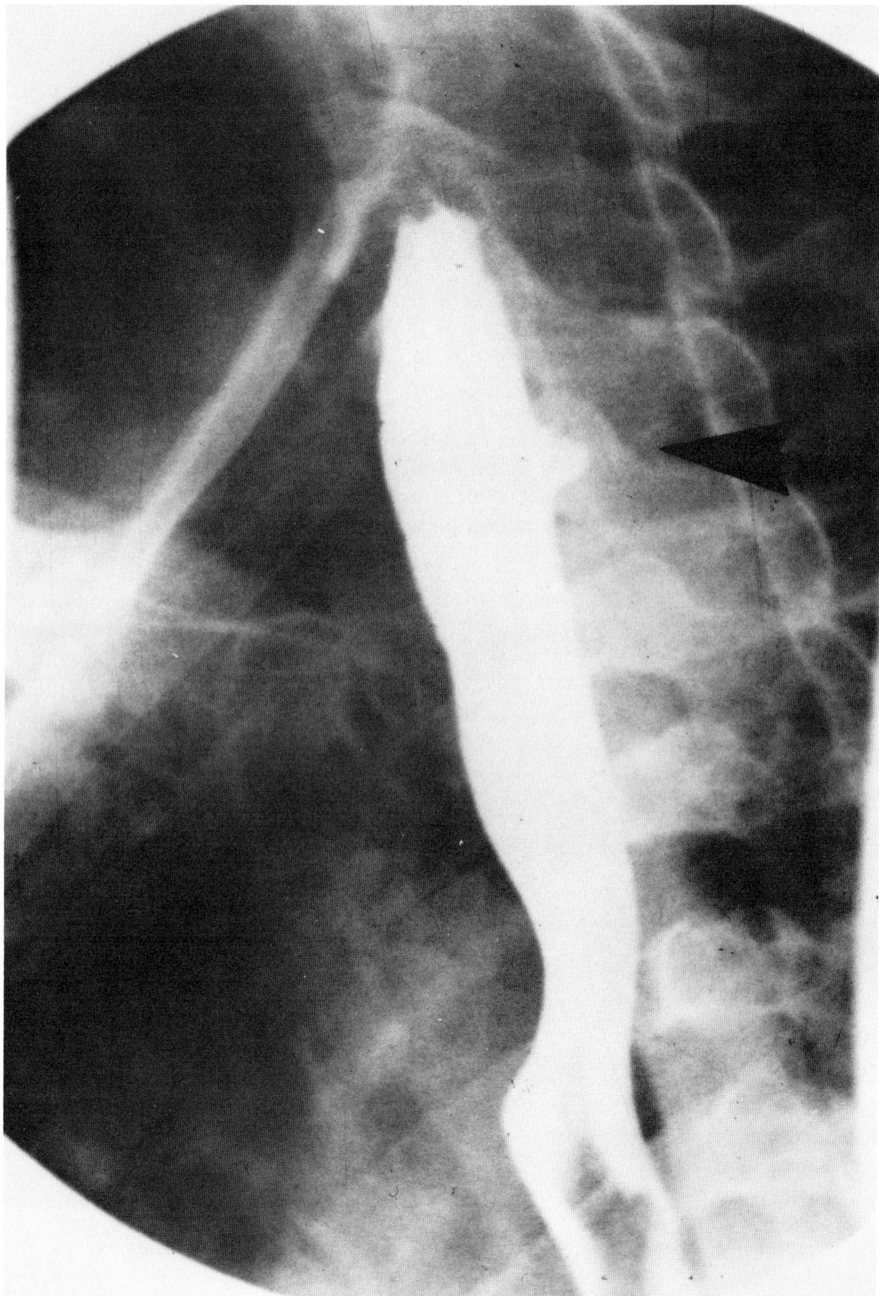

Figure 20.12. Upper One-third Esophageal Diverticulum
Radiograph of Mr. Z. (Case 8) shows a small lateral diverticulum, which gave rise to neck pain radiating to the ear. The diverticulum arose from the upper one-third of the esophagus below the level of the cricopharyngeal muscle. This structure contrasts with cricopharyngeal diverticula which protrude through a posterior weakened zone immediately above the cricopharynx.

The source of his neck pain has not been explained. However, this may have been a traction diverticulum secondary to previous neck injury because its base was attached to strands of fibrous scar. Similar diverticula have been recently reported in the literature (31).

Case 9. Mr. S., age 26, presented with recurrent respiratory infection and with dysphagia and odynophagia. Radiologically he had a small traction diverticulum and a bronchoesophageal fistula (32) (Fig. 20.13). Division of the diverticulum corrected the dysphagia and brought an end to his respiratory infections. This diverticulum resembled those described at the carinal level and differed only in the level at which the esophageal wall adhered to local pulmonary structures. A lymph node at the base of the diverticulum contained a caseating granuloma from which acid-fast bacilli were isolated. In its mode of production this structure corresponds to the classic traction diverticulum.

Esophageal diverticula form a diverse group and each requires careful investigation. The surgeon can choose definitive therapy only after he has evaluated associated motor disorders.

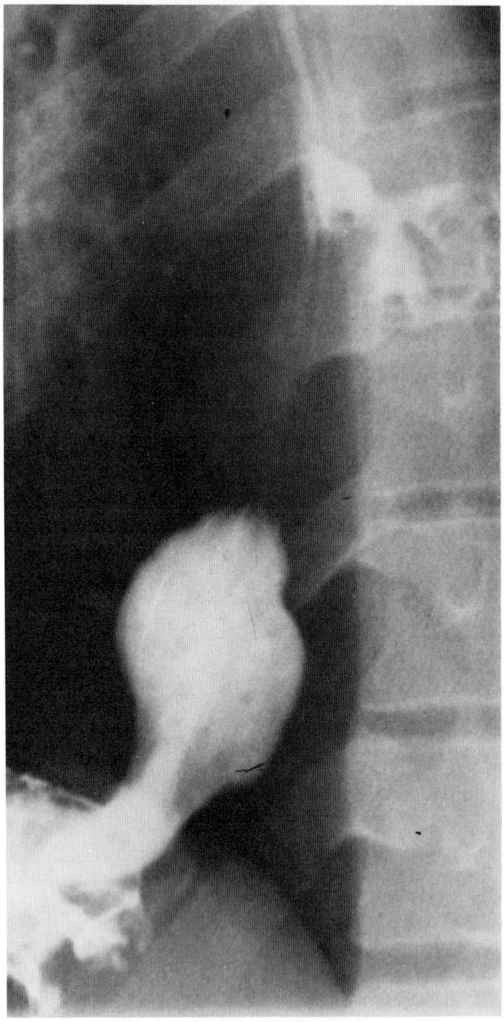

Figure 20.13. Traction Diverticulum with Bronchial Fistula

Mr. S. (Case 9) had a diverticulum which was lower than usual and incorporated a tuberculous lymph node. He also had an esophagobronchial fistulous tract. At operation the diverticulum and fistula were visualized and divided, with resolution of respiratory and esophageal symptoms.

References

1. Rokitansky, C.: Spindelformige Erweiterung der Speisrohrf. Med. Jahrb. d.k.k. Osterr. Staates, *21:* 219, 1840.
2. Law, S. W., and Overstreet, J. W.: Pulsion diverticula of the mid-thoracic esophagus. J. Thorac. Cardiovasc. Surg., *48:* 855, 1964.
3. Ellis, F. H., Jr., Schlegel, J. F., Lynch, V. P., and Payne, W. S.: Cricopharyngeal myotomy for pharyngo-esophageal diverticulum. Ann. Surg., *170:* 340, 1969.
4. Goodman, H. I., and Parnes, I. H.: Epiphrenic diverticula of esophagus. J. Thorac. Surg., *23:* 145, 1952.
5. Habein, H. C., Jr., Moersch, H. J., and Kirklin, J. W.: Diverticula of the lower part of the esophagus; clinical study of 149 non-surgical cases. Arch. Intern. Med., *97:* 768, 1956.
6. Allen, T. H., and Clagett, O. T.: Changing concepts in the surgical treatment of pulsion diverticula of the lower esophagus. J. Thorac. Cardiovasc. Surg., *50:* 455, 1965.
7. Harrington, S. W.: Surgical treatment of pulsion diverticula of thoracic esophagus. Ann. Surg., *129:* 606, 1949.
8. Franklin, R. H., Kay, R. G., Sigman, H. H., and LeBrun, H.: Large oesophageal diverticulum simulating achalasia of the cardia. Br. J. Surg., *50:* 889, 1963.
9. Gatklin, J., Bloch, R., and Sundgren, R.: Intraphrenic esophageal leiomyoma associated with diverticula preoperatively diagnosed by angiography. Acta Radiol. [Diagn.] (Stockh.), *16:* 673, 1974.
10. Cross, F. S., Johnson, G. F., and Gerein, A. N.: Esophageal diverticula; associated neuromuscular changes in the esophagus. Arch. Surg., *83:* 525, 1961.
11. Plous, E., Freedman, J., and Wolfe, P. L.: Carcinoma within a lower esophageal (epiphrenic) diverticulum. J. Thorac. Cardiovasc. Surg., *47:* 129, 1964.
12. Effler, D. B., Barr, D., and Groves, L. K.: Epiphrenic diverticulum of the esophagus; surgical treatment. Arch. Surg., *79:* 459, 1959.
13. Joseph, W. L., Katz, R. I., Levin, P. A., and Longmire, W. P., Jr.: The diagnosis and treatment of esophageal diverticula. Ann. Thorac. Surg., *3:* 375, 1967.
14. Henderson, R. D., Ho, C. S., and Davidson, J. W.:

Primary disordered motor activity of the esophagus (diffuse spasm). Ann. Thorac. Surg., *18:* 327, 1974.

15. MacCarty, R. L., Dukes, R. J., Strimlan, C. V., Dines, D. E., and Payne, W. S.: Radiographic findings in patients with esophageal involvement by mediastinal granuloma. Gastrointest. Radiol., *4:* 11, 1979.

16. Wallace, R. P.: Traction diverticulum of esophagus (roentgenographic demonstration; symptoms noted in series of 26 patients). Arch. Intern. Med., *60:* 454, 1937.

17. Schick, A., and Yesner, R.: Traction diverticulum of esophagus with exsanguination; report of case. Ann. Intern. Med., *39:* 345, 1953.

18. Lerner, M. A., and Katz, R.: A new syndrome of left vocal cord paresis and esophageal diverticulum due to mediastinal fibrosis. A.J.R., *125:* 193, 1975.

19. Kaye, M. D.: Oesophageal motor dysfunction in patients with diverticula of the mid-thoracic oesophagus. Thorax, *29:* 666, 1974.

20. Mendl, K., McKay, J. M., and Tanner, C. H.: Intramural diverticulosis of the oesophagus and Rokitansky-Aschoff sinuses in the gallbladder. Br. J. Radiol., *33:* 496, 1960.

21. Braun, P., Nussle, P. B., Roy, C. C., and Cuendet, A.: Intramural diverticulosis of the esophagus in an eight-year-old boy. Pediatr. Radiol., *6:* 235, 1978.

22. Creely, J. J., and Trail, M. L.: Intramural diverticulosis of the esophagus. South. Med. J., *63:* 1257, 1970.

23. Montgomery, R. D., Mendl, K., and Stephenson, S. F.: Intramural diverticulosis of the oesophagus. Thorax, *30:* 278, 1975.

24. Fee, B. E., and Dvorak, A. D.: Intramural pseudodiverticulosis of the esophagus. Neb. Med. J., *61:* 9, 1976.

25. Rahle, G., Wilbert, L., Lankisch, P. G., and Huttemann, U.: Intramural esophageal diverticulosis. Acta Hepatogastroenterol (Stuttg.), *24:* 110, 1977.

26. Overbeek, J. J. M., Edens, E. T., Gökemeijer, J. D. M., and Broker, F. H. L.: Intramural diverticulosis of the esophagus. Laryngoscope, *88:* 1671, 1978.

27. Weller, M. H., and Lutzker, S. A.: Intramural diverticulosis of the esophagus associated with postoperative hiatal hernia, alkaline esophagitis and esophageal stricture. Radiology, *98:* 373, 1971.

28. Castillo, S., Aburashed, A., Kimmelman, J., and Alexander, L. C.: Diffuse intramural esophageal pseudodiverticulosis. New cases and review. Gastroenterology, *72:* 514, 1977.

29. Jancu, J., and Marvan, H.: Multiple diverticula of the esophagus. Am. J. Gastroenterol., *60:* 408, 1973.

30. Clements, J. L., Abernathy, J., and Weens, H. S.: Atypical esophageal diverticulae associated with progressive systemic sclerosis. Gastrointest. Radiol., *3:* 383, 1978.

31. Cooper, R. A.: Lateral diverticulum of the cervical esophagus. J.A.M.A., *242:* 415, 1979.

32. Balthazar, E. J.: Esophagobronchial fistula secondary to ruptured traction diverticulum. Gastrointest. Radiol., *2:* 119, 1977.

CHAPTER 21

Mixed Motor Disorders of the Esophagus

A variety of esophageal motor disorders will be discussed in this chapter. Some are very rare and are mentioned only for completeness, some have minor or absent associated symptoms and others are normal variations of age and pregnancy. Recognition of these motor changes is important in diagnosis, but also in the differential diagnosis of major esophageal motor disorders.

These diseases can be classified as primary when related to neurogenic or myogenic failure and secondary when related to endogenous or exogenous esophageal irritation.

Among these mixed motor disorders neurogenic primary diseases are most common. Included for discussion are the diabetic and alcoholic esophagus, motor changes of Parkinsonism, hereditary spastic ataxia, neural damage from ganglion destruction and neurologic stimulation from endogenous hormonal release and secondary to the toxin release of tetanus.

Diabetes

The gastrointestinal manifestations of diabetes include delayed gastric emptying and slow transit time in the small bowel (1). The esophageal component of diabetic neuropathy, which has been recognized only recently, rarely produces significant symptoms.

In random studies of patients with diabetes, the motor abnormality, which can be demonstrated radiologically and manometrically, does not produce symptoms and bears no relationship to the patient's age, the duration of the diabetes or the presence of other gastrointestinal abnormalities (2). Radiologic (3) and manometric studies show extensive motor changes throughout the esophagus. The pharyngeal motor wave is of low amplitude but the cricopharynx functions normally. In the body of the esophagus, there is an increase of disordered motor activity, a decrease in the motor response to deglutition and a reduction in the amplitude of peristalsis. Gastroesophageal junctional tone is reduced and the relaxation in response to deglutition is poor (4–8). These well-developed findings almost certainly reflect vagal degeneration secondary to diabetic neuropathy.

Case 1. Mrs. G., age 62, had a 2-year history of diabetes that was well controlled by diet and insulin. She developed mild retrosternal burning discomfort and intermittent dysphagia to solid food. The initial radiologic studies of her stomach and esophagus were reported as normal. However, manometric studies showed a totally respiratory-negative gastroesophageal junction, and moderate low-amplitude lower esophageal disordered motor activity. We considered that these motor changes were related to a hiatal hernia and gastroesophageal reflux and concluded that the component which vagal neuropathy may have contributed was masked by the effects of reflux.

Further radiologic studies demonstrated a small hiatal hernia and free reflux. Treatment by diet, bed elevation and antacids relieved her symptoms completely.

Although initial radiologic studies were normal, her investigation was pursued because, by itself, diabetic neuropathy did not account for her distress. Once the diagnosis of gastroesophageal reflux was made, specific therapy gave satisfactory relief of symptoms.

Case 2. Mr. R., age 41, had had severe and poorly controlled diabetes for 25 years. He had peripheral neuropathy and severe diabetic retinopathy.

Dysphagia, heartburn and reflux were his presenting symptoms. Radiologically reflux was present and a small hiatal hernia. Endoscopically he had an inflamed but nonulcerated esophagus. Manometric studies showed a low tone poorly relaxing high pressure zone (HPZ) compatible with reflux. In the body of the esophagus disordered motor activity (DMA) was very severe and of low amplitude with a mirror image pattern similar to achalasia. In the extreme upper esophagus a few peristaltic motor waves were present (Fig. 21.1). Such a severe motor abnormality was not considered compatible with reflux alone.

Surgical correction of reflux has relieved his symptoms; however, follow-up manometric studies have not shown the improvement in motor function which would be expected if reflux were the primary cause of his DMA. This man's motor disorder is considered to be secondary to his diabetic neuropathy.

Although diabetic vagal neuropathy produces manometric and radiologic changes in the esophagus, it does not by itself result in esophageal symptoms. When associated with reflux the neurologic damage may augment reflux motor abnormalities and can then be an additive factor in symptom production.

Alcoholic Neuropathy

Esophageal motor changes are found in alcoholic patients but, unlike diabetics, the motor changes are seen primarily in those with a peripheral neuropathy (9). These motor changes by themselves do not produce symptoms and are recognized only after careful radiologic and manometric study. Pharyngoesophageal function is normal and motor changes, if present, are most marked in the distal esophagus; here, there is an increase in the disordered motor activity but normal function is preserved in the gastroesophageal junctional zone (9). Although this is not proved, the motor changes are probably secondary to vagal degeneration. Like the diabetic patient, the alcoholic with esophageal motor changes requires no treatment and if he has symptoms they are usually secondary to gastroesophageal reflux and should be traced accordingly.

Parkinsonism

Esophageal symptoms are not usually associated with Parkinsonism. In his original publication, "An Essay on the Shaking Palsy," in 1817, Parkinson (10) stated—"so much are the actions of the muscles of the tongue, pharynx and c. impeded by impaired action and perpetual agitation, that the food is with difficulty retained in the mouth until masticated: and then as difficultly swallowed." The abnormality described by Parkinson is at the cricopharyngeal level; however, difficulties also arise with motor function in the body of the esophagus (11). Although the majority of Parkinson patients have cricopharyngeal and pharyngeal symptoms, a small number also complain of food

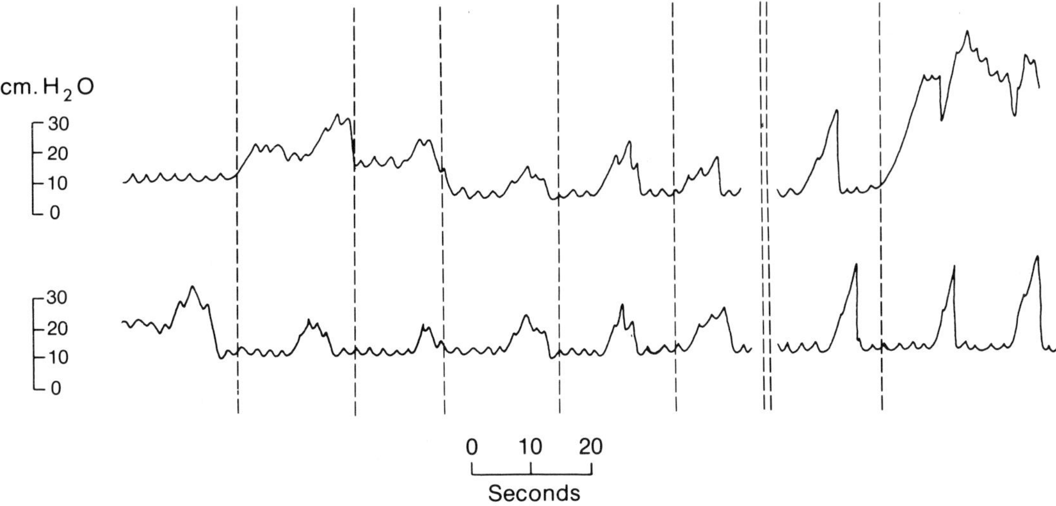

Figure 21.1. Diabetic Neuropathy and Hiatal Hernia

Mr. R. (Case 2) has gastroesophageal reflux and severe diabetic neuropathy. Manometrically his HPZ was of low tone with poor relaxation. In the body of the esophagus there was severe low amplitude disordered motor activity with peristalsis present only in the upper one-third. These motor changes are too marked to be secondary to reflux and must also reflect neural damage.

obstruction in the distal esophagus and lesions have been found in the dorsal vagal nuclei (12).

Hereditary Spastic Ataxia

This is a rare autosomal dominant disease (13). Reports of esophageal symptoms are limited. In one family minor motor abnormalities were reported in 4 of 5 affected subjects and 1 patient had dysphagia with a radiologically dilated and atonic esophagus. Manometrically there was low amplitude DMA in the body of the esophagus. The Mecholyl test was negative. These motor changes were considered to represent vagal degenerative changes.

Ganglion Destruction

Destruction of ganglia by infiltrating malignancy or amyloid has been reported as a cause of secondary esophageal motor change.

Esophageal Motor Disorders Associated with Malignancy

Kelley (14) has described motor disorders in esophageal and proximal gastric malignancy which appear to be nonspecific and to reflect local invasion of the distal esophageal wall and partial obstruction. The motor pattern includes reduced gastroesophageal junctional tone and reduced relaxation in response to deglutition. The body of the esophagus shows excessively powerful contractions, which are usually synchronous and of prolonged duration (Fig. 21.2).

Although not specific to malignancy, this motor pattern may alert the surgeon to the need for careful investigation to exclude malignancy. In some patients with submucosal malignancy at the gastroesophageal junction, the radiologic changes may mimic achalasia (15); here manometric evaluation is particularly useful.

The following cases illustrate the potential value of motor studies in the detection of malignancy.

Case 3. Mrs. B., age 46, had a 6 months' history of progressive dysphagia and, on radiologic examination, had an obstructing lesion at the gastroesophageal junction (Fig. 21.3). Endoscopy on two occasions demonstrated the obstruction but showed no evidence of active inflammation prox-

imal to it. Bouginage was attempted, but the stricture was considered undilatable by endoscopic techniques. Repeated biopsies and brushing produced no evidence of malignancy. On manometry, a tracing from the body of the esophagus showed a severe high-amplitude motor disorder that was distinctly different from the low-amplitude disturbance seen with gastroesophageal reflux (Fig. 21.2). We considered that malignancy was the most likely diagnosis and subsequently this was confirmed at operation. Here manometric studies, although not diagnostic, provided useful information and directed us toward an exploratory operation and subsequent resection.

Case 4. The experience of Mr. D. was described (p. 168) to illustrate the difficulty in distinguishing between achalasia and malignancy. He had developed progressive dysphagia over a 2-year period and was thought to have achalasia. Because the radiologic studies showed some esophageal dilation and a tapered lower esophagus (Fig. 21.4), bouginage was attempted and after it failed he had a feeding gastrostomy.

Manometry showed a diffuse, low-amplitude motor disorder in the body of the esophagus but normal proximal esophageal peristalsis. This finding excluded achalasia and attention then was directed to the undilatable stricture. Although endoscopy and biopsy had not produced a positive tissue diagnosis, open biopsy at operation confirmed that this man had a linitis plastica. Resection of the stomach gave 2 years of excellent palliation.

These two cases illustrate the importance of precise diagnosis. Although manometry did not make a specific diagnosis in either case, the evidence provided by the tracings altered our approach to therapy and led to definitive surgical treatment.

Amyloid

Amyloid involvement of the gastrointestinal tract may produce a variety of clinical and radiologic manifestations. Involvement of the esophagus can destroy the ganglion cells of the myenteric plexus and result in an atonic esophagus, mimicing achalasia or scleroderma (16–18). In extreme cases, dysphagia may become a dominant symptom with resultant weight loss of general debility.

Idiopathic Intestinal Pseudoobstruction

Idiopathic intestinal pseudoobstruction (IIP) is characterized by recurrent intestinal obstruction. The bowel is noted to be dis-

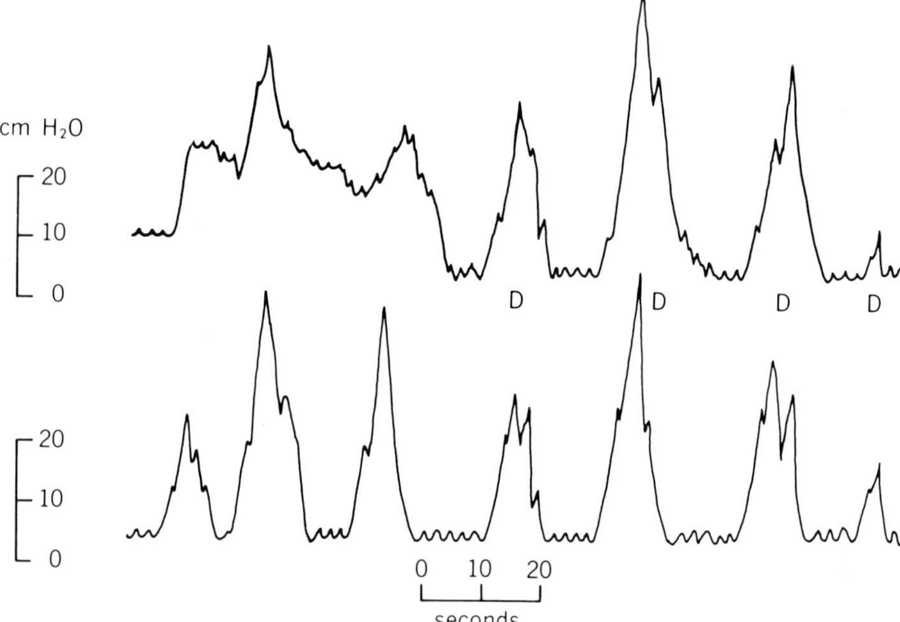

Figure 21.2. Disordered Motor Activity and Carcinoma of Esophagus
In manometry of Mrs. B. (Case 3), the gastroesophageal junction was able to relax and motor waves in the body of the esophagus were of high amplitude and prolonged duration (D). The waves are distinctly different from those seen in reflux and suggest that the distal obstruction was not a peptic stricture and hence was likely to be due to a malignancy.

tended, but there is no mechanical source of constriction (19). Secondary bacterial overgrowth may result in steatorrhea and chronic malnutrition.

Abnormalities of esophageal motor function have been described in patients with IIP, and these changes include loss of HPZ relaxation and loss of peristaltic motor activity in the body of the esophagus. The Mecholyl test is reported to be occasionally positive. These motor changes when present must be differentiated from scleroderma or achalasia. The motor changes strongly suggest a neurogenic disorder.

Although these findings are of great interest, the disorder of IIP is very rare, and the esophageal manifestations have not yet been fully studied.

Idiopathic Vagal Nerve Degeneration

We have seen two patients who presented with idiopathic unilateral recurrent nerve paralysis and severe secondary disordered esophageal motor activity.

Case 5. One patient, Mrs. C., age 60, had a classic manometric pattern of achalasia in the lower two-thirds of the esophagus with normal gastroesophageal tone. The gastroesophageal junction did not relax and showed low-amplitude disordered motor activity. Peristalsis was present and the upper one-third of the esophagus and the pharyngoesophageal junction and pharynx both functioned normally (Fig. 21.5). No gastric acid was secreted in response to the Hollander test.

This patient has good evidence of vagal paralysis—recurrent nerve palsy and one negative Hollander test. She has developed an achalasia-like pattern of motor activity in the lower esophagus, which probably is secondary to the vagal nerve lesion.

Chronic Endogenous Cholinergic Stimulation

The hormone gastrin is released from the gastric antrum under the influence of vagal stimulation and alkalinization. This hormone has a cholinergic stimulating effect which may influence HPZ tone.

In patients with Zollinger-Ellison (20) syn-

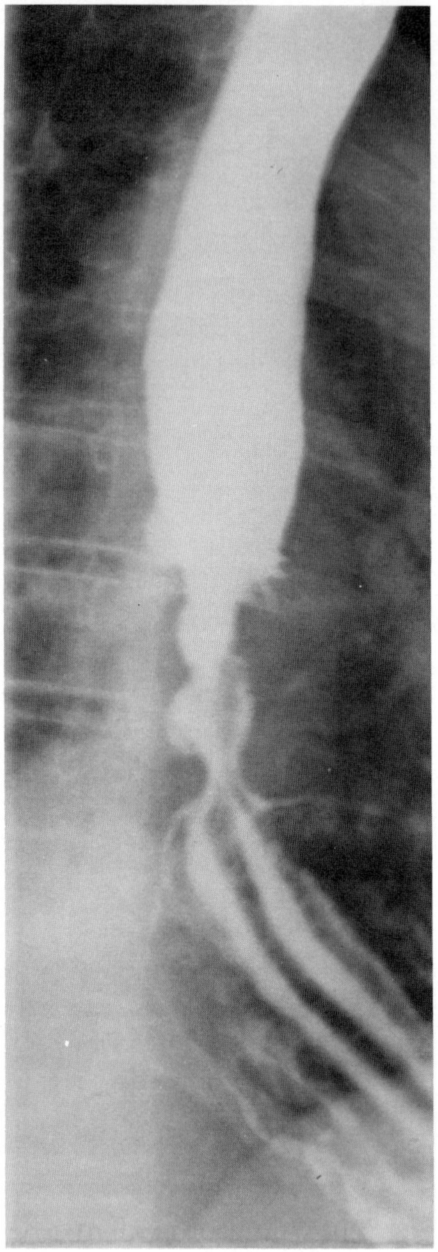

Figure 21.3
Mrs. B. (Case 3) had a lower esophageal carcinoma. Endoscopy had shown a stricture without inflammation, but brushing and direct biopsy had not produced a positive tissue diagnosis. Barium swallow shows a hiatal hernia and irregular stricture at the gastroesophageal junction. This radiologic study suggests but does not confirm malignancy.

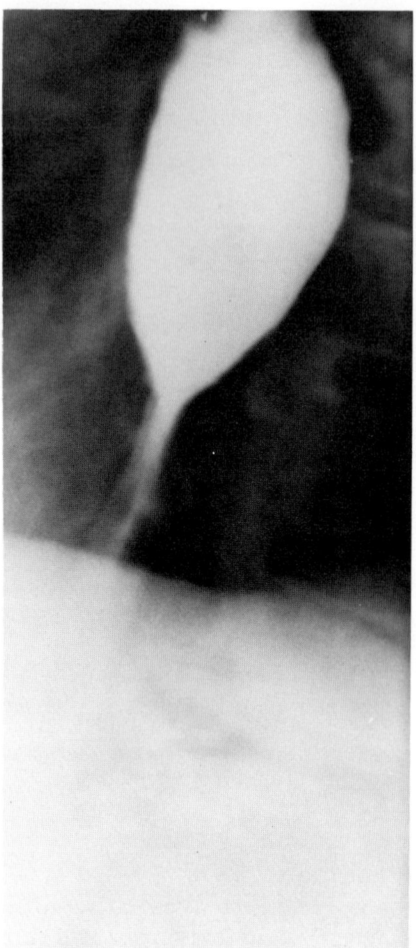

Figure 21.4. Carcinoma of Fundus of Stomach with Esophageal Obstruction
Mr. D. (Case 4) presented with progressive dysphagia of 2 years' duration. A radiologic diagnosis of achalasia was made, and he was treated inappropriately by dilatation. Later manometry showed normal peristalsis, and endoscopy did not provide a tissue diagnosis. Subsequently thoracotomy confirmed the presence of malignancy.

drome and in patients with pernicious anemia (21), there is a chronic elevation of serum gastrin levels. Manometric studies in patients with Zollinger-Ellison syndrome have demonstrated that the HPZ tone is above normal and shows an augmented response to intravenous pentagastrin. In patients with pernicious anemia, despite the high serum gastrin levels the HPZ tone is low, and they have less response to pentagastrin than that found in normal subjects.

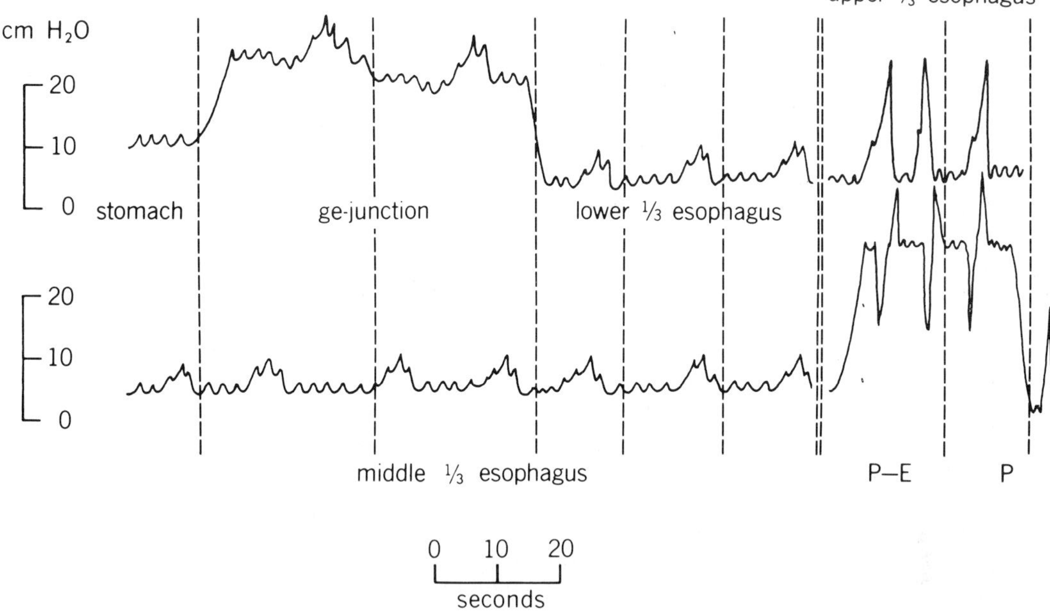

Figure 21.5. Idiopathic Vagal Nerve Degeneration
Mrs. C., age 60, has an idiopathic left recurrent laryngeal nerve palsy and a negative Hollander test. Esophageal symptoms developed abruptly following the onset of the nerve palsy. The lower esophagus shows the motor pattern characteristic of achalasia, but the proximal one-third retains peristaltic activity. P, pharynx; P-E, cricopharynx; ge, gastroesophageal.

These motor changes are of interest; however, they have not been associated with clinical symptoms.

The Esophageal Response to Infection

The esophageal response to infection varies with the infecting agent. With most bacterial and viral infections motor change is related to inflammation; however, some infections have a neurogenic effect from toxin stimulation or from neural destruction.

Classification

Primary: Neural—Nerve destruction:
　　　　　　Chagas' disease
　　　　　—Neural stimulation:
　　　　　　Tetanus
Secondary: Bacterial—Secondary infection:
　　　　　　Pemphigus
　　　　　　Epidermolysis
　　　　　　bullosa
　　Fungal—*Monilia*
　　Viral—Chickenpox virus

Chagas' Disease

This disease is confined mostly to South America (22–24). It is transmitted by the redaviid bug which bites mostly children and after a blood meal will defecate near the site of injury. It is the feces which contains the *Trypanosoma cruzi* responsible for Chagas' disease. An acute illness follows and if the child survives then an enlarged heart, megacolon or megaesophagus may follow 30 to 40 years later.

Parasites damage the esophageal ganglion cells resulting in loss of motor power and progressive esophageal dilatation. The disease in many ways mimics achalasia both in symptoms and in radiologic and manometric features.

Up to 35 per cent of people with chronic Chagas' disease develop abnormal esophageal radiology. Staging of the disease is based on the extent of esophageal dilatation: Stage I below 4 cm diameter; Stage II 4 to 7 cm; Stage III 7 to 10 cm; and Stage IV greater than 10 cm maximal diameter. As in achalasia, symptoms tend to change with increasing esophageal dilatation. In Stages I and II food obstruction and acute regurgitation may be present; in Stage III and IV obstruction, night regurgitation and aspiration of infected esophageal content may lead to secondary respiratory infection.

Manometrically changes usually start in the body of the esophagus with loss of propulsive motor waves. Both the smooth and striated muscles may be involved. As the disease progresses the HPZ becomes involved with reduced or absent relaxation. In the early stages the motor findings will vary; however, once both the body and HPZ are completely involved the motor changes may be indistinguishable from achalasia.

Treatment recommendations are similar to those in achalasia. Bag dilatation is commonly used in Stages I and II; Heller myotomy is reserved for Stages III and IV and for those who fail to respond to dilatation.

Tetanus

Dysphagia may be the presenting symptom in 30 per cent of patients with tetanus (25). Cephalic tetanus (26) involves primarily the muscles of deglutition and the pharynx. Radiologic studies in such patients show spasm of these muscles and a normal distal esophagus (27). Manometric studies, although they have not been reported, would probably show involvement of the skeletal muscle portion of the upper esophagus, cricopharynx and pharynx.

Bacterial Infections

Bacterial infections of the esophagus are rare and mostly are seen as a secondary infection in patients with pre-existing esophageal ulceration or malignancy. These would occur, for example, in patients with esophageal involvement from pemphigus (28) or epidermolysis bullosa (29).

The infectious component will produce secondary inflammatory motor change with low amplitude disordered motor activity. I have seen similar motor changes in patients with adjacent intrathoracic abscesses giving rise to edema and inflammation of the esophageal wall.

Fungal Infections

The only common fungal infection is monilia esophagitis (*Candida albicans*) (30, 31). Rarely blastomycosis and coccidiomycosis have been implicated (32). Monilia infections almost exclusively occur in patients with pre-existing and debilitating disease or patients on long-term steroids and antibiotics.

The infection presents with pain and dysphagia which may be severe (33–35). Oral monilia (thrush) is usually also present, allowing a direct visual diagnosis from recognition of the typical white spots on the roof of the mouth and pharynx.

Radiology of the esophagus demonstrates an extensive ulcerative process in the esophagus, and the mucosa is irregular and shaggy in appearance. Endoscopic evaluation shows an extreme degree of ulceration much more severe than that seen with reflux induced esophagitis.

Manometric evaluation has not been previously reported because of its lack of diagnostic specificity. I have studied two such patients presenting with atypical symptoms not clearly recognized before study. In both patients despite extensive ulceration, the esophageal motor pattern was well preserved with a minor degree of low amplitude DMA. This observation suggests that the disease is predominantly mucosal and the muscle of the esophagus is relatively free of inflammation.

Nystatin (Micostatin) is the medication of choice and is effective in the management of the uncomplicated monilia infection. Occasionally these patients have stricture. When dilatation is required for stricture, it should be done with extreme care since the esophageal wall is not as thickened as in reflux esophagitis and perforation is a significant risk.

Viral Infection

Viral infections (36–38) occur in the esophagus and have been described as a complication of chickenpox. There are no reported motor changes, although secondary DMA from inflammation almost certainly occurs and would account for the described dysphagia.

Infections produce their motor effect either by direct neural involvement or by secondary inflammation. The only specific motor abnormality is that produced by Chagas' disease.

Rare Esophageal Disorders

Behçet's disease is a systemic disorder characterized by oral and genital ulceration, arthritis and thrombophlebitis (39). In rare instances it is associated with esophageal ulceration. In one patient described by Arma and colleagues (40), the esophageal motor studies resembled those seen in achalasia and, subsequently, Heller myotomy produced complete resolution of the dysphagia. This appears to be the only patient with Behçet's disease reported to date who had esophageal manometric studies.

Case 6. Mrs. N., age 59, is similar to the patient reported by Brodie and Ochsner (41). She had nonspecific esophageal ulceration, a midesophageal stricture but a normal distal esophageal mucosa. Motor changes were of a secondary type and the gastroesophageal junction, although reduced in tone, continued to relax in response to deglutition (Fig. 21.6). In this patient, correction of an associated hiatal hernia with reflux and continued dilatation of the esophagus improved the esophageal symptoms, but the ulcerative process has continued during the 3 years of follow-up (Fig. 21.7).

To date, experience with Behçet's disease is too limited to allow us to characterize the esophageal motor disorder associated with it.

Giant Esophagus

The dominant symptom in giant esophageal muscular hypertrophy and dilatation is progressive and severe dysphagia. In one such case (42), the esophageal muscle was 3 cm thick and muscular changes extended into the proximal stomach. Resection of the esophagus and proximal stomach gave effective relief of symptoms. No manometric studies were done in this patient; therefore, the motor defect has not been characterized.

Systemic Amyloidosis

Dysphagia has been reported in systemic amyloidosis and it also may be present when such patients have a normal barium swallow. Again no manometric data are available to clarify the nature of the defect.

Esophageal Myopathies

Thyrotoxic Myopathy

Little attention has been paid to the dysphagia described in patients with thyrotoxic myopathy. Fischer and colleagues (43) have described increased disordered motor activity in the body of the esophagus in these patients. Further studies are necessary to clarify the significance of these motor changes and to determine whether or not they produce symptoms.

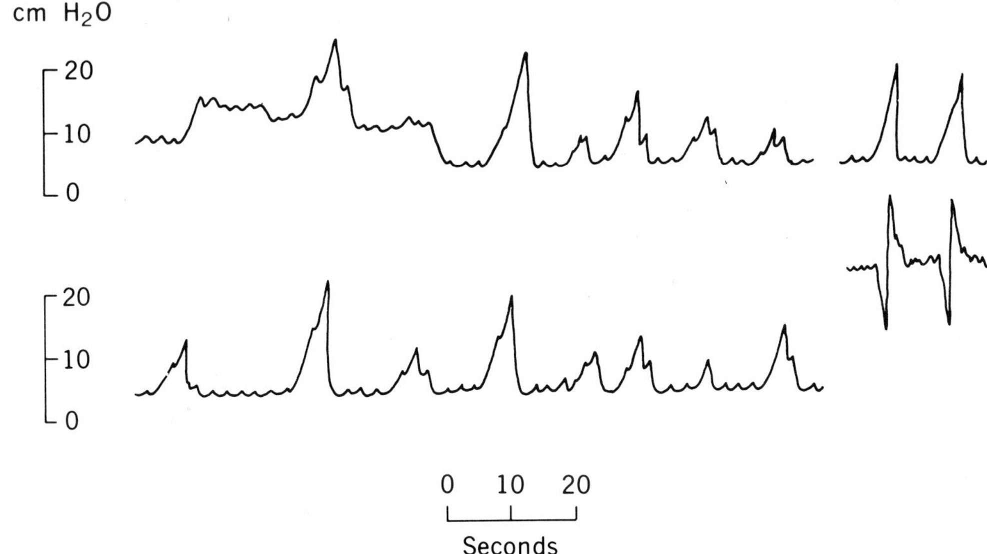

Figure 21.6. Behçet's Disease
Mrs. N. (Case 6) shows decreased tone in a gastroesophageal junction, which relaxes in response to deglutition. The body of the esophagus shows a severe disorder of motor activity with low-amplitude motor waves. The pharyngoesophageal junction and pharynx are normal. This woman has Behçet's disease, but the manometric findings are not specific.

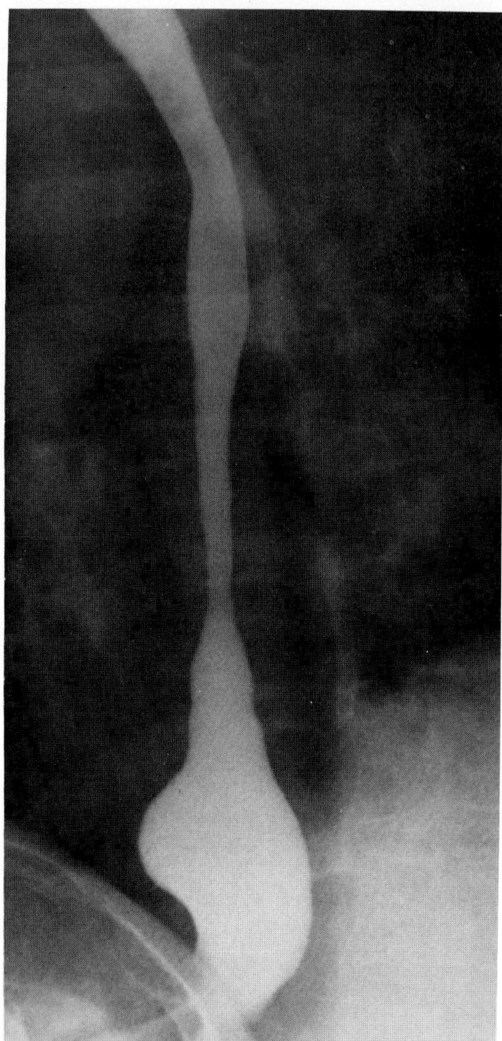

Figure 21.7. Behçet's Disease of Esophagus Behçet's disease, a rare disorder, occasionally involves the esophagus. This patient (Mrs. N., Case 6) has a severe esophageal stricture that has been controlled by repeated dilatation. Reflux was controlled by gastroplasty; this did not prevent further ulceration in the midbody of the esophagus.

Myotonia Dystrophia

Myotonia usually involves the skeletal muscle esophagus; however, motor abnormalities in the lower esophagus have also been described (44).

Variations in Normal Esophageal Motor Function

All motor abnormalities detected on manometry do not necessarily indicate disease because the motor function of the human esophagus varies markedly with age. In the neonate, the gastroesophageal junction has a low tone which gradually increases during the first 6 days of life (45). Motor waves in the neonate have been described as progressing from the esophagus into the proximal stomach. In most young children, the junction behaves as if it is located above the physiologic diaphragm and has only a short intra-abdominal segment.

Esophageal motor function in the adult may be altered by pregnancy. In the early months, gastroesophageal reflux is sufficiently common to be considered normal (46).

It has been shown that HPZ tone falls when progesterone is used in the oral contraceptive pill (47). During pregnancy there is a progressive fall in HPZ tone which reaches its lowest level at 36 weeks gestation and returns to normal following delivery (48–50).

Old age is characterized by progressive deterioration in esophageal motor function and increasingly disordered motor activity. These changes may become pronounced enough to simulate major esophageal disorders such as achalasia, scleroderma or reflux esophagitis (51, 52).

Motor disorders in old age should be interpreted with caution because the physician may be tempted to assign these to the aging process and to refuse investigation in the mistaken belief that they are not reversible and, even if a specific disease process were recognized, to withhold definitive treatment because he considers the patient unfit for major surgical correction. These attitudes are mistaken because conservative therapy vigorously applied or surgery carefully selected may bring great symptomatic relief.

Case 7. Mrs. U., age 78, had been in excellent health until 2 years before admission when she developed profound dysphagia. She described her symptoms poorly, denying major pharyngoesophageal dysphagia and complaining chiefly of difficulty with solids at the gastroesophageal junctional level. Her family doctor, an astute observer, first noted that she held food in her mouth for a long time and swallowed repeatedly with each mouthful. After each swallow she coughed and frequently choked severely.

She would admit to only mild and infrequent retrosternal burning which was not a source of major distress. During this 2-year period she had lost 60 pounds, but despite this remained mentally active and could walk about and do her housework unassisted.

Each of three radiologic studies showed only a severe motor incoordination. The third study, done to assess food obstruction and to visualize the defect in swallowing, confirmed the existence of major obstruction at the pharyngoesophageal junction and demonstrated a small hiatal hernia in the lower esophagus.

Manometry showed a low-tone gastroesophageal junction and total low-amplitude disordered motor activity. The pharyngoesophageal junction was abnormal—i.e., there was an incoordination between the pharyngeal motor wave and the point of maximal cricopharyngeal relaxation.

Endoscopy showed a stricture at the gastroesophageal junction that was not recognized previously and severe ulcerative esophagitis distributed in a linear and patchy fashion throughout the entire length of the esophagus.

The esophagus was dilated with Malloney bougies up to Fr #60 and her dysphagia improved immediately. The patient maintained this improvement and has gained weight steadily on a regimen of antacids and bed elevation.

This elderly woman clearly shows the importance of careful evaluation, and illustrates how much can sometimes be gained from complete investigation.

References

1. Katz, L. A., and Spiro, H. M.: Gastrointestinal manifestations of diabetes. N. Engl. J. Med., *275:* 1350, 1966.
2. Vela, A. R., and Balart, L.: Esophageal motor manifestations in diabetes mellitus. Am. J. Surg., *119:* 21, 1970.
3. Vix, V. A.: Esophageal motility in diabetes mellitus. Radiology, *92:* 363, 1969.
4. Mandelstam, P., and Lieber, A.: Esophageal dysfunction in diabetic neuropathy-gastroenteropathy; clinical and roentgenological manifestations. J.A.M.A., *201:* 582, 1967.
5. Horgan, J. H., and Doyle, J. S.: A comparative study of esophageal motility in diabetics with neuropathy. Chest, *60:* 170, 1971.
6. Mandelstam, P., Siegel, C. L., Lieber, A., and Siegel, M.: The swallowing disorder in patients with diabetic neuropathy-gastroenteropathy. Gastroenterology, *56:* 1, 1979.
7. Langille, D., Brown, B. S., Sidorov, J. J., Baillie, R., and Hayne, O.: The esophagus in diabetes mellitus; cinefluorographic and manometric observations. J. Can. Assoc. Radiol., *22:* 124, 1971.
8. Hollis, J. B., Castell, D. O., and Braddom, R. L.: Esophageal function in diabetes mellitus and its relation to peripheral neuropathy. Gastroenterology, *73:* 1098, 1977.
9. Winship, D. H., Caflisch, C. R., Zboralske, F. F., and Hogan, W. J.: Deterioration of esophageal peristalsis in patients with alcoholic neuropathy. Gastroenterology, *55:* 173, 1968.
10. Parkinson, J.: *An Essay on the Shaking Palsy.* MacMillan, London, Sherwood, Neely, and Jones, 1817.
11. Eadie, M. J., and Tyrer, J. H.: Alimentary disorders in parkinsonism. Aust. Ann. Med., *14:* 13, 1965.
12. Eadie, M. J.: The pathology of certain medullary nuclei in parkinsonism. Brain, *86:* 781, 1963.
13. Walker, J., Singer, K., and Baker, P.: Disorders of esophageal motility in a family with hereditary spastic ataxia. Neurology, *19:* 1212, 1969.
14. Kelley, M. L., Jr.: Intraluminal manometry in the evaluation of malignant disease of the esophagus. Cancer, *21:* 1011, 1968.
15. Henderson, R. D., Barichello, A. M., Pearson, F. G., Mugashe, F., and Szczepanski, M.: Diagnosis of achalasia. Can. J. Surg., *15:* 190, 1972.
16. Sage, M. R., Hall, P., and Williams, D. R.: The radiological and pathological features in a case of secondary amyloidosis involving the gastrointestinal tract. Austalas. Radiol., *22:* 42, 1978.
17. Brody, I. A., Wertlake, P. T., and Laster, L.: Causes of intestinal symptoms in primary amyloidsis. Arch. Intern. Med., *113:* 512, 1964.
18. Monteiro, J. G.: The digestive system in familial amyloidotic polyneuropathy. Am. J. Gastroenterol., *60:* 47, 1973.
19. Schuffler, M. D., and Pope, C. E., 2d: Esophageal motor dysfunction in idiopathic intestinal pseudoobstruction. Gastroenterology, *79:* 677, 1976.
20. Isenberg, J. I., Csendes, A., and Walsh, J. H.: Resting and pentagastrin-stimulated gastroesophageal sphincter pressure in patients with Zollinger-Ellison syndrome. Gastroenterology, *61:* 655, 1971.
21. Isenberg, J. I., Csendes, A., and Walsh, H. J.: Gastroesophageal sphincter pressure in pernicious anaemia and Zollinger-Ellison syndrome. Lancet, *1:* 972, 1971.
22. Earlam, R. J.: Gastrointestinal aspects of Chagas' disease. Am. J. Dig. Dis., *17:* 559, 1972.
23. Bettarello, A., and Pinotti, H. W.: Oesophageal involvement in Chagas' disease. Clin. Gastroenterol., *5:* 103, 1976.
24. Ferreira-Santos, R.: Aperistalsis of the esophagus and colon (megaesophagus and megacolon) etiologically related to Chagas' disease. Am. J. Dig. Dis., *6:* 700, 1961.
25. Edrington, E. B.: Dysphagia as the initial symptom of tetanus; treatment with toxoid. South. Med. J., *59:* 1333, 1966.
26. Jaffari, S. M.: Cephalic tetanus. Indian Pract., *19:* 389, 1966.
27. Weider, D. J., and Tingwald, F. R.: Dysphagia as initial and prime symptom of tetanus; report of a case. Arch. Otolaryngol., *91:* 479, 1970.
28. Foroozan, P., Enta, T., Winship, D. H., and Trier, J. S.: Loss and regeneration of the esophageal mucosa in pemphigoid. Gastroenterology, *52:* 548, 1967.
29. Schuman, B. M., and Arciniegas, E.: The management of esophageal complications of epidermolysis bullosa. Am. J. Dig. Dis., *17:* 875, 1972.
30. Andrén, L., and Theander, G.: Roentgenographic appearances of esophageal moniliasis. Acta Radiol. (Stockh.), *46:* 571, 1956.
31. Woods, J. W., Manning, I. H., and Patterson, C. N.: Monilial infections complicating the therapeutic use of antibiotics. J.A.M.A., *145:* 207, 1951.
32. Vantrappen, G., and Hellemans, J., Eds.: *Diseases of*

the Esophagus. Springer-Verlag, New York, 1974.
33. Sheft, D. J., and Shrago, G.: Esophgeal moniliasis; the spectrum of the disease. J.A.M.A., *213:* 1859, 1970.
34. Hold, J. M.: Candida infection of the oesophagus. Gut, *9:* 227, 1968.
35. Grieve, N. W.: Monilial oesophagitis. Br. J. Radiol., *37:* 551, 1964.
36. Pearce, J., and Dagradi, A.: Acute ulceration of the esophagus with associated intranuclear inclusion bodies; report of four cases. Arch. Pathol., *35:* 889, 1948.
37. deSa, D. J.: Chickenpox oesophagitis (Letter to Editor). Br. Med. J., *1* (6116)*:* 858, 1978.
38. Johnson, H. N.: Visceral lesions associated with varicella. Arch. Pathol., *30:* 292, 1940.
39. Berlin, C.: Behçet's disease as a multiple symptom complex; report of ten cases. Arch. Dermatol., *82:* 73, 1960.
40. Arma, S., Habibulla, K. S., Price, J. J., and Collis, J. L.: Dysphagia in Behcet's syndrome. Thorax, *26:* 155, 1971.
41. Brodie, T. E., and Ochsner, J. L.: Behçet's syndrome with ulcerative oesophagitis; report of the first case. Thorax, *28:* 637, 1973.
42. Wall, M. H., Espinas, E. E., Silver, A. W., and Byron, F. X.: Giant esophagus; an unusual case of massive idiopathic hypertrophy and dilatation of the esophagus and proximal stomach. Ann. Thorac. Surg., *4:* 60, 1967.
43. Fischer, R. A., Ellison, G. W., Thayer, W. R., Spiro, H. M., and Glaser, G. H.: Esophageal motility in neuromuscular disorders. Ann. Intern. Med., *63:* 229, 1965.
44. Hughes, D. T., Swann, J. C., Gleeson, J. A., and Lee, F. I.: Abnormalities in swallowing associated with dystrophia myotonica. Brain, *88:* 1037, 1965.
45. Gryboski, J. D., Thayer, W. R., Jr., and Spiro, H. M.: Esophageal motility in infants and children. Pediatrics, *31:* 382, 1963.
46. Payne, W. S., and Olsen, A. M.: *The Esophagus.* Lea & Febiger, Philadelphia, 1974.
47. Van Thiel, D. H., Gavaler, J. S., and Stremple, J.: Lower esophageal sphincter pressure in women using sequential oral contraceptives. Gastroenterology, *71:* 232, 1976.
48. Schulze, K., and Christensen, J.: Lower sphincter of the opossum esophagus in pseudopregnancy. Gastroenterology, *73:* 1082, 1977.
49. Van Thiel, D. H., Gavaler, J. S., Joshi, S. N., Sara, R. K., and Stremple, J.: Heartburn of pregnancy. Gastroenterology, *72:* 666, 1977.
50. Fisher, R. S., Roberts, G. S., Grabowski, C. J., and Cohen, S.: Altered lower esophageal sphincter function during early pregnancy. Gastroenterology, *74:* 1233, 1978.
51. Zboralske, F. F., Amberg, J. R., and Soergel, K. H.: Presbyesophagus; cineradiographic manifestations. Radiology, *82:* 463, 1964.
52. Leenhardt, P., Pelissier, M., and Thevenet, A.: L'oesophage du vieillard. Montpellier Med., *45:* 14, 1954.

Study of the wide spectrum of motor disorders in the esophagus continues to produce major additions to our understanding of this organ. Continued pursuit and careful investigation of these disorders should lead in future to more accurate diagnosis and more effective treatment.

The purpose of this book has been to organize and rationalize the approach to the investigation and treatment of esophageal motor disorders. If the patient's symptoms arise from the esophagus, a cause for these symptoms can almost always be found. Once the diagnosis is established, a rational course of management will produce, in most patients, a satisfactory improvement or total relief of distress.

The aim of therapy is to restore normal function and to allow the patient to eat without distress. Successful therapy will return the patient to the state described by G. Eckstein in *The Body Has a Head* (Harper & Row, 1970):

"All of the delights reaches not much further than the mouth, reaches the point where we think, isn't that nice, and the next instant something agreeable has gotten away from us. As the delight disappears further into the digestive tube and from the mind it leaves a callous sense of well-being that persists until drowsiness supervenes."

Index

(Page numbers in **boldface** type refer to illustrated pages
for the entries.)